Introducing New Treatments for Cancer

PRACTICAL, ETHICAL AND LEGAL PROBLEMS

Edited by
C. J. Williams
CRC Medical Oncology Unit,
Southampton University Hospitals,
Southampton, UK

JOHN WILEY & SONS
Chichester · New York · Brisbane · Toronto · Singapore

Copyright © 1992 by John Wiley & Sons Ltd
Baffins Lane, Chichester
West Sussex PO19 1UD, England

Other Wiley Editorial Offices

John Wiley & Sons, Inc., 605 Third Avenue,
New York, NY 10158-0012, USA

Jacaranda Wiley Ltd, G.P.O. Box 859, Brisbane,
Queensland 4001, Australia

John Wiley & Sons (Canada) Ltd, 22 Worcester Road,
Rexdale, Ontario M9W 1L1, Canada

John Wiley & Sons (SEA) Pte Ltd, 37 Jalan Pemimpin #05-04,
Block B, Union Industrial Building, Singapore 2057

Library of Congress Cataloging-in-Publication Data

Introducing new treatments for cancer: practical, ethical, and legal
  problems / edited by C. J. Williams.
      p.   cm.
  Includes bibliographical references and index.
  ISBN 0 471 93113 6 (cloth)   ISBN 0 471 93445 3 (paper)
  1. Cancer—Treatment—Moral and ethical aspects. 2. Clinical
trials—Moral and ethical aspects.   I. Williams, C. J. (Christopher
John Hacon)
  [DNLM: 1. Clinical Trials. 2. Ethics, Medical. 3. Neoplasms—therapy.
  QZ 266 I599]
RC270.8.I58   1992
174'.25—dc20
DNLM/DLC
for Library of Congress   91-24553
                                                                      CIP

British Library Cataloguing in Publication Data

A catalogue record for this book is
available from the British Library

ISBN 0 471 93113 6 (cloth)   ISBN 0 471 93445 3 (paper)

Typeset by Dobbie Typesetting Limited, Tavistock, Devon
Printed in Great Britain by Biddles Ltd, Guildford, Surrey

Cancer

Contents

Contributors

D. Craig Allred
Department of Pathology, University of Texas Health Science Center at San Antonio, Texas, USA

Karen Antman
Dana Farber Cancer Institute, Massachusetts, USA

Colin B. Begg
Department of Epidemiology and Biostatistics, Memorial Sloan-Kettering Cancer Center, New York, USA

Jesse A. Berlin
Clinical Epidemiology Unit, University of Pennsylvania School of Medicine, Pennsylvania, USA

George Blackledge
Medical Research Department, ICI Pharmaceuticals, Macclesfield, UK

Renzo Canetta
Pharmaceutical Research Institute, Bristol-Myers Squibb Company, Wallingford, Connecticut, USA

Stephen K. Carter
Pharmaceutical Research Institute, Bristol-Myers Squibb Company, Lawrenceville, New Jersey, USA

Gary C. Chamness
Department of Medicine/Oncology, University of Texas Health Science Center at San Antonio, Texas, USA

Gary M. Clark
Department of Science/Oncology, University of Texas Health Science Center at San Antonio, Texas, USA

Alan S. Coates
Department of Clinical Oncology, Royal Prince Alfred Hospital, New South Wales, Australia

Rory Collins
Clinical Trial Service Unit, Oxford University, Oxford, UK

Genevieve Decoster
Department of Clinical Research, F. Hoffman-La Roche Ltd, Basel, Switzerland

Richard Doll
Clinical Trial Service Unit, Oxford University, Oxford, UK

Claire Gilbert Foster
Centre of Medical Law and Ethics, King's College, London, UK

Michael A. Friedman
Cancer Therapy Evaluation Program, National Cancer Institute, Maryland, USA

Charles Hamilton
Department of Radiotherapy, Royal South Hants Hospital, Southampton, UK

Eduard E. Holdener
Department of Clinical Research, F. Hoffman-La Roche Ltd, Basel, Switzerland

Alison L. Jones
Department of Medicine, Royal Marsden Hospital, Surrey, UK

Bengt Jönsson
Department of Economics, Stockholm School of Economics, Stockholm, Sweden

Göran Karlsson
Department of Health and Society, Linköping University, Linköping, Sweden

Frank Lawton
Department of Obstetrics and Gynaecology, King's College Hospital, London, UK

Carol M. Lim
Department of Clinical Research, F. Hoffman-La Roche Ltd, Basel, Switzerland

Stephen Lock
Royal College of Physicians, London, UK

Richard R. Love
Department of Human Oncology, University of Wisconsin–Madison, Wisconsin, USA

David Machin
Medical Research Council, Cancer Trials Office, Cambridge, UK

William J. Mackillop
Ontario Cancer Treatment and Research Foundation, Kingston Regional Cancer Center, Ontario, Canada

William McCulloch
US Bioscience Incorporated, Pennsylvania, USA

William L. McGuire
Department of Medicine/Oncology, University of Texas Health Science Center at San Antonio, Texas, USA

Jonathan Montgomery
Faculty of Law, University of Southampton, Southampton, UK

Claude Nicaise
Pharmaceutical Research Institute, Bristol-Myers Squibb Company, Connecticut, USA

George A. Omura
Comprehensive Cancer Center, University of Alabama, Birmingham, USA

Brian O'Sullivan
Ontario Cancer Institute, Princess Margaret Hospital, Toronto, Canada

Michael J. Palmer
Ontario Cancer Treatment and Research Foundation, Kingston Regional Cancer Center, Ontario, Canada

Mahesh K. B. Parmar
Medical Research Council, Cancer Trials Office, Cambridge, UK

Richard Peto
Clinical Trial Service Unit, Oxford University, Oxford, UK

Trevor J. Powles
Department of Medicine, Royal Marsden Hospital, Surrey, UK

Carol F. Quirt
Ontario Cancer Treatment and Research Foundation, Kingston Regional Cancer Center, Ontario, Canada

Marcel Rozencweig
Pharmaceutical Research Institute, Bristol-Myers Squibb Company, Wallingford, Connecticut, USA

Philip S. Schein
US Bioscience Incorporated, Pennsylvania, USA

R. John Simes
Department of Clinical Oncology, Royal Prince Alfred Hospital, New South Wales, Australia

Tony Smith
British Medical Association, BMA House, London, UK

Robert Souhami
Department of Oncology, University College Hospital, London, UK

Sally Stenning
Medical Research Council, Cancer Trials Office, Cambridge, UK

Lesley Stewart
Medical Research Council, Cancer Trials Office, Cambridge, UK

Charles Stiller
Childhood Cancer Research Group, University of Oxford, Oxford, UK

Atul K. Tandon
Department of Medicine/Oncology, University of Texas Health Science Center, Texas, USA

Martin H. N. Tattersall
Department of Cancer Medicine, Royal Prince Alfred Hospital, New South Wales, Australia

Graham Thorpe
Countess Mountbatten House, Moorgreen Hospital, Southampton, UK

Jeffrey S. Tobias
Department of Radiotherapy and Oncology, University College Hospital, London, UK

Victor Tunkel
Faculty of Law, University of London, London, UK

Frank Wells
Association of the British Pharmaceutical Industry, London, UK

Christopher J. Williams
CRC Wessex Regional Medical Oncology Unit, Southampton University Hospitals, Southampton, UK

Introduction

Cancer is the second leading cause of death in the Western world and results in even greater loss of years of life than cardiovascular disease. Despite encouraging improvements in the care of individual tumours many patients are incurable and the need for effective new therapies is as great as ever. The idea for this book came from my own experience of some of the problems of trying to introduce potential new treatments into routine clinical practice.

Perhaps the most important step in developing a successful new treatment is that made by the basic scientist(s) who identifies or hypothesizes a new approach. Discussion of this process is *not*, however, the remit of this book— we are here concerned with the problems of taking a treatment from the pre-clinical stage into the patient and hopefully into routine clinical practice.

My original plan for the structure of the book was relatively simple, with 12 or so moderately long chapters on topics such as ethics and the management of different types of clinical trials. However, as the book developed it quickly became evident that this is an increasingly complex field where there are many viewpoints and vested interests. This led to an evolutionary change in the book's structure so that there are over 30 relatively short chapters—the international cast list representing lawyers, ethicists, social scientists, statisticians, pharmacologists, journal editors, pharmaceutical company physicians, radiotherapists, medical oncologists and specialists in continuing care. Although most chapters have deliberately not been heavily referenced (suggested reading is included) a few seem to be better served by a more "academic" approach and are thus fully referenced.

To date cancer researchers have done a reasonable job in identifying treatments of *major* benefit to patients. However, changes in funding, the increasingly direct involvement of pharmaceutical companies and the academic pressures on research clinicians are making development of new treatments increasingly difficult. This is compounded by the enormous costs of such an undertaking and the consequent high price of new drugs. An additional major problem has been that up until now clinical trials have not been large enough to identify treatments producing modest but important effects (a 10% improvement in survival for instance). Only recently, as clinicians appreciated that dramatically effective new therapies are unlikely, have we woken up to the need to define what is best current therapy. This information will provide a basis for optimizing conventional treatment and will be the appropriate control for testing new treatments. Implicit in the desire to achieve these ends is the need for very large clinical trials which produce results that have a narrow confidence interval.

Clearly this exercise in developing new treatments includes many individuals. By far and away the largest group are the patients who are included in trials and for this reason the first section of the book is concerned with legal and ethical aspects of clinical trials and with patient attitudes to such therapy. Two central sections are concerned with a variety of problems peculiar to various types of clinical trials. The fourth section discusses the relatively new areas of treatment of pre-malignant conditions and of cancer prevention programmes. The last section covers the reporting of and dissemination of information about new treatments.

Since the book is aimed at a wide audience (more than mirroring the breadth of its contributors) I have asked authors to provide a short biography so that readers from one discipline may better appreciate the background of the writer of each individual chapter. Because of the large number of chapters I have written introductory notes for each section—the views expressed therein, some of which may be regarded as contentious, are my own and do not necessarily reflect those of individual contributors to that section.

The aim of this book is to draw attention to the complex problems that we face in trying to improve cancer treatments. Only by awareness and dialogue can we improve the current poor state of affairs. Although the situation can be improved by changes in attitudes on the part of clinicians, many of the problems have ethical, legal and political dimensions that must be tackled. The role and relationship of pharmaceutical companies with clinical research and governmental bodies remains ambiguous. They need to be redefined in a way that stresses the importance of clinical research as a tool for benefiting patients and the community. Individual researchers must examine their own goals and should plan future clinical research in such a way that it is most likely to give a clear and useful answer to the question being posed. Lastly, statutory bodies should reassess their potential role in licensing new cancer therapies. Up until now there has, rightly, been much stress on good clinical practice in phase I and II trials. What has been lacking is willing acceptance of and need for a much simpler approach to large-scale phase III trials to define the clinical role of new agents.

Chris Williams

Section I

ETHICS AND CONSENT

Notes on Section I

This introductory section brings together eight chapters which are essentially concerned with ethical and legal aspects of clinical trials. Some of the variation in practice around the world is tackled, though the principles are obviously applicable worldwide.

Chapter 1, by **Victor Tunkel**, discusses the legal position of clinical research in Britain. He writes very much from the lawyer's standpoint and potentially as the "patient's friend". The most contentious part of this chapter is his view on the possibility that consent to treatment for phase I studies may not be fully valid. There is no doubt that the chances of *real* benefit for patients in a phase I study of a new drug are exceedingly low (see Chapters 10 and 11). It is also true that many dying patients (those usually suitable for such studies) may find it difficult to make a rational decision and to give consent free from undue pressure. However, his suggestion, based on the views of Kennedy and Grubb (*Medical Law*, 1989), that the law might not *allow* patients to consent to what is essentially a non-therapeutic treatment in phase I studies of a new cytotoxic drug is sure to provoke argument.

He (rightly, to my mind) raises the important issue of no fault compensation though also points out some of the problems encountered in applying this in legal systems based on case law. On the subject of per capita payments he sees little wrong in law or ethics provided that the research ethics committee knows and allows them. This opinion is partially supported by Jonathan Montgomery writing on the effect of international variation in law and ethics. In the section on conflict of interest he suggests that the researcher should make a "full and frank disclosure" of their interests including per capita payment—presumably this might include telling the patient. This principle is one that I would suggest is rarely applied and in the third chapter (summary of a Royal College of Physicians report on research involving patients) the working party specifically states that "per capita payments to doctors are unethical" and go on to say that "even fees paid to an institution may lead to undue pressure to recruit patients". In addition, to the potential for abuse of patients consequent upon per capita payment there is a real risk that it may reduce the size of the trial and thus its usefulness. I have personally been invited to participate in a trial where there was per capita payment. Because of the insistence of a high level of

Introducing New Treatments for Cancer: Practical, Ethical and Legal Problems. Edited by C. J. Williams
© 1992 John Wiley & Sons Ltd

recompense on the part of clinicians the company concerned was forced to restrict accrual to the study to a maximum of 140 patients—a grossly inadequate number to answer the question being tested. Such an approach means that everyone potentially loses out—apart from the researcher receiving the per capita payment.

This is a very difficult area since research is expensive and in the current climate is unlikely to be paid for out of routine clinical budgets. Payment of *specific* additional costs to an institution is more acceptable than payment to individual researchers, but care must be exercised when employing doctors or nurses for a specific project. If their salary depends on income from per capita payment there is an obvious risk that patients will be pressurized to join trials in order to secure their job. Funding of such personnel should ideally be made on a lump sum basis before the study starts—an act of faith on the part of the pharmaceutical company. An alternative way to fund per capita payments would be for pharmaceutical companies to pay monies into a central research fund which would administer payment. However, this adds an extra layer of bureaucracy and does not overcome the pressure on the clinician to enter as many patients as possible.

Jonathan Montgomery (Chapter 2) discusses variation in practice around the world and suggests that protocols should be designed so that they match the ethical and legal criteria of the strictest country—the doctrine of the *strongest* link. While this may be true for many trials, there is room for flexibility in large-scale simple studies (see Souhami, Chapter 13) where the initial protocol is not restrictive. Surely such trials can abide by local ethical practice and do not need to insist on uniformity. One bar to this may be where journals refuse to publish or national statutory bodies do not accept data where there has *not* been formal written "informed consent" by the patient. However, it is worth pointing out that informed consent does not always result in a trial considered to be ethical by the majority of clinicians. For instance, in a recent controlled trial published in the *New England Journal of Medicine* patients receiving cisplatin were randomized to receive no antisickness drugs or a new drug. Not surprisingly, since it is well known that nearly all patients vomit after cisplatin therapy the new drug was better than no antisickness treatment at all. This paper was roundly condemned by experts in the field as unethical since moderately effective antisickness drugs which were already available were withheld from patients in the control arm. They felt the appropriate study was to compare the new drug with conventional antisickness treatments. However, partly because patients gave "consent" the study was considered acceptable to the *New England Journal of Medicine* (a highly prestigious publication) and the trial also provided very important data for drug registration with the Food and Drug Administration (FDA) in the United States (which often insists on comparison with a no-treatment control). The registrational requirements of the FDA and to a lesser extent other national statutory bodies have become of paramount importance. However, they remain bureaucratic and rigid, often only appearing to assess data needs for registration when studies have been completed. More appropriate would be extensive *discussion* between regulatory body, pharmaceutical company and research clinicians *before* phase I, II and pivotal trials start. This need not become so stultifying that innovation is squashed; rather, scientifically valid studies can be designed from the outset. At present rigid criteria and a lack of early consultation result in time wasting and in some cases inappropriate research.

Chapter 3 is a summary of a report of the **Royal College of Physicians** which was written to provide a framework upon which clinicians could base ethical research. Although it certainly was not the aim of the report, some critics have claimed that it is proscriptive, restrictive and will injure the ability of researchers to carry out clinical trials. Professor Michael Baum has been prominent in discussion of trial ethics and particularly consent. A meeting in London in the spring of 1991 discussed the subject of consent and ethics in clinical research to see if the whole process of consent to clinical trials can be made to work more effectively for the patient and physician. One radical suggestion is based on the notion that clinical research has changed the doctor–patient relationship. Normally, the patient comes to the doctor requesting and consenting to any treatment that might cure them of their ill. In the case of clinical trials the doctor approaches the patient as supplicant asking them for their consent to inclusion in a clinical trial. It has been suggested that this role reversal has caused much of the conflict over consent. One way out of this situation is to use the device employed by some teaching hospitals with regard to medical students. Such hospitals explain to patients that they may on admission choose to sign a document allowing medical students to see them or alternatively sign a form forbidding this. In the case of routine therapy patients usually consent to treatment that their doctor recommends—in the case of hospitals conducting clinical trials patients could be asked to sign for consent to inclusion in *any* clinical trial being carried out in that hospital or alternatively they may choose to refuse to consent to *any* trial. Clearly, if such a system were introduced research ethics committees would need to scrutinize any protocol very closely before giving approval. Even so it may be that such blanket approval should exclude special studies such as phase I and II trials of new cytotoxic agents. However, it could be an ideal tool for large-scale studies comparing standard therapies—there are clearly logical inconsistencies when a patient going to one or another clinician may be offered different treatments and consent is accepted as implicit in the relationship. However, the same patient consulting a third physician who is comparing these two standard therapies will be required to give full informed consent—a process described by Michael Baum as "double standards".

There is a large degree of paternalism in this radical suggestion—the notion that it is very often in the patient's interest for the clinician to run the show.

Chapter 4 by the Oxford trials group (**Rory Collins, Richard Doll and Richard Peto**) argues against some of the restrictive elements of the Royal College of Physicians report and similar documents. They use the large ISIS-2 study as an example of their approach, which employs the uncertainty principle (see Chapter 13), encourages individual approaches to consent and emphasizes large numbers in trials (also see Chapter 13). A cornerstone to their arguments is that ethical standards applicable to normal clinical practice should apply to clinical research—a theme propounded by Michael Baum (as discussed above), who pointed out the existence of "double standards". Some of the same themes are taken up in Chapter 5 by **Jeffrey Tobias** which quotes the reaction of the late Dr Franz Ingelfinger (editor of the *New England Journal of Medicine*) on finding out that he had oesophageal cancer. In his case he found it easier to deal with his illness if he had someone to make the decisions for him—an idea that many cancer patients would subscribe to. Despite this, as Dr Tobias states, more patients these days want to play a positive role in making decisions regarding their treatment. This has in the United States and to a lesser extent in other Western countries led to patients treated outside of trials wishing extensive discussions before treatment decisions are made. Thus the choice for patients attending a hospital which takes part in clinical trials could be threefold: (1) blanket acceptance to inclusion in any trial without discussion; (2) refusal of any trial without discussion; or (3) full discussion of any trial before acceptance or refusal.

These new suggestions will lead to much discussion and will generate strong feelings on both sides; however, this only goes to illustrate that ethics are not set in tablets of stone but are an evolving and responsive set of values.

The chapters by Collins and his colleagues, Tobias and by **Tattersall and Simes** (Chapter 6) outline some of the disadvantages of the current rather rigid ethical system. Most importantly the research of Tattersall and Simes and of others suggests that the process of informed consent can in itself heighten anxiety in individual patients. It may also discourage patient accrual—which in a clinically important trial may harm the community by delaying or reducing the chances of demonstrating that the therapy being tested is beneficial (Chapter 4).

Despite their reservations, the authors of Chapters 5 and 6 conclude that patients should be given the opportunity to consent to treatment in clinical trials though they recommend a "caring and sensitive consent process tailored to the individual's needs"—much as employed in the British part of the ISIS-2 trial (Chapter 4).

Guardianship of the current ethical system is the remit of research ethics committees. **Claire Gilbert Foster** discusses those in Britain in Chapter 7. Their function is similar to that in other Western countries though there are variations internationally. One of these has been the freedom for British research ethics committees to go their own way, there being no national or legal framework for such committees. Because of this there is an unwelcome (?) variation in the way such committees run. This can be especially troublesome in the case of large-scale multicentre trials as attested to by Jonathan Montgomery. One solution put forward has been the formation of a national ethics committee, though Dr Gilbert Foster points out some of the pitfalls of this approach and argues for consideration of a national association of research ethics committees. Such an approach may raise standards and give a more uniform approach though it would not necessarily overcome all the problems of national or international studies. It would, however, be a useful resource for difficult problems and would serve as a forum for discussion of areas of concern. For instance, reservations have recently been expressed in Britain about the policy of some ethical committees of turning down applications on the grounds that they are unethical because of the high cost of the treatment being tested, the argument being that an expensive new treatment will take away resources from other valuable areas of medicine—an act which would be unethical.

Stephen Lock (Chapter 8), who is the editor of the *British Medical Journal*, argues that journals have a role in ensuring that research is ethical. International journals of this type have an important function in leading and reporting on ethical debate—an area regarded by many doctors as dry and not of relevance to them. Such journals need to make such topics far more readable and of real importance to individual doctors. As well as this function, journals need to take an ethical view on papers submitted to them, though Stephen Lock points out that they do not have all the facilities to act as a policeman. It has been suggested (Begg and Berlin, Chapter 24) that one way around publication bias is to have researchers submit their research protocol to a journal before starting the trial. If approved the journal then guarantees to publish the trial on completion. In a similar way ethics could be assessed before the trial is begun. This "upside-down" approach is discussed more fully in the introductory notes for Section V.

A further concern of Dr Lock is the need for a bio-ethics research committee. He argues cogently for this to be separate from any national research ethics committee that may be formed; with regard to cancer such a committee appears to be immediately relevant because of the potential for *gene therapy*. This is at present only a gleam in the eye of researchers but the first embryo attempts at genetic manipulation in cancer are already being reported. The National Institutes of Health (NIH) in the United States approved in July 1990 two research protocols that could allow scientists to treat human cancer by inserting foreign genes into patients' cells. The chairman of the NIH's Recombinant DNA Advisory Committee (RAC) described this as the "first vote for true human gene therapy".

These trials are based on work by Rosenberg and his colleagues at the NIH first published in the *New England Journal of Medicine* (30 August 1990). This showed that insertion of retroviral genes into patients' genes was feasible. The researchers now want to use the technique in malignant melanoma and in a rare genetic immune deficiency syndrome. Florence Antione commenting in the *Journal of the National Cancer Institute* (5 September 1990) notes that "gene therapy has been controversial and a number of groups have resisted its implementation. To ensure that the research is conducted with the greatest safety and that no social, moral, or medical ethics are violated, the NIH has subjected these trials to the most comprehensive and thorough reviews possible". Despite this, it seems likely that the debate will continue.

1 Legal Aspects of Clinical Trials in the United Kingdom

The general theme of this book is the problems which have to be overcome in the conquest of disease and, specifically, cancer. The other contributors examine the scientific, ethical and practical problems which workers in this field know they must tackle. It might be thought quite unnecessary and unfortunate that they should be further handicapped by legal obstacles. The law in this area does not mean to impede medical advance. It is merely fulfilling its most basic function: trying to hold an acceptable balance between legitimate conflicting interests. Patients have rights (as, in a sense, now also do animals and human embryos) and therefore health professionals and drug manufacturers have correlative duties. The adjustment of the balance between, for example, doctors' and patients' interests is a fine one and may be altered from time to time by legislation or by decisions of the courts. It may also vary considerably from one country to another. This last complication, the disparate legal and ethical requirements of different countries and their different legal systems may at times be tiresome for researchers and manufacturers whose activities transcend national boundaries. The current tendency, and especially now in Europe, is for the different legal cultures and their practitioners to draw more closely together. This gives hope of more uniform attitudes and practice in, among others, the medico-legal field. For the present, however, it should be understood that one country may allow experimentation which another forbids; that a brief survey can only summarize the law in broad terms; that this summary is mainly of UK law, with a glance or two sideways at other jurisdictions; and that in this medico-legal area much of the law remains ill defined and speculative.

THE OVERLAP OF LAW AND ETHICS

Experimentation on humans necessarily involves both legal and ethical problems. The World Medical Association in its well-known Declaration of Helsinki tried to set out what are the proper aims and limits of human experimentation. The Declaration has no legal status but insofar as it has been widely approved and adopted by national medical bodies it may be

Introducing New Treatments for Cancer: Practical, Ethical and Legal Problems. Edited by C. J. Williams
© 1992 John Wiley & Sons Ltd

taken as sound guidance to which prudent practitioners should adhere. It is, and is expressed to be, subject to local requirements applicable to the researcher; and these may be more (or occasionally less) stringent. General guidelines of this sort are admissible in evidence in court in order to establish current standards, so as to raise, or, as the case may be, resist, a suggestion of negligence or unprofessional conduct. They might even be used to support an allegation of negligence against an ethics committee by suggesting that it had failed to ensure conformity with current standards of care. But in neither case would a proven departure from the guidelines in itself conclusively constitute negligence. That is a question of law, to be determined by a court applying the standards of the time and the place.

MEDICAL ADVANCE VERSUS RISK

Some risk is inevitable in experimentation on humans, whether it be of adverse reaction or deterioration through non-treatment. A balance has to be maintained between the advancement of medical knowledge and the protection of subjects. This need to balance benefit and risk is a recurring theme in the Declaration of Helsinki. But the point of balance may be movable. In particular, where acute or advanced disease is present, the testing of more drastic or less proven therapies may be justifiable on a balance-of-risks principle. Experimentation on cancer patients adds a further dimension to this, especially in phase I and phase II trials, where not only is no benefit to be expected but there is also a distinct possibility of adverse side-effects. It will be helpful for us first to consider the position of clinical trials in general; then to see the special problems of trials of new treatments for cancer.

HUMAN SUBJECTS

For purposes of the law we should recognize at least three distinct categories of subjects. (Children, mentally disordered and unconscious subjects are not relevant here and are omitted.)

(a) Healthy volunteers, often recruited from among students, medical staff, pharmaceutical company employees, etc. They are usually paid for their services and given express legal rights by a written agreement (see further below). The Royal College of Physicians in their guidelines on *Research on Healthy Volunteers* (October 1986) expressed reservations about the recruiting of junior colleagues, students and the unemployed for this purpose.

(b) Patients for whom the research has no direct therapeutic relevance. Usually they are under treatment for some unconnected complaint, and provide a convenient population or control group for comparison. However, cancer patients may come into this category where a new treatment needs to be tested but is thought not to offer any benefit to any actual subject participating.

(c) Patients for whom the research has therapeutic relevance. The great majority of phase III studies are done on these subjects. "Therapeutic" in this context includes placebo treatment and adjuvant therapy.

It is important to emphasize that all of the above subjects must be volunteers. No one may be subjected to experimentation without their knowledge and consent. For this purpose knowledge calls for a positive informative process by the researcher; consent is a positive formal response by the subject. I emphasize this because of a tendency of some clinicians to conflate them into one transaction.

THE PROBLEM OF "INFORMED CONSENT"

There is a well-known conflict between what patients feel they have the right to know and what practitioners think suffices to tell them. This has given rise to a body of case-law, mostly following surgical mishaps. In some states in the USA and in Canada, a more "rights-based" approach has led to the conclusion that if the patient was not told of virtually every risk, his consent was not valid and the operation itself was therefore tortious. (If so, it would be regarded as an assault and thus actionable though nothing went wrong.) In England, the courts are more willing to leave the amount of information to be measured according to the judgment of the medical profession. Even so, one cannot be said to consent to something unless one knows its main implications. In the case of experimental drugs, appliances, techniques, etc., that means that the intended subject must be told of the physical facts— what they will have to do or have done to them, and its likely discomforts; and of any special risks known to be involved. The problem with any newish drug is that on the one hand not all the risks are known or, indeed, knowable; on the other, to list every foreseeable risk may be a bit academic as well as an unnecessary discouragement to volunteers.

So how much does the UK researcher have to say to sufficiently inform? According to the cases (all concerning surgery), the subject must be told of material risks, i.e. those more-than-remote risks which a responsible body of practitioners in that speciality would think it appropriate to warn a prudent, inquiring patient. The leading cases are *Bolam* v. *Friern Hospital Management Committee*, [1957] 2 All ER 118, on the standard of the general duty of care of a doctor to his patient; and *Sidaway* v. *Governors of Bethlem*

Royal Hospital, [1985] AC 871 and *Gold* v. *Haringey Health Authority*, [1987] 2 All ER 888 on the extent of the doctor's duty to inform of risks. How the principles laid down in these cases transfer to the experimental situation is not clear, but insofar as we are dealing with a novel therapy which, in a sense, the patient may not need, and which may not be known to be beneficial, and whose side-effects are as yet undiscovered, the duty on the researcher to inform should be considered at least as extensive as that of the surgeon.

THE INFORMING AND CONSENTING PROCEDURES

These distinct procedures must be carried out properly for the protection not only of the subject but also of the investigator and the authority. The information should be in writing, in plain, brief and down-to-earth English. Ethics committees spend an undue amount of time rewording and sometimes rewriting clinicians' attempts to enlighten potential subjects. Investigators should appreciate the need to do this effectively, not for the sake of literacy but of legality. Perhaps connected with this is the inclination of some investigators to give mere verbal information. This may be justified in very trivial cases (e.g. merely taking a small blood sample) but in any substantial procedure there should be a written patient information sheet so that there can be no conflict of evidence in any subsequent dispute. Moreover the patient or his family need something to take away with them, which also has the name of someone responsible and a 24-hour phone number. See Chapters 5 and 6 for further discussion of this point.

THE REALITY OF CONSENT

Consent is not valid if it results from undue pressure. It is perhaps unavoidable that a patient in hospital will feel some psychological pressure to cooperate, especially if gravely ill. The informing process must therefore be to some extent a de-pressurizing. It has to be made clear that it is an experiment (with or without therapeutic relevance, as the case may be); that he or she is under no obligation to volunteer; that refusal to do so will not affect conventional treatment; that he may drop out of the project at any time. If a patient needing treatment is to receive a placebo, he must be told of this possibility (in lay language: a "dummy pill" or "inactive substance"). If this means a spell of, in effect, non-treatment, this may raise ethical problems which, with all these other aspects, will have to be considered by the ethics committee—similarly with randomizing between two or more existing treatments. The clinician may think these are equally effective and might have been chosen for the particular patients anyway, and that no ethical issue therefore arises. Nevertheless a patient has the right to know he is being randomized rather than being given the individual consideration he expects. Some lawyers argue that since randomization may mean that a doctor gives some patients a less promising or appropriate treatment, or no treatment at all, or (in a double-blind test) that he doesn't know which treatment, he is in breach of his overriding duty to do his medical best for his patient. However, I would suggest that such randomized tests are acceptable in law and ethics provided the patient knows he may be randomized, and what this means. It is therefore especially important that the patient is clearly told that he may be given a placebo, or non-treatment, or even a temporary "wash-out" phase during which he will be deprived of his regular treatment. It is not just the fact, but the significance of these things that needs to be understood by the patient if he is to be regarded as fully consenting. Some further aspects of randomizing between novel unproven treatment and non-treatment are considered below.

THE CONSENT FORM

The form which the patient signs should be a quite separate document, retained by the researcher. Most authorities have a standard form and this is probably preferable to individual researchers' own efforts at drafting. It ought really to refer specifically to the patient information sheet as having been read, explained and understood. As mentioned earlier, in the case of healthy volunteers there is usually a full-blown bilateral agreement.

PER CAPITA PAYMENTS

There is nothing wrong in law or ethics for a researcher to be paid by a sponsor on the basis of numbers subjected to the trial, so long as the financial details were fully disclosed in the application to the ethics committee and not disapproved by them. In such cases the researcher must be even more conscientious than usual to ensure that he does not unduly influence subjects into volunteering. The General Medical Council has said that it is unethical for any reward to be accepted which could influence the researcher's assessment of the drug or procedure on trial.

CANCER TREATMENT TRIALS: SOME SPECIAL CONSIDERATIONS

What has been outlined above applies to clinical trials involving new treatments for cancer as it does to other trials. However, there may be a wider scope to trials applied to cancer patients. As with other drugs, a new cancer drug must undergo phase I studies (see Chapters 10 and 11) to ascertain maximum dosage and tolerance. Where the new drug is cytotoxic— expressly designed to destroy tissue—an exceptional dilemma is posed for both law and ethics. However thoroughly it has been tested in preliminary studies, there has to be a first use on human subjects: first in phase I to find out the dosage range, and only after that in phase II to see if it works.

Clearly, with a trial of this nature, healthy volunteers cannot be used. The practice is to select cancer patients who have not responded to the standard treatments, and to give them doses starting with the ineffective minimal and rising to the unacceptably toxic. In this way the optimum dose acceptable to a wide range of patients may be discovered. The trouble is that not only at the two extremes but throughout the dosages given there may be no real expectation of any benefit (Chapter 11); and, at the higher dosages at least, there is the certainty of detriment.

That being so, the trial, although not unrelated to the patient's condition, cannot be regarded as therapeutic and the patient must be so told. What is more difficult is to fulfil the further requirement of informing the patient as to possible side-effects when, in the nature of things, these cannot be known. Yet according to all the authorities, the patient's consent will only be genuine and valid if so fully informed. Moreover, from a purely practical point of view, the researcher is more than usually at risk of legal liability: for whilst in the normal way, a cancer patient whose condition deteriorates may find it very difficult to establish that his treatment or non-treatment was a cause, it would be comparatively easy to attribute a toxic overdose reaction to its cause; and since, unlike, say, the side-effects of routine radiotherapy, it was totally unnecessary and unasked for, there could be heavy legal liability to the patient (or his estate) if his prior consent was not effective.

The matter does not stop even there. We are bordering upon an area where the law does not allow a subject to consent. It is well known that there are some medical or pseudo-medical procedures which in law cannot be consented to. Some of these are specific crimes, of which no more need be said. Others are procedures which are known to be wholly detrimental to the subject. (In their earliest days, heart transplants came close to this and, indeed, were declared illegal in some countries.) The law allows doctors to take risks with patients, even the most outside chances. But it doesn't allow patients to consent to undergo certain harm with no balancing benefit. In the new standard work *Medical Law* (1989), Kennedy and Grubb, writing of non-therapeutic research on patients, say

> Ordinarily, a doctor's duty of care for his patient would preclude his engaging in non-therapeutic research on such a person. This is because it would be difficult to show that it was in the best medical interests of the patient—who is by definition, ill—to be exposed to additional interventions which are not designed to aid in his treatment. There may, of course, be circumstances in which a patient with a minor illness may volunteer to take part in non-therapeutic research. If the proposed research carries no demonstrable risk of harm to the patient nor will it affect deleteriously the patient's condition, then it may be

that the patient may lawfully be party to non-therapeutic research. In our view, however, the evidence of absence of risk would have to be clear and compelling.

The authors then go on to stress that in such cases, which they describe as rare, there must be full voluntariness, in the sense of absence of any form of pressure; full disclosure of material risks, answering any questions truthfully; and a limit to the degree of risk posed, namely, it should not exceed a minor increase over minimal. If any of these criteria is not met the procedure would not be lawful, and therefore a battery, irrespective of the actual outcome and, of course, of the purported consent.

This is an area where the law has not laid down hard and fast rules in advance. The best that a lawyer can hope to do is to accurately predict judicial response to a hypothetical case. If the above authors are correct it seems that many phase I trials of cytotoxic drugs cannot lawfully be carried out on human subjects. But this could be just one more instance of the mutual unawareness of doctors and lawyers as to each others' doings. Perhaps the way forward is that a wider legal acceptation of non-therapeutic experimentation in these cases will eventually emerge, the conditions of which will include:

(1) the subjects must be patients who are very seriously ill, and who know this;
(2) they have not responded to conventional treatment;
(3) a promising new drug is available, applicable in general to their condition, but it has not been tested, or sufficiently tested;
(4) it is made quite clear to the patients that the drug is not expected to have any benefit for them, but that the knowledge gained could benefit future patients;
(5) they are told of all known and foreseeable risks, including death if that be the case.

A patient-information and consent form should set out these points in the plainest language. It would be prudent to have it explained to and signed by a close relative as well as the patient. If after this explanation a patient consents, still entertaining the hope of benefit, it would be self-induced. There is no harm in hoping, provided that the patient has not been encouraged to think fatalistically, i.e. that he will be no worse off for agreeing to the trial.

Whether this procedure will be regarded as producing consent effective in law remains to be tested. It is doubtful if anything less than this could suffice. Graham Thorpe, in Chapter 16, argues from the standpoint of the clinician that research on the dying patient can be ethical and in some cases desirable. This may well be so, and no doubt judges would be slow to interfere with what can be shown to be desirable medical research, provided such ethical safeguards have been applied as can be applicable. If so, it seems that we may need to add a further category of human subject to the three mentioned on pages 10–11 above:

(d) Patients whose condition, in the present state of knowledge, is terminal; and who know this; and who are willing to undergo the most drastic trials fully aware that these cannot help them, can only make them worse, and can only be for the possible benefit of others. (I realize that I am depicting the worst-possible situation, but that is necessary for purposes of the present discussion.) It may be that the law would respect such decisions of self-sacrificing subjects while of course continuing to protect ordinary patients and healthy volunteers from unduly harmful non-therapeutic experiments, as at present. We will presumably find out only when the representatives of a self-sacrificed patient after his or her death try to sue for unnecessary pain and suffering and possible life-shortening that the deceased underwent. This may sound a somewhat unlikely cause of action but there are a lot of these nowadays, especially in the medico-legal area!

PHASE II STUDIES

With phase II studies of a cytotoxic drug, what has been established in Phase I as the optimum dosage range may be tried on a wide selection of cancer patients. At this stage there will presumably be some therapeutic justification, even if, with a disease as intractable as cancer, the chances of positive benefit in any specific case remain small. On that assumption the above cautionary words do not necessarily apply. It is the familiar balance-of-risks situation considered already.

OTHER TRIALS OF CANCER TREATMENTS

Two other types of trial of cancer treatments may be mentioned here as perhaps raising legal or ethical problems. The first concerns adjuvant therapy. Here patients who, having been treated apparently successfully, are thought to be at moderately high risk of recurrence are asked to undergo continuing preventive chemotherapy. What statistics there are suggest that a relatively small proportion of patients benefit; and that many, whether they benefit or not, suffer unpleasant (or worse) side-effects which may be short term or long term. So, with benefit uncertain (and unprovable), and the unavoidable adverse effects, this might be thought to pose legal or ethical problems similar to those considered under phase I above. However, it would be fair to regard the use of adjuvants as therapeutic, notwithstanding patients may be randomized as to whether they receive the adjuvant or not.

The second type of trial is also of preventive treatment, but with the aim of anticipating cancer in subjects who do not as yet have it (see Chapters 22–24).

These potential patients are identified as being at high risk because, for example, they have a pre-malignant condition or on account of their family history. To see if this new treatment works there have to be trials with the subjects randomized to treatment/non-treatment.

These two types of preventive trial raise two of the most frequently debated questions concerning the trial of a new treatment where none was previously available. As to the new treatment, the doctor must believe, on reasonable grounds, that it may work; and must give full information to enable the patient to make a free choice whether to undergo it and also to withdraw at any stage. As to the non-treatment of patients (or, in the second case, potential patients) the rule is that they should continue to receive the normal treatment. In these cases, however, there may not be any, save for close observation and regular checks, which they will presumably get as untreated controls. The frequent objection to randomization, that the doctor is not doing the best for his or her patient, does not apply here—at least until the effectiveness of the new treatment is established.

That being so, and always provided there is fully informed consent, these procedures do not seem to raise especially new questions not already inherent in randomizing and in balancing risks of unproven remedies against risk of serious illness occurring or recurring.

LOCAL RESEARCH ETHICS COMMITTEES

Local research ethics committees (LRECs) are supposed to exist and to meet regularly in every health district in the UK (see Chapter 7). Every proposed study, experimental procedure, survey, questionnaire or whatever should be submitted to the LREC for its prior approval. (That this is not yet a nationwide legal requirement is surprising. It ought to be included in every clinician's terms of appointment.)

Unlike in the USA, where, in major hospitals, researchers' projects go for evaluation first to a scientific committee and only then to an ethics committee, in the UK the LREC is expected to do both jobs. For scientific matters beyond their ken, the LREC is supposed to make its own inquiries or to co-opt further experts. New guidelines have recently been published in draft by the Department of Health to indicate what the Department considers appropriate for the composition and procedure of LRECs, and their ethical criteria. However, these are advisory only: every LREC is independent and entitled to impose its own procedures and standards. Even so, certain ethical and legal principles must be universal and consistent. Informed consent is one. It is vital that it is properly and effectively obtained along the lines suggested above, in order to protect the patient and so that researchers and their employing authority should not be unnecessarily at risk of legal claims for foreseeable adverse effects.

THE RIGHTS OF ADVERSELY AFFECTED SUBJECTS

What if, following the experimental procedure, a subject suffers an adverse condition, allegedly in consequence? In what circumstances is a claim, or rejection of a claim, justified? The special position of cancer patients who are willing to be subjected to high doses of a new cytotoxic drug has been considered already. What follows is concerned with the more typical subject and the general run of drugs and other trials.

(a) Causation: for any claim, whatever its legal basis, to succeed, causation must first be established. Proof of cause and effect to the level of scientific certainty is not called for; it suffices to show that the experiment was the cause more probably than not. Even so, this may involve difficult scientific speculations as well as legal problems.

Inevitable deterioration or mere lack of improvement are clearly excluded. More difficult are composite causes; a predisposing condition which was not known to be an exclusion criterion; or a concurrence of two or more independent causes at least one of which has nothing to do with the experiment. Such cases have to be determined on their peculiar facts. Where a clinician has been in any way negligent (e.g. in not observing the protocol) in such a way as to materially increase the risk of mishap, the law may be more willing to infer this to be a cause—it need not be *the* cause in the sense of sole cause. If, however, there is no such negligence apparent, a patient or healthy volunteer who proves the experimental treatment to be one, but only one, of two or more possible causes will fail: *Wilsher* v. *Essex Area Health Authority,* [1988] 1 All ER 871. In USA the courts may be more indulgent to plaintiffs in this situation, e.g. in requiring a careless defendant to disprove causation: *Sindell* v. *Abbott Laboratories* (1980), 607 P.2d 163.

It follows that it matters little whether clinician or drug manufacturer can be shown to be at fault unless that fault is causally relevant to the condition complained of. Finally, there is the issue of no-fault liability. The *Pearson Report* (Royal Commission on Civil Liability and Compensation for Personal Injury) in 1978 recommended a scheme for the UK but it has not been introduced. If it ever is, and is applied to medical mishaps, it will still require causation to be established.

(b) Assuming causation is established or admitted, the rights of injured subjects then depend on their legal status.

(1) Healthy volunteers: the normal practice is for the sponsor of a research project to accept strict liability for any resulting injury. For example the form of contract recommended by the Association of the British Pharmaceutical Industry (ABPI) to its members in their *Guidelines for Medical Experiments in Non-Patient Human Volunteers* (1988) states:

8. The company sponsoring the study confirms that . . . (iii) In the event of my suffering any significant deterioration in health or well-being caused directly by my participation in the study, compensation will be paid to me by the company.

Similarly, a new draft contract prepared by solicitors for Hampstead Health Authority in 1988 says:

In the event that any Volunteer suffers any deterioration in health (including any harmful susceptibility to toxicity) as a result of his/her participation in the Test, . . . the Manufacturer shall be obliged to pay him/her compensation for injury to health or resulting in death.

In both these contracts the sponsor, contracting directly with the subject and accepting no-fault liability, is liable once causation is established to pay whatever figure a court would assess as the damages.

(2) Patients submitting to non-therapeutic experiments: in principle there is no reason why the above contracts should not be extended to these patients. In practice the tendency has been to regard patients as in a separate category, less protectable than healthy volunteers. Sponsors do not often contract directly with them. A legal opinion which accompanied the Hampstead draft contract, mentioned above, suggests that as patients in this category are no less volunteers than healthy volunteers are, they should be contracted with in the same way. If so, the same no-fault liability would extend to them. However, the ABPI guidelines allow only for "non-patient volunteers" who are to be recruited by general notice rather than by direct approach. This seems to exclude patients of any sort. Likewise the 1986 Report of the Royal College of Physicians *Research on Healthy Volunteers*: "although it may be scientifically appropriate to use patients as control subjects for a condition from which they do not suffer, they should still be regarded as patients and not as healthy volunteers".

So, in the likely event of their having no contractual rights against the sponsor, patients in this category must prove fault on someone's part and their rights would be similar to those of the third category next to be considered. In passing, it should be mentioned that the medical protection bodies which insure doctors against negligence claims do so only in respect of negligence in treatment of patients. Non-therapeutic experiments done negligently do not appear to be covered by their policies. With the recent assumption of so-called Crown indemnity, whereby health authorities now act as insurers in respect of their employees' due performance, this may make little practical difference in most cases, since the trial would be in the course of the clinician's normal employment. It could still be significant where, for example, the trial or some of it is done outside an NHS hospital. With their acceptance of indemnity it would be opportune for health authorities to make it a condition of employment that a clinician does no research trials on patients without first getting LREC approval. With such a term in their contract, an authority would be entitled to say that, notwithstanding Crown indemnity, an unapproved trial would be at the clinician's risk.

(3) Patients submitting to therapeutic experiments: these are the least protected by the law in this country. If any carelessness, whether by sponsor or clinicians, or any unjustifiable withholding of risk information, etc., can be shown to be probably the cause of the proven adverse condition, they have a claim against the party concerned. Negligence, very broadly, means failure to reach a standard of care thought appropriate to the circumstances and based on what was or ought to have been foreseen. Furthermore, if in the course of employment an employee negligently causes harm, the employer (e.g. health authority) may be made liable vicariously. Where, however, a patient suffers side-effects or deterioration through, for example, some previously unknown and undiscoverable property of an experimental drug or device, then, as mentioned above, he has no legal remedy against anyone; because no one has negligence liability to the patient, or strict liability by contract with him.

It is true that sponsors of trials do contract with the clinician or health authority to indemnify them against claims for non-negligent injury. But on the assumption that no one is shown to be negligent, no one is liable to the patient; in other words, there is nothing much for the sponsor to indemnify against. This seems very unfair to the patient who has been injured partly in the interests of medical advance and partly in those of commercial profit. One wonders why they are not informed that they volunteer at their own risk of unforeseeable injury; and whether, if they were, they would volunteer so readily!

When I have mentioned this lack of protection to clinicians, they have sometimes suggested that they could ask the drug company or other sponsor to add to their contract a clause stating that in the event of the patient suffering injury (or serious injury, or whatever) the company would bear full no-fault liability. The trouble is that, first, the drug companies won't agree to this and, indeed, the ABPI actually tells them not to; and, second, even if they did, it would not give the patients any rights—in England, at least—because of our doctrine of privity of contract.

THE PRIVITY PROBLEM

English law says that parties to a contract get rights and duties as a result; but that no one else, not being a contracting party, can get any rights under it. This strict doctrine applies in most other common law countries, e.g. Canada, Australia, New Zealand, Nigeria. The notable exception is the USA, where for over a century a third party has been able to enforce rights in a contract made for his benefit. In countries whose law is based on Roman law (mainland Europe and South Africa) a stipulation in favour of a third person may be enforceable by him. Back in England, however, the effect is that if a sponsoring company were to contract with the investigator that in certain circumstances the company would compensate patients who suffered unforeseeable ill-effects, a patient so affected, being an outsider to the contract, could not make the company honour its promise. The investigator could sue the drug company but would only recover nominal damages, having suffered no personal ill-effects or loss.

There are several legal means of getting over this problem and giving the patient rights directly against the company. But any of them requires the company's agreement, and the ABPI in its guidelines *Clinical Trials: Compensation for Medicine-induced Injury* (1983) recommends the opposite:

> where injury is attributable to a medicine in a clinical trial, the ABPI recommends . . . that the following guidelines should be accepted without legal commitment . . . (a) the company should favourably consider the provision of compensation for personal injury . . . (c) compensation should only be paid for the more serious injury of an enduring and disabling character.

There is considerable scope here for patient power; drugs trials need willing subjects, but why should they volunteer if they are given nothing in return, and especially no rights to compensation for unforeseeable injury? This raises the interesting question whether there is a duty, on the part of investigators under instruction from the ethics committee, to warn patients of this "legal risk". If they were so warned, it would bring indirect pressure to bear on the sponsors to do what I suggest conscience requires.

The new Department of Health guidelines now under discussion point in this direction, but rather feebly. In paragraph B.8 LRECs are told that they should

> seek confirmation that any company conducting a patient or healthy volunteer study will accept responsibility for "no-fault" compensation.

This presumably means something more than mere moral responsibility for injury induced by their drugs, for that exists anyway. So in every proposed trial the LREC must lean on the investigator applicant to lean in turn on his sponsor to bind themselves to strict liability to subjects. For reasons given earlier, this can't be legally effective unless the company contracts direct with the patients. It is therefore disappointing to find the Department's same guidelines referring with apparent approval to the ABPI guidelines of 1983, quoted above, which precludes legal liability, even for serious injury, where fault cannot be established. More serious than this inconsistency is the underlying lack of purpose in the Department's approach. It is unfair, as well as ineffectual, to ask individual, disparate, uncoordinated LRECs to square up to the pharmaceutical industry. An LREC which tries to impose such conditions on sponsors is likely to find that projects are taken to less-demanding districts. If the Department of Health want, quite rightly, sponsoring companies to bear strict liability for unforeseeable mishaps, they should have the resolution to implement this as national policy, not leave it to local enterprise. In the words of the RCP report of 1984 paragraph 16: "There remains the lacuna of the injury occurring in the absence of fault. The major issues of liability will have to await solution on a national basis and there is nothing that individual Ethics Committees can do about them."

THE NEW LAW OF PRODUCT LIABILITY

There is now a further extension to the legal rights of subjects, taking the law beyond its previous sticking-point of negligence liability. In 1985 the European Community by its Product Liability Directive 85/374/EEC required every member state to impose liability, irrespective of negligence or fault, upon producers and importers into the EC of defective products which do injury or damage. "Product" includes drugs (it was the thalidomide disaster that gave the impetus leading to the Directive) and probably blood products. "Defect" includes inadequate warnings or instructions as well as in chemical content. The UK complied by passing the Consumer Protection Act 1987. However, the EC left to member states the freedom to allow or disallow producers a defence of indiscoverability, often called the "state of the art" defence.

The response of member states so far is patchy. At the time of writing, several have still not legislated at all. Denmark, Greece and Luxembourg do not allow any such defence. France and Spain are still thinking about it. Germany looks like it will not allow its drug manufacturers to raise the defence. As for the UK, the Act by s.4(1)(e) allows manufacturers a defence if they prove (onus on them):

> that the state of scientific and technical knowledge at the relevant time was not such that a producer of products of the same description as the product in question might be expected to have discovered the defect if it had existed in his products while they were under his control.

So it seems that the manufacturers will succeed if they can show that a hypothetical painstaking manufacturer at the relevant time (i.e. the time of supplying the drug or device) would not have known and could not, by research, be expected to have discovered it. This UK formulation, however, has been frowned upon by the European Commission, who see it as a widening of the very narrow defence permitted by their Directive, from in effect "indiscoverability" to "not reasonably discoverable". The UK may therefore yet be challenged over this non-compliance and have to tighten its law. For the present, however, the practical application of this defence will depend upon the attitude of UK courts when cases come to be litigated. Bearing in mind that existing notions of duty of care, causation and remoteness of damage may continue to influence the courts, subjects injured by undiscoverable defects may be little better off than formerly. As it stands s.4(1)(e), apart from reversing the burden of proof, seems to make UK product liability for drugs comparable with that in the USA. There, despite strict liability for most products, the California Supreme Court has ruled that prescription drugs manufacturers are liable only if negligent: *Brown* v. *Superior Court* (1988), 44 Cal.3d 1049; 245 Cal. Rptr 412; 751 P.2d 470. By contrast Australia is now considering reforming its law by a new Trade Practices Bill which would not require any defect to be established at all, and would allow a defence only if it could not have been discovered that the goods would act as they did.

CONCLUSIONS: VARIATIONS AND IMBALANCES

With even ethical standards at variance, it is too much to hope that differing national laws will be assimilated for the purposes of clinical trials. Investigators in each country must seek up-to-date guidance on what is required of them.

The law should be a help, not a hindrance, to the progress of medical science and the development of new therapies. But it also has to provide reasonable safeguards for the subjects of necessary experimentation. Less than complete protection for patient subjects may seem to give investigators and the pharmaceutical industry more freedom of action and margin of error. But this is a short-term and illusory advantage if it leads to a reluctance of patients to volunteer. Even if it does not, it is wrong that patients are ever experimented on at their own risk, and terribly wrong that they are not warned of this. The balance between the blameless investigator, authority and sponsor on the one hand, and the blameless injured patient on the other, is not an even balance. He should have a legal right to full measure of compensation, not just a hope of an ex gratia hand-out. Why not tell the patients and let them decide?

NOTE ADDED IN PROOF

Since this chapter was written, the Department of Health has issued in final form the guidelines for Local Research Ethics Committees (August 1991), discussed as in draft in the chapter. Paras 3.17–3.19 deal with the question of compensation of subjects of experiments who suffer non-foreseeable injury. There is no improvement in the feeble proposals for protecting subjects mentioned above.

The guidelines pay no heed to the Royal College of Physicians' report "Research Involving Patients" (January 1990) which in its Chapter 11 deplores the present situation and recommends improvements "to meet the justified expectation that compensation will be forthcoming for injury" without any requirement to prove negligence.

ABOUT THE AUTHOR

Victor Tunkel LLB (Nottingham), Barrister (Gray's Inn): Senior Lecturer in Law, Faculty of Laws, Queen Mary and Westfield College, University of London. Formerly Lecturer in Law, University of Bristol, and Visiting Lecturer, universities of Reading and Buckingham. Tutor, Council of Legal Education Inns of Court School of Law (Bar School). Lay Member of Local Research Ethics Committees. Contributor of occasional medico-legal articles to the *British Medical Journal*, *The Lancet*, *Criminal Law Review*, etc.

2 Law and Ethics in International Trials

JONATHAN MONTGOMERY

While researchers will usually be familiar with the legal framework governing trials in their home countries and acquainted with the customs of the ethics committees which scrutinize their work, the design of international trials raises new considerations. This paper explores three such areas: the law and ethics of consent, the role of ethics committees, and issues relating to compensation for subjects injured by mishaps.

Three major factors must be considered when establishing an international research programme. The first is the variation in factors external to the trial which may make the comparison of data unreliable. Examples might include the recruitment of subjects. In some countries subjects may be predominantly poor because other economic classes rely on private physicians without an interest in research for their care. Such factors must be taken into account in developing research methodologies in order to ensure the scientific validity of results. Research which will not yield scientifically rigorous data will rarely be ethical, because there will be few benefits to outweigh the risks of detriment to the research subjects. Detailed consideration of this type of problem is beyond the scope of this paper.

The second factor peculiar to designing international research relates to the legal and ethical requirements laid down by each of the countries in which it is proposed to run the trial. In part this problem is a practical one. Researchers need to ensure that they have followed the proper procedures in terms of licences and ethics committee approval. However, it also raises methodological considerations. Clearly, in order to enable results to be comparable it is necessary to ensure that the way in which research is carried out is as uniform as possible. However, the legal and ethical restrictions on permissible research will vary between countries.

Some may not permit trials without fully informed consent from the research subjects; others will rely primarily on ethics committees to protect patients and may find less extensive disclosure of risks acceptable. The need for uniformity requires that the design of the project be compatible with the most restrictive of the relevant countries' frameworks. Provided that it is acceptable to this then it will also be adequate, indeed more than adequate,

Introducing New Treatments for Cancer: Practical, Ethical and Legal Problems. Edited by C. J. Williams
© 1992 John Wiley & Sons Ltd

to satisfy the others. This paper cannot deal in detail with all the variations in approach of the world's legal systems, but it seeks to illustrate the problem by reference to the examples taken from North America and Europe.

The third varying feature which needs to be taken into account when designing international research relates to liability for accidents occurring during the trial. In some jurisdictions liability will only arise where someone can be shown to be at fault, for example by failing properly to inform the subject or culpably ignoring known contraindications (see Chapter 1). In others liability may "strict", i.e. the researcher, or manufacturer of a drug, may be liable to compensate the victims of accidents even where they were not at fault. Perhaps they could not have been expected to foresee or prevent the mishap occurring. Nevertheless, the accident was caused by their activities and under a strict liability system this is sufficient to lead to an obligation to compensate the injured research subject. In both these cases, no payments need be paid unless an accident occurs but researchers might need to build the possibility of liability into their costings (this could be done by insuring against the risk of accidents occurring).

In yet other legal systems compensation may be provided by a general scheme which compensates the victims of accidents even where no individual can be held responsible. This is sometimes called no-fault compensation. Such schemes can be funded in a number of different ways. Sometimes the state may provide the funding. In other cases researchers may be obliged to insure against the risk. It may be made a condition of the licensing of a drug for use that the manufacturers belong to an insurance scheme. This will give rise to costs which will be incurred even if no accident can be connected to the product in question. Again these costs would need to be taken into account when funding is secured for the research. This chapter cannot hope to provide a detailed account of all the relevant systems, but will explore these questions using concrete examples.

The aim of this chapter is therefore to draw the attention of researchers to the questions which need to be asked about variations in the law and regulatory practice between different countries. This should enable potential pitfalls to be avoided at an early stage in research design and reduce the risk that projects are frustrated by unexpected legal difficulties.

NATIONAL AND INTERNATIONAL STANDARDS OF ETHICS

Consideration of the standards of research ethics applied across the world needs to be divided into two sections. The first is purely procedural, dealing with whose approval needs to be sought, and at what point it is necessary to secure it. The second relates to the substantive principles of ethics which will be used by the relevant bodies to determine whether the research should be authorized.

WHOSE APPROVAL SHOULD BE SOUGHT?

The first thing which will need to be ascertained by any researcher designing an international trial will be whether formal approval is required for all stages of the trial. In the UK drug trials need no licensing for phase I, but need a clinical trial certificate for phases II and III from the Committee on Safety of Medicines (CSM) [1]. Finally, a medicine cannot be marketed without a product licence. Other countries, however, have formal requirements relating to the phase I stage. Examples include the USA where new drugs cannot be used even on an investigational basis unless the Food and Drug Administration (FDA) has been notified of specified information and has not objected within 30 days. Trials intended to be partly carried out in America would therefore need to file the relevant "Notice of Claimed Investigational Exemption for a New Drug" with the FDA prior to phase I trials, even though no application need be made to the UK CSM at this stage.

In addition to discovering whether formal approval is required at every stage, researchers will also need to identify the bodies from whom approval must be sought. Some systems may require national approval instead of, or in addition to, permission from local ethics committees. Further, sometimes national approval may be conditional on prior authorization from local committees; in other cases local committees may only consider cases after trials have received approval at a national level. Consequently, inquiries must be made about the appropriate procedures in each of the countries where it is proposed to carry out the trial.

In some cases responsibility for seeking approval may be left to those carrying out the research rather than being tackled at the initial design stage. This will be the most convenient way forward for countries, such as the UK in respect of phase I trials, where the only approval needed is that of a local ethics committee. Individual researchers are likely to know the requirements of their local committees already and be well placed to present and justify the proposal. Where national approval is required, however, it is likely to save time and the duplication of effort if authorization is obtained at an early stage prior to the recruitment of individual researchers.

Once the appropriate bodies have been identified it may also be necessary to discover something about their powers and composition. In the context of international trials, it is even more important than usual to seek to anticipate the questions which are likely to be asked by ethics committees. If the trial is to be run in different countries at approximately the same time, it is vital that its progress is not delayed. Committees may not meet frequently, and the risk of having to resubmit the proposal at a later meeting should be reduced as much as is possible. Most systems seek to ensure that the groups entrusted with the responsibility of scrutinizing research proposals contain lay members, health care professionals and scientists (see Chapter 6). It may be wise for researchers to prepare their proposals with this variation of interests in mind. Information may need to be presented in more than one form in order to cover the expected concerns of each of these groups. Similarly, researchers should ensure that the committees which they approach are permitted to authorize the type of research proposed. Some research may be exempt from the need for approval at one or more levels, but alternatively it may be the case that committees are only allowed to consider low-risk research or research on certain categories of subject. Research on prisoners, for example, may well be subject to a different regime than applies to general hospital patients.

WHAT PRINCIPLES WILL BE APPLIED?

A distinction should be drawn in considering the principles which ethics committees and licensing authorities will apply between the rules which limit the powers of those bodies and the ethical guidelines which they will use in order to decide whether to permit research. If an objection to the trial is based on a rule of the first type, then the design will have to be changed. If the concern is of the second class, then a better explanation of the researchers' position might suffice to persuade the body to change its mind.

Where a piece of research contravenes the first category of rules, the authority will have no choice but to refuse to allow it to proceed. An example might be a proposed phase I trial which did not inform the research subjects that they were being subjected to an experimental procedure which was not intended to improve their health. Most legal systems will limit such procedures to volunteers and if this is the case an ethics committee could not lawfully authorize non-consensual research. It would be irrelevant that the committee thought that the research was ethical because they would have no power in law to authorize an illegal experiment.

In most cases, however, the concern will be less with the legal limits of permissible research than with the ethical principles which are applied. Here the ethics committee must decide not whether it *could* authorize the trial, but whether it *should* do so. While there may be significant variation between countries in respect of the rules which govern the lawfulness of research procedures, the ethical principles which are applied are likely to be drawn from the same sources and therefore enshrine similar values. Nevertheless, there will remain differences of detail.

The scope for variation is considerable and is inevitably coloured by sociological and political factors. Some cultures trust scientists and health professionals more readily than others. Further, laws can change rapidly and researchers should be wary of accepting old accounts of the law without checking that there have not been new developments. In order to illustrate the nature of the problem a more detailed look at variations in the laws of consent will be offered in the next section of this chapter. First, however, it is appropriate to consider the internationally accepted ethical guidelines which have been developed since the Second World War.

The revelation of the abuses of Nazi scientists led to the drawing up of the Nuremburg Code in 1947. This contained ten principles which were to be satisfied before experimentation on human subjects could be justified. They included the need for consent and the right of withdrawal, the avoidance of unnecessary suffering, the use of human subjects only where other sources of knowledge had been exhausted, and proportionality between the risks to the research subjects and the benefits expected to accrue from the experiment. These principles still dominate thinking on the ethics of medical research.

The World Medical Association has produced further guidance, set out in the Declaration of Helsinki (originally 1964, revised in 1975 and 1983). This Declaration adopts the Nuremburg principles but also introduces an important new distinction—that between clinical and non-clinical research. The basis for the distinction is enshrined in paragraph 6 of Part II of the revised Helsinki Declaration:

> The physician can combine medical research with professional care . . . only to the extent that medical research is justified by its potential diagnostic or therapeutic value for the patient.

Where doctors choose a novel therapy because they believe it to be the best care available, this should be governed by the law relating to treatment, not that dealing with research. Research is only problematic because there may be a conflict between the interests of the patient/subject and those of the researcher. Research which is at the expense of an individual patient's treatment must be carefully scrutinized. But doctors should not be prevented from providing the best care they can because of heavy-handed regulation. In cases of non-clinical (or "purely scientific") research further safeguards are needed. The Declaration of Helsinki therefore obliges researchers to withdraw subjects from their trials if they believe that to continue would harm them.

It is probable that the principles set out in these two international statements will be used by all research committees. All international trials should therefore be designed with them in mind. In addition, however, there will usually be more detailed guidelines drawn up in each country. In the UK the most important of these have been produced by the Royal College of Physicians. Two working party reports have been produced: *Research on Healthy Volunteers* (1986) and *Research Involving Patients* (1989). In addition the college has published *Guidelines on the Practice of Ethics Committees Involved in Medical Research Involving Human Subjects* (2nd edition, 1989) (see Chapter 3). Draft guidance has also been produced by the UK Department of Health. Any researcher seeking approval of a trial in the UK would clearly be well advised to bear this guidance in mind. It does not bind the committees, but it will usually be taken into account. Other assistance is also available, for example the Association of the British Pharmaceutical Industry has provided *Guidelines for Medical Experiments in Non-Patient Human Volunteers* (1988).

Similar documents are likely to be available in most countries with developed mechanisms for regulating scientific and health care practice. In the USA the Department of Health and Human Services has produced regulations which are formally applicable only to research funded by the Department, but which in practice are much more widely influential than this position requires. Much of the material in these documents will be similar, but any person seeking to ensure that the same trial can be conducted in a number of countries would be well advised to consult the appropriate documents setting out the principles which advise ethics committees on their responsibilities. The best sources of information as to the existence of such documents are probably the professional organizations or health departments of the countries in question.

THE LAW OF CONSENT

The principle of voluntary co-operation by research subjects is central to the framework set out in the international documents. It is also fundamental to most legal frameworks governing research on human subjects. Variations in the laws of consent between different jurisdictions therefore provide a good example of the way in which legal systems differ and illustrate the point by reference to what is probably the most important area of law. Three different approaches to the law of consent will be outlined here, but researchers should not rely on this account for practical advice on their projects. They should ensure that they obtain up-to-date information about the details of the rules prevailing in the relevant countries when carrying out research. This piece is intended to demonstrate the sort of questions which they would need to ask, not to provide a law manual.

PROFESSIONAL STANDARDS TESTS

In some countries, including England, the judges have shown themselves peculiarly reticent to scrutinize the work of the medical profession. The reason for this reluctance is a combination of belief in the altruism of doctors and respect for their expertise [2]. Even in the area of consent the English courts have declined to adopt the view that patients are entitled to know everything [3]. Instead they have treated the law of informed consent as raising exactly the same issues as any other malpractice claim, i.e. whether the doctor in question acted in a way acceptable to a responsible body of professional practitioners.

Where this approach to standards of informed consent is used, a court seeking to determine whether a researcher has acted properly will proceed by calling expert witnesses to give evidence as to standard practice. In most cases, the fact that standard practice has been followed will be sufficient legal justification for the researcher's actions because it will show that they have not been 'negligent' in carrying out their duty to consider the interests of the research subjects. The judges usually reserve the right to declare some standard practices unlawful, but rarely exercise it. In essence, therefore, the law reinforces professional standards rather than imposing different rules upon them. If this approach to the law prevails, then the process of getting ethics committee approval would generally show that the design of the trial met the required legal standards. Provided the trial was carried out as approved, it is probable that the law will have been complied with.

It is unclear whether any legal system would apply such an unrestrictive principle to consent to research. Even in England, where the judiciary are particularly beneficent to the medical profession, it is generally held that this approach would be modified in the context of research (see Chapter 1). It must be said, however, that there is yet to be an English case on the point and no prediction can claim infallibility. The distinction drawn by the Helsinki Declaration between clinical and non-clinical research might well be used. Where research is intended to benefit the research subject directly it will be more plausible to suggest that the issues are the same as those arising in the course of ordinary treatment. In cases of non-therapeutic research it is likely that one of the two other models will prevail.

TESTS BASED ON WHAT THE SUBJECT WANTS TO KNOW

Most legal systems scrutinize the practice of health professionals in relation to consent more closely than the first model would allow. They recognize the vulnerability that follows from the relative ignorance of patients, and to an even greater extent research subjects. Consequently, they seek to ensure that this imbalance of knowledge is remedied by obligations to inform the patient of risks, side-effects and alternatives. The greater a system's commitment to individualistic or rights-based arguments the more onerous these obligations are likely to be. This approach to the problem emphasizes the quality of the patient's decision—asking whether the consent given was sufficiently informed.

A problem arises as to whether the test to be applied should be objective or subjective. A subjective test would ask whether this particular research subject has been told everything which they personally would want to know. The researcher would then need to find out what sort of risks each individual subject was concerned about. This is the approach taken by West German law [4].

The burden placed on researchers by a subjective test is uncertain in scope and in the common law countries (those whose law derives from England and the USA) it is more usual to use an objective test. This requires a researcher to tell the subjects everything which a reasonable subject would be expected to want to know. This would usually be combined with the opportunity to ask questions, to which the researcher would be expected to give full and honest answers. Thus in a Canadian case the court stated that the subject should be told of "all the facts, probabilities and opinions which a reasonable man might be expected to consider before giving his consent" (*Halushka* v. *University of Saaskatchewan* (1965), 53 DLR 2d.436, 444).

The final aspect of consent law which should be mentioned here relates to deliberate non-disclosure. In the context of consent to treatment it is common for legal systems to develop a concept of the "therapeutic privilege". This permits physicians to withhold information when they believe that it would damage the patient's health to disclose it. This means that even where the usual test would require a piece of information to be given to a patient it may be legitimate to fail to do so in the patient's own interests. The exact scope of this principle varies considerably. In the context of research, however, it is very unlikely that a justification of "therapeutic privilege" will be recognized. In the treatment context a patient's health might suffer if they were scared out of accepting treatment, but the research subject's health is not at risk by refusing to participate.

TESTS BASED ON THE CONFLICT OF RESEARCHERS' AND SUBJECTS' INTERESTS

The third approach begins not with the quality of the subject's consent but with the position of the researcher. In the context of treatment the patient and the doctor are assumed to have the same aim—to make the patient well. Research is different. The interest of the researcher is in discovering new information. There is a risk that this may conflict with the interests of the research subject in their own safety. Indeed it is probable that the research subject will be taking risks in order to benefit others. The researcher is therefore caught on the horns of a dilemma. At the same time they are responsible for the efficiency of the research and the safety of the subjects— responsibilities which may conflict.

This problem is not restricted to the context of medical science. Professional advisers in any area may often find that the interests of a client conflict with those of the adviser, or those of another client of the adviser. In these areas the solution has been to require them to make a "full and frank disclosure" of their interests even when there is only a potential (not actual) conflict of interests. This ensures that the client is able to appreciate the position.

If the professional fails to make such a disclosure they are responsible for any prejudice to their clients' interests.

This approach is also applicable in the context of medical research. Researchers may be required to put all the information they have about the risks before the subject, so that it is absolutely clear that they have not placed their own concerns above the safety of the subject. The Nuremburg Code goes this far and requires *all* information to be shared with the patient. This has been adopted in the USA (Department of Health and Human Services, *Regulations on Protection of Human Subjects* 45 CFR 46 (1983), *Whitlock* v. *Duke University* (1986), 637 F. Suppl. 1463). The conflict of interests test may also be combined with the reasonable patient test, as it was in the Canadian case discussed above, so that the researcher is required to disclose everything which a reasonable subject might wish to know.

PROBLEMS WITH SPECIAL GROUPS OF POTENTIAL SUBJECTS

The general rules applied in any legal system are likely to be subject to variation in respect of some groups of research subjects. These are likely to be those who are incapable of giving fully informed consent either because of a permanent incapacity or because of the existence of a higher than usual degree of vulnerability. The most obvious examples of the former are children and people with mental disorders or mental handicap. The latter type of case might include prisoners, who are reliant on the continued goodwill of the prison medical services and may feel pressurized into consenting against their better judgment. Members of the armed forces may be in a similar position.

Some commentators argue that such groups can never be used in research without breaching ethical and even legal requirements [5]. Certainly it is probable that special legal rules will apply to safeguard their welfare. In particular, it would usually be thought necessary to exhaust the possibilities for research on competent subjects before using subjects who cannot give valid consents themselves. Researchers wishing to draw subjects from such groups should ensure that they inquire about special rules. It should be noted that even the definitions of these groups may differ between jurisdictions. For example, a child who can understand the nature of the choice involved in becoming a research subject would be competent to consent to research in England, while in other countries there are age-based limits. The age limits may vary considerably.

LIABILITY FOR MISHAPS

The range of legal approaches to compensation for the victims of research-related accidents was outlined in the introduction to this chapter. In many cases there will be no special rules in relation to research. Compensation will be payable on the same basis as it would for malpractice in the course of treatment. It is generally accepted, however, that research subjects should be better protected than patients. Unlike patients they shoulder an increased burden of risk for the benefit of others, not themselves. In addition more volunteers may be encouraged to come forward if they are confident that if the worst were to happen, and their altruism were to expose them to injury, they will at least receive compensation.

This section is designed to introduce the general shape of compensation systems so researchers can understand the principles on which they work. The details of the law of any particular country may vary considerably, but in most cases the best way to protect a researcher from liability for mishaps is through insurance rather than scrutinizing the legal rules. See Chapter 1 for further discussion of this area.

FAULT-BASED LIABILITY

In order to obtain compensation in a fault-based system, the injured research subject would have to establish three things: (1) that the researcher or manufacturer being sued had breached the appropriate legal standards of conduct; (2) that the injury suffered by the subject was caused by the failure to reach the required standard; and (3) what the injury is "worth" in financial terms. Each of these steps has its own problems.

The standards in issue will vary. There will be problems of law, such as those discussed in the context of consent—what are the rules to be applied? These will not necessarily be very clear. If the law requires a researcher to avoid being negligent it may be necessary to determine what the usual practice of researchers is before the standard can be identified. There will also be problems of fact. It may not be clear whether or not the standards were honoured in a particular case. The victim of the accident will need to establish exactly what happened. They may have been unconscious at the time the accident happened. The researchers may not remember what occurred in relation to one subject amongst a large study.

The second step, proof of causation, can also present major problems. Research is usually carried out precisely because no one really knows how things work. If the condition of a patient taking part in a trial deteriorates, is this a result of the drug being tested or the original condition being treated? Unless the patient can establish that it is the former they will not get compensation. Very often no one will know one way or the other. If so the person injured will go uncompensated.

If the first two hurdles are overcome, there is still the question of how much compensation is payable. This will be determined by the nature of the injury. So far as common types of injury are concerned, most systems have a rough tariff scale to determine how much they are worth. Loss of earnings will be added in, as will the cost of meeting future needs. A lump sum will usually be arrived at, payable once and for all, but in some jurisdictions smaller amounts may be payable on a continuing (perhaps annual) basis.

STRICT LIABILITY

Under a strict liability system the accident victims will need to prove only the second and third of the steps discussed above. They must show only that the injury was caused during the research to overcome the equivalent of (1). Nevertheless, the difficulties of the final two steps remain, and the existence of strict liability by no means guarantees compensation. It is quite common to find that strict liability exists for injuries caused by defective goods. Member states of the European Community are required to have laws whereby the producers of defective products, including drugs, are made strictly liable for accidents. In many countries, such as England under the Consumer Protection Act 1987, this position is mitigated by the existence of defences which reintroduce some elements of fault. Thus a manufacturer who shows that an accident could not have been avoided whatever they did will not be liable. This means that there may be no clear line between fault-based laws and strict liability. In principle, however, a research subject who is the victim of an accident during a trial should have a greater chance of receiving compensation through strict liability than where proof of fault is necessary.

NO-FAULT LIABILITY

The intention of no-fault schemes is that they avoid the pitfalls of litigation. An injured person should receive support when only the third step discussed above is established. In practice, however, it is likely that causation will still have to be shown. In addition an accident victim may have to produce evidence of the circumstances in which the accident happened. This is because most no-fault schemes apply only to particular types of injury, such as the New Zealand scheme which applies to those caused by "medical misadventure". Thus the research subject seeking compensation in New Zealand will have to go through the same step (2) as with a fault-based system, and will have to prove that the events constituted "medical misadventure"—an exercise different from step (1) as described above, but in many ways equivalent to it. Thus it is clear that no-fault schemes are less simple than might be imagined.

In terms of the liability of the researcher, it is necessary to ascertain two things about countries where a no-fault scheme exists. The first relates to the way in which it is funded. Some schemes are funded from a levy on the practitioners or manufacturers whose work they cover (e.g. the Swedish Pharmaceutical Insurance Scheme). In such cases the cost of this levy will be part of the overheads of the research. The second matter which should be investigated concerns the co-existence of fault and no-fault systems. Sometimes the existence of no-fault compensation may exclude liability through the courts. In others a researcher might be liable in both the courts (when at fault) and also under a no-fault scheme, although an individual claimant may have to choose either one avenue or the other.

THE IMPORTANCE OF DOCUMENTATION AND INSURANCE

The main impacts on research design concern costing and record keeping. All litigation raises difficulties of proof and written evidence may be crucial in establishing whether a researcher acted properly or not. This would include carefully drafted consent forms and notes. Researchers should ensure that if an accident does occur the fullest possible records are made as soon as is practicable. The paperwork is not imbued with any kind of magic, but it makes life considerably easier.

It is important that researchers ensure that they will not be personally faced with a large bill for damages. The easiest way to deal with liability for mishaps is to insure against having to pay them. The cost of this insurance is a component of the overall cost of the research project and should therefore be included in funding applications. Alternatively, the organizations funding research may prefer to offer an indemnity to researchers whereby they undertake to meet any legal liabilities which arise. In some cases insurance cover or indemnity might be provided by a researcher's institution or employer rather than by the funder of a particular project. This latter approach has major attractions for international research, in that it will prevent the need for the intricacies of compensation systems to be taken into account by the person designing the overall trial.

CONCLUSION

This chapter has not provided a manual of the law relating to research in different countries. Instead, it has sought to outline in general terms the range of variation between legal systems. This should enable researchers to identify what sort of questions should be asked to establish the necessary details. The successful design of international trials will probably depend on a mixture of initial central planning and delegation. Individual researchers in different countries will usually be able to ensure that the research is carried out in accordance with local legal requirements, provided that the overall design is workable in accordance with all the models of ethical and legal requirements discussed. Local variation will not then jeopardize the overall study. Insurance against financial liability is probably best sorted out locally wherever possible and it should be made clear where this is the case, so that local researchers cannot seek to claim indemnity against the original designer. Most of all, researchers should ensure that it is clear who takes responsibility for complying with local legal requirements.

REFERENCES

1. Teff H (1984) Regulation under the Medicines Act 1968: a continuing prescription for health. Modern Law Rev 47: 303–323
2. Montgomery J (1989) Medicine, accountability and professionalism. J Law Society 16: 319–339
3. Montgomery J (1988) Power/knowledge/consent: medical decision making. Modern Law Rev 51: 245–251
4. Shaw J (1986) Informed consent: a German lesson. Int Comp Law Quarterly 35: 864–890
5. Giesen D (1988) International medical malpractice law. Martinus Nijhoff, London, pp 569–573

FURTHER READING

Areen J et al, (1984) **Law, science and medicine**. Foundation Press, New York (with annual supplements), Ch 6
Bankowski Z, Howard-Jones N (eds), (1982) **Human experimentation and medical ethics**. Council for International Organizations of Medical Sciences, Geneva
Dworkin G, (1987) Law and medical experimentation. University of Monash Law Review, 13: 189
Giesen D, (1988) **International medical malpractice law**. Martinus Nijhoff, London, pp 564–604
Kennedy I, Grubb A, (1989) **Medical law: text and materials**. Butterworths, London, Ch 11
Nuremburg Code (1947)
World Medical Association (1964) **Declaration of Helsinki** (revised 1975 and 1983) WMA, Helsinki

ABOUT THE AUTHOR

Jonathan Montgomery has been a lecturer in the Faculty of Law at the University of Southampton since 1984. His main research interests lie in the fields of the law relating to health, health care and to the family. He has written numerous articles in legal periodicals on these matters. He is co-author of *Nursing and the Law* (Macmillan, 1989) and co-editor of the *Encyclopedia of Health Services and Medical Law* (Sweet & Maxwell, looseleaf). He teaches health care law in the law and medical faculties at Southampton and regularly provides lectures and workshops for health professionals on legal matters. He is a member of the Ethics Advisory Committe of the British Paediatrics Association.

3 Research Involving Patients

SUMMARY AND RECOMMENDATIONS OF A REPORT OF
THE ROYAL COLLEGE OF PHYSICIANS*

SUMMARY

The careful study of disease as it occurs in patients, and the equally careful scrutiny of the effects of treatment, are an indispensable part of the continuing process of improving the efficiency of diagnosis and the effectiveness of treatment. Most patients realise that experience gained from their own case may contribute to their personal benefit or to that of society and, if asked, readily agree to take part in research into their condition. Accordingly, a patient who willingly participates in research has the status of a volunteer similar to that of a healthy person so that some of the questions relating to selection, consent, conduct of research and compensation in the event of injury are similar to those addressed in the College's report on *Research in healthy volunteers*, published in 1986. It is important to realise, however, that the patient is in a position of at least partial dependence which may affect the degree of voluntariness of collaboration, and also that there is a risk that enthusiasm on the part of the researcher could lead to undue persuasion or incomplete declaration of the facts. Furthermore, the patient's ability to give consent to participate in research may be impaired by illness. For these and other reasons, the College has prepared a separate report addressing the special problems of *Research involving patients*.

A balance has to be struck between the benefits which may flow from properly conducted research, and the risk of infringing the autonomy, or of causing harm to the individual patient. The report provides guidance for all concerned—including patients, researchers, doctors, nurses and other health workers, sponsors of research, Research Ethics Committees and the institutions in which research takes place. The general public, too, may find this report useful.

This report should be read in conjunction with the second edition of the College's *Guidelines on the practice of ethics committees in medical research involving human subjects*, which is being published at the same time as this

*Published by permission of the Royal College of Physicians (*Journal of the Royal College of Physicians*, 1990, 24: 10–14). Copies of the full report (and other related reports) are available from the Royal College of Physicians, 11 St Andrew's Place, London NW1 4LE, UK.

Introducing New Treatments for Cancer: Practical, Ethical and Legal Problems. Edited by C. J. Williams
Published 1992 by John Wiley & Sons Ltd

report. The *Guidelines* describe the contribution and working of medical Research Ethics Committees and are designed to assist those committees in their work. Necessarily, many of the issues are common to these two publications, particularly those concerned with consent given by patients to participate in a research study, and the conduct and monitoring of research on human subjects.

This report considers all forms of research in patients, whether they involve the study of treatment which may benefit individual patients (therapeutic research) or the acquisition of knowledge which can be of no immediate benefit to the patient (non-therapeutic research). The discussion of medical research in this document includes research involving surgical procedures. It does not include fetal tissue.

Particular attention is paid to potentially vulnerable groups of patients such as unborn babies, children, elderly people, patients suffering from mental illness or handicap, and patients in custody. The report also gives consideration to special cases such as research in severely ill or unconscious patients, or research into sudden unexpected events in which it may be difficult to obtain consent for the investigation. Arrangements for compensation in the event of injury occurring as a result of participating in research are also considered, as is the need to protect the patient's confidentiality.

RECOMMENDATIONS

Research involving patients is in the interests of patients and of society and should proceed without unnecessary impediment. Certain safeguards are, however, necessary to protect the patient from suffering physical or emotional harm or breach of confidentiality in the course of research.

ROLE OF RESEARCH ETHICS COMMITTEES

1. All research involving patients should be approved by a local Research Ethics Committee. This applies to research undertaken in hospitals and in other institutions, research conducted in general practice and elsewhere in the community and research carried out by doctors and non-medical health or other workers. Recommendations on the composition and function of Research Ethics Committees are set out in Chapter 4 of the full report.

ASSESSING THE AIMS, QUALITY, RISKS AND BENEFITS OF RESEARCH

2. The Research Ethics Committee should be satisfied that the question addressed by the research activity is a worthwhile one and Research Ethics Committees should examine the overall design of proposed research that comes before them.
3. Research Ethics Committees must assess whether, in proposed research, the risk or inconvenience caused to the patient is justifiable in relation to the value of the information sought.
4. Research Ethics Committees and investigators have a duty to ensure that the risks inherent in proposed research have been reduced to the minimum necessary to achieve the research objective.
5. Investigators must ensure that the study protocol effectively excludes special groups of patients in whom the risk of participation would be particularly great.
6. As a general rule, research involving patients should not incur risk greater than minimal. An exception to the general rule may be justified where there is great potential benefit to the individual participating in therapeutic research (that is, research which offers the prospect of direct benefit to the patient taking part). Non-therapeutic research involving greater than minimal risk might be approved by a Research Ethics Committee but only under rare circumstances where: (i) the risk of the research procedure is still very small in comparison to the risks already incurred by the patient as a consequence of the disease itself; (ii) the disease under study is a serious one; (iii) there is great potential benefit in terms of the importance of the knowledge gained; (iv) there is no other means of obtaining the knowledge; and (v) the subject understands well what is involved and wishes to participate.

SELECTION OF PATIENTS AND USE OF MEDICAL RECORDS

7. Any list of patients' names should be confidential to the person or institution responsible for its construction.
8. Where records are used as a starting point in the recruitment of patients, the person who approaches the patient should normally be the individual who was responsible for the clinical care at the time that the patient's relevant case records were generated.
9. Research work based upon scrutiny of medical records should continue without unnecessary impediment, but great care is required to avoid causing harm or distress to patients or their relatives, particularly through breach of confidentiality. Research which will involve access to personal medical records should receive approval by the local Research Ethics Committee.

RECRUITMENT OF PATIENTS

10. Arrangements should be made to exclude patients who may be at increased risk from proposed research procedures.
11. Excessively frequent requests to patients to participate in research should be avoided.
12 Patients should be invited to participate in research as volunteers in the same way as healthy individuals are invited to volunteer.
13. In the course of inviting a patient to participate in research, an investigator must make it clear that the patient is free to decline to participate without giving a reason, that a decision to decline will be accepted without question or displeasure and that the patient will then be treated as though the matter had not arisen and without any disadvantage to future care.
14. The patient participating in research should understand that he will remain free to withdraw at any time, that no reason need be given for the withdrawal, that the withdrawal will be accepted without question, without incurring displeasure and without any disadvantage to future care.

CONSENT

15. Patients should know that they are taking part in research.
16. Research involving a patient should only be carried out with the patient's consent. We have found it necessary to describe exceptions to this general rule in the case of some innocuous observations of behaviour, research based on anonymous specimens or on medical records and some research into unheralded emergencies.
17. The simple procedure of seeking oral consent after an oral explanation may need to be supported by additional measures.
    (i) *A Patient Information Sheet* may be used to back up the oral description of what is involved.
    (ii) *Time to reflect* may be arranged to allow the patient to consider the question of enrolment.
    (iii) *Written consent* may be sought.
    (iv) *A third party* may act as adviser or friend to the patient.
    (v) *Witnessed consent* may be a useful alternative in patients with impaired capacity to comprehend.
    (vi) *Special arrangements* are necessary in the case of patients who may have impaired capacity to comprehend (e.g. children, the mentally handicapped and patients with mental illness).
18. Research involving minimal risk or greater than minimal risk should be described in a Patient Information Sheet which is given to patients when they are invited to participate and retained by them. The Information Sheet should be submitted to the Research Ethics Committee for approval.

19. The use of written consent and a consent form is recommended in research projects associated with minimal or more than minimal risk or with significant discomfort. The Consent Form should be submitted to the Research Ethics Committee for approval.

RESEARCH INVOLVING CHILDREN

20. Research which could equally well be done on adults should never be done on children.
21. Children should be consulted when the question of their participation in research arises.
22. Even if an investigator believes that a child is capable of giving consent the approval of a parent or guardian should be obtained before any research procedure is contemplated on a child under the age of 16 years. It may also be desirable to obtain parental consent in some older children.
23. Where the research is for the benefit of children generally, and the child is incapable of giving consent, the investigator can properly rely on the consent of a parent or guardian. If, when the parental approval has been obtained, a child objects to the procedure itself, the investigator and the parent or guardian should reconsider whether it is appropriate to proceed.

RESEARCH INVOLVING THE MENTALLY HANDICAPPED

24. Research should never be carried out in mentally handicapped patients which could equally well be undertaken in adults who are not mentally handicapped.
25. Research in mentally handicapped patients should be limited to that which is related to mental handicap.
26. Research in mentally handicapped patients is subject to the usual constraints affecting all research in patients.
27. Many mentally handicapped patients are capable of giving consent but consideration should be given to the use of simple tests of competence and to the use of "two part" consent forms in which the first part comprises a test. Even if consent is forthcoming it is good practice to obtain the consent of the next-of-kin after proper explanation of the intended research. A strong ethical case can be made out for therapeutic and non-therapeutic research involving only minimal risk in mentally handicapped patients not competent to give consent. The best guidance might be that there should be agreement by close relatives and that the individual should seem to consent to the procedure, but the legal status of such research remains uncertain.

RESEARCH INVOLVING THE MENTALLY ILL

28. Research should never be carried out in mentally ill patients which could equally well be undertaken in adults who are not mentally ill.
29. Research in mentally ill patients should be limited to that which is related to the mental illness.
30. Research in mentally ill patients is subject to the usual constraints affecting all research in patients. Most patients with mental illness are competent to make up their own minds as to whether they wish to take part in research and to comprehend the implications of the research.
31. The Research Ethics Committee must be convinced that the inclusion of patients who are incompetent to give consent is acceptable and that it arises because the research is specifically directed to the condition of patients who might be incompetent.
32. Where competence is in doubt or absent, due to psychosis, dementia or other causes, and in all patients detained under the Mental Health Act irrespective of competence, a procedure which seeks what is in effect a mixture of consent by the patient and consent by a relative or nominated individual may be the most satisfactory arrangement. The same considerations affect therapeutic and non-therapeutic research in mentally handicapped and mentally ill individuals who are incompetent to give consent; the legal status of such research is at present uncertain.

RESEARCH INVOLVING PRISONERS

33. Research should not be undertaken solely in prisoners who are patients unless the fact of being imprisoned is itself an essential component of the research topic.

RESEARCH INVOLVING SEVERELY ILL PATIENTS

34. Where the severity of a patient's illness renders him incompetent to give consent to participate in research the principles which should apply resemble those applicable to mentally handicapped and mentally ill patients.
35. In research involving severely ill patients the researcher should obtain as competent consent as possible. No patient who refused or, if incapable of refusing, resisted should be included or continued in research. A near relative should be informed of the nature of the research and the details of what is involved and should concur. In general, the patient should be told about the participation in research later, when he recovers sufficiently to comprehend. The same considerations that affect therapeutic and non-therapeutic research in mentally handicapped individuals who are incompetent to give consent may also apply in

mentally ill patients incompetent to give consent; the legal status of such research is at present uncertain.

RESEARCH INVOLVING PREGNANT PATIENTS

36. Research in pregnant patients should only be undertaken if pregnancy is an essential part of the research.
37. Research into pregnancy and childbirth requires special consideration since two individuals, mother and child, are inevitably involved and the rights and concerns of the father may need to be taken into account.

RESEARCH INVOLVING ELDERLY PATIENTS

38. The participation of elderly patients in research is desirable. Elderly patients present special problems because of their altered metabolism, the frequency of multiple ailments, and their reduced tolerance of invasive procedures. In general, elderly patients should be assumed to be competent to give consent unless there is evidence to the contrary. It should not be thought that, because of their age, they need to know any less about the intended research than a younger patient.

INITIATION OF RESEARCH WITHOUT CONSENT

39. There are some circumstances in which it is justifiable to initiate research without the consent of the patient. *These are described in detail in the full Report*. Such circumstances do not affect the duty of the investigator to obtain the prior approval of the Research Ethics Committee in the usual way.

INDUCEMENTS TO PATIENTS

40. Improved care should not be offered as an inducement to participate.
41. Payments to patients are generally undesirable but are occasionally acceptable in studies which are lengthy and tedious. Payments to patients should not be for undergoing risk and should not be such as to persuade patients to volunteer against their better judgement.
42. Any payments to be made to patients should be reviewed by the Research Ethics Committee.

INDUCEMENTS TO RESEARCHERS

43. Personal expenses incurred by a doctor in the course of undertaking research involving patients may be reimbursed by the sponsor of the research. It is proper for doctors engaged in research to be paid a fee

for their services but doctors should not be paid a fee for carrying out research work in sessions for which they are already being paid from another source.

44. The physician responsible for the project or trial is responsible for informing his employer of payments, for ensuring that proper accounting procedures are adopted with independent audit and for fulfilling all legal requirements. Financial arrangements should be made through the finance office of a health authority or a university and the accounts supervised by the financial officers.

45. Payments made to doctors must be reasonable in terms of the time and effort given to the trial and openly declared.

46. Payments made to doctors on a *per capita* basis (i.e. according to the number of patients that they recruit to a study) are unethical. Even fees paid to an institution on a per capita basis may lead to undue pressure to recruit patients.

47. All financial arrangements and also *ad hoc* payments should be divulged to Research Ethics Committees.

48. In the conduct of "post-marketing surveillance" of medicines, the Guidelines drawn up between the Association of the British Pharmaceutical Industry, the British Medical Association, the Committee on Safety of Medicines and the Royal College of General Practitioners should be followed.

RANDOMISED CONTROLLED THERAPEUTIC TRIALS

49. The randomised controlled therapeutic trial has proved extremely valuable as a tool for examining the effectiveness of treatments and we give special attention to it because of its importance and because of the special ethical issues it raises. We discuss amongst other things the use of placebo treatments, double-blind procedure and randomisation. Detailed recommendations are set out in Chapter 7 of the main report.

CONDUCT OF RESEARCH

50. The ordinary requirements of patients—both medical and others—should not be neglected in the course of the involvement in research and the identity of the person in overall clinical charge of the patient's care must be clear.

51. Where research activities will be delegated by the investigator, the investigator should delegate only to individuals who have the necessary skills and experience.

52. The confidentiality of personal data must be preserved during the conduct of research.

53. The rights of patients, other doctors and sponsors to have access to the results of research require special consideration.
54. The results of research should be published free from any interference by financial sponsors of the research.

MONITORING THE CONDUCT OF RESEARCH

55. Research Ethics Committees should require investigators in charge of approved research projects to submit a brief report of progress at least annually.
56. Investigators should be requested to send copies of any published reports to the Research Ethics Committee.
57. Ways in which patients and health workers may approach the Research Ethics Committee when there is concern about the conduct of research should be devised and made known. It will sometimes be appropriate for this information to be included on the Patient Information Sheet.

ARRANGEMENTS FOR COMPENSATION

58. Although the chances of harm coming to patients in the course of carefully conducted research are very small, it is important that proper arrangements are made to compensate patients in the event of such harm occurring.
59. Bodies that sponsor research, including both publicly funded bodies (such as the Research Councils, the Department of Health and the National Health Service) and the pharmaceutical industry, should now so arrange their affairs as to implement the principle that injury due to participation in research sponsored by them or conducted by their staff with the approval of a Research Ethics Committee shall be compensated by a simple, informal and expeditious procedure.
60. In the event of any significant injury the patient must be entitled to receive compensation regardless of whether there may or may not have been negligence or legal liability on any other basis.

ACKNOWLEDGMENTS

The College thanks all those organisations and individuals who gave oral and written evidence. Their names are given in the full report.

MEMBERSHIP OF THE WORKING PARTY

Sir Raymond Hoffenberg, KBE MD FRCP (*Chairman*)
R. A. L. Brewis, MD FRCP (*Honorary Secretary*)
C. Chantler, MD FRCP
A. L. Diamond, LLM
C. J. Dickinson, DM FRCP
R. H. T. Edwards, FRCP
D. R. Laurence, MD FRCP
Katherine Levy, MB
Lavinia W. Loughridge, FRCP
Lady Lovell-Davis, MA
Miss D. Marks-Maran, SRN
Lord McColl, FRCS
Mrs Renée Short, Hon MRCP, Hon FRCPsych
W. van't Hoff, FRCP

IN ATTENDANCE

D. A. Pyke, CBE MD FRCP (*Registrar*)
D. B. Lloyd, FCCA (*Secretary*)
Ann Cowell (*Working Party Secretary*)

4 Ethics of Clinical Trials

RORY COLLINS, RICHARD DOLL and RICHARD PETO

THREE MAIN RECOMMENDATIONS

I. As long as therapeutic trials are appropriately governed by the "uncertainty principle", current ethical guidelines for medical research should RESTORE the distinction that previous guidelines made between (a) therapeutic trials and (b) other types of research involving patients

This distinction was made very clearly in the 1963 MRC ethical guidelines [1], and was particularly emphasized by, among others, Sir Harold Himsworth, then Secretary of the MRC.

A related recommendation stresses similarities between patient care out of trials and in trials that may not be shared by other types of research involving patients: *Ethical guidelines should avoid applying unnecessarily "double standards" to the ethics of routine medical care and to the ethics of therapeutic trials.*

Patients do not cease to be human if they are not in a randomized trial; hence, the amount of informed consent, non-negligent liability, etc., that is humanly appropriate outside a randomized trial may not be greatly different from that which is appropriate in a randomized trial—and, of course, vice versa.

The 1963 MRC guidelines, in distinguishing between therapeutic trials and other research procedures, said that "The former fall within the ambit of patient care and are governed by the ordinary rules of professional conduct in medicine; the latter fall within the ambit of investigations on volunteers." The present recommendation, however, is not that guidelines for routine medical care and for trials should necessarily be the same, but merely that ethical guidelines should consider separately the requirements for routine medical care, for therapeutic trials that are governed by the "uncertainty principle" (see below), and for other research involving patients.

II. For ethical reasons, medical research needs to generate reliable answers

In therapeutic trials this implies that both systematic errors (i.e. biases) and random errors (or, at least, standard deviations) in the measured effects of treatment should be small in comparison with the size of therapeutic effect

Introducing New Treatments for Cancer: Practical, Ethical and Legal Problems. Edited by C. J. Williams
© 1992 John Wiley & Sons Ltd

that may well have to be measured [2]. This requirement often entails the need for proper randomization of really large numbers of patients [3]. *Unnecessary obstacles to randomization or to large numbers may lead to many thousands of future patients being inappropriately treated.*

III. For ethical reasons, the design of trials should in general be governed by the "uncertainty principle"

A statement of this follows, in a form that might be adapted routinely into many trial protocols.

Uncertainty

A fundamental trial eligibility criterion is that no patient should be entered if the responsible physician and/or the patient are for any medical or non-medical reason(s) *reasonably certain* that one of the treatments that might be allocated would be inappropriate, in comparison with some other treatment that could be offered to this patient in the trial or outside it. In particular, patients can be entered only if the responsible physician is *substantially uncertain* as to which of the trial treatments would be most appropriate for this particular patient. (Likewise, patients cannot remain on their allocated treatment if for any reason(s) the responsible clinician and/or the patient should become reasonably certain that to do so would be inappropriate.)

REASONS UNDERLYING THESE RECOMMENDATIONS

The fundamental ethical consideration that should underlie both routine medical treatment and medical research is respect for the individual patient as a human being. Discussions of what might be the various practical implications of this one fundamental consideration have led to the drafting of various sets of ethical guidelines, for treatment or for research.

Traditionally, ethical guidelines for *treatment* and for *research* have been considered separately, because routine treatment is generally held not to involve any important interests other than those of the patient (or, in the case of private practice, the doctor and patient), while research may sometimes involve extraneous interests that could, at least in principle, distort the doctor–patient relationship to the detriment of the patient. Research itself, however, consists of a wide variety of activities, some of which (e.g. certain physiological investigations) are not expected to be of any medical value to the patient, and others of which (e.g. the randomized comparison of two standard forms of treatment) are.

Although the fundamental ethical consideration that should underlie the randomized comparison of treatments is the same as that which should underlie all other types of medical research and of routine medical treatment, the practical implications may be importantly different. Indeed, in many important respects the ethical considerations for trials comparing different treatments have more in common with routine medical treatment than with other types of medical research. This is the reason for our fundamental recommendation that ethical guidelines should be considered separately not just for *two* circumstances (routine treatment, and research) but for *three*:

(1) medical treatment with no research;
(2) randomized treatment trials that are governed by the "uncertainty principle"; and
(3) other medical research.

In some respects the ethical guidelines that eventually evolve for (2) and for (3) may resemble each other, but in some important respects they will differ. To the extent to which they do eventually resemble each other, no harm has been done by first considering them separately. To the extent to which they should differ, however, harm may be done to research and/or to patients by failing to consider these differences. At present, for example, patients entering trials may be subjected to inhumane, and therefore unethical, "consent" procedures that would certainly be considered humanly inappropriate (i.e. unethical) in ordinary medical practice.

To clarify these points, a recent practical example will be described in some detail.

PRACTICAL EXAMPLE: ISIS-2 TRIAL OF STREPTOKINASE IN ACUTE MYOCARDIAL INFARCTION

History

Fibrinolytic treatments such as streptokinase (SK) were developed about 40 years ago, and the first small randomized trial of intravenous SK in acute myocardial infarction (MI) was published more than 30 years ago, in 1959. During the 1960s and 1970s about two dozen small trials of intravenous SK were published (total: 6000 patients). Taken separately, their results were not persuasive, and by 1981 such fibrinolytic treatment was used routinely in fewer than 1% of UK patients presenting to hospital with acute MI. Similarly, US medical experts in 1981 described SK as being "dangerous and ineffective", and it was rarely used.

A systematic overview of the results of these previous trials did, however, indicate a significant mortality reduction [4]. To determine whether an effective treatment was routinely being withheld from patients, two large simple trials comparing routine treatment versus routine treatment plus SK were therefore organized: one from Italy (GISSI [5]) and one from Britain (ISIS-2 [6]), with overlapping committee membership.

   Eligibility for randomization was defined not in terms of enzymes, symptoms, ECG or any other fixed aspects, but by the *"uncertainty principle"*.

(1) If the responsible physician is, for *any* reason(s), *"reasonably certain"* that trial treatment (i.e. SK or placebo in ISIS-2) is *indicated* for a particular patient then that patient is not eligible for the trial.
(2) If the responsible physician is, for *any* reason(s), *"reasonably certain"* that trial treatment is *contraindicated* for a particular patient then that patient is not eligible for the trial.
(3) But, all remaining patients (i.e. those for whom the responsible physician is *"substantially uncertain"* *whether or not to recommend* trial therapy) are eligible for randomization.

In ISIS-2, all non-trial treatments—including, if the doctor ever became "reasonably certain" that this was appropriate, open-label (non-trial) active SK—were wholly at the discretion of the doctor, and if at any stage the doctor became "reasonably certain" that the trial treatments should be interrupted (e.g. because of allergy or bleeding) then this was to be done.

The uncertainty principle in other trials

Analogous principles could underlie many other trials, both in vascular and in neoplastic disease, and they ensure that no patient is ever denied (or given) any treatment that the responsible physician is "reasonably certain" to be appropriate (or inappropriate). In such studies there is an approximate parallelism between good science and good ethics: randomization is both uninteresting and unethical if it is already known by those directly responsible for patient care that one particular trial treatment is less appropriate than some other (trial or non-trial) treatment, but may be interesting and ethical otherwise. (Now that it is known how effective SK is at preventing death (see below), it may in retrospect seem strange that doctors were happy to randomize some patients to placebo, but at the time the chief problem was to encourage them to be happy to randomize at least some patients to active SK.)

What sort of "consent" was it appropriate to seek in ISIS-2?

The median time between pain onset (which usually occurred at home) and randomization in the coronary care unit was only 5 hours. Patients were therefore often shocked, frightened, in pain, and in many cases sedated.

Many were randomized at night, and the longer the delay before trial treatment began the less likely it was to save their lives. (Indeed, an average delay of 20 minutes would have resulted in about ten extra deaths among those allocated active treatment in ISIS-2 [6].) How much information should have been imposed on them? Should the high risk of death over the next few days have been stressed *to everybody*, along with the possible hazards of treatment (which is what would be needed for fully informed consent), or should at least *some* patients chiefly have been offered care and reassurance? And, what should the information have consisted of—the collective misjudgment of the medical profession at the time as to the expected benefits of SK, or what?

ISIS-2 consent in the UK

The UK protocol [7] stated that:

> the degree and timing of consent is entirely a matter for individual doctors to decide for individual patients in the light of local requirements and advice from any relevant ethical committees. This will result in a wide range of practices, ranging from formal written consent at one extreme, through various degrees of verbal consent, to, at the opposite extreme, some vague mention of the trial intended merely to offer patients an easy opportunity to *initiate* any discussion they want.

In other words, doctors should speak to patients as seemed *humanly* appropriate. Presumably some errors of judgment may have occurred that led to inappropriately inadequate discussions for some and inappropriately detailed discussions for others, but the aim was to do whatever was considered best for each *individual* patient by the people directly responsible for their care. Moreover, in Britain even any written consent was generally fairly brief (see Appendix 1).

ISIS-2 consent in the USA

By contrast, consent in the USA was a formal procedure that most doctors considered humanly inappropriate. (In discussions during the planning of ISIS-2 in the USA, objections to the inhumanity of the proposed consent procedures were answered by the comment that the aim was to protect the doctor, not to protect the patient, and that if protection of the doctor from lawyers harmed the patient then that was the price one had to pay for doing studies in the USA.) The US protocol [8] stated that:

> procedures for obtaining informed consent will have been determined by the Institutional Review Board or Human Subjects [sic] Committee of each hospital: in most instances, written informed consent will be required.

In fact, written consent was always required, even though the US consent document was a preposterous imposition on a medical emergency. This is reproduced in Appendix 2 to illustrate what had to be read to the person who was acutely ill. (Try reading the first paragraph or two of the "Risks and Discomforts" section to an imaginary patient!)

Effects on UK and US recruitment

Perhaps partly because of the inhumane US consent procedure, recruitment into ISIS-2 was far less rapid in the US (where only 400 patients were randomized) than in the UK (where 6000) were. This is despite an approximately equivalent degree of apparent interest by cardiologists in the two countries at the start of the study.

Many deaths due to the US informed consent procedure

If the USA had recruited as fast as the UK then the trial would have ended six months earlier, and since the eventual ISIS-2 results have transformed medical practice (improving the treatment of several hundreds of thousands of patients a year worldwide, thereby avoiding a few tens of thousands of unnecessary deaths), that six-month delay means that about 10 000 unnecessary deaths are directly due to whatever it was that slowed recruitment into ISIS-2 in the USA. Apart from the consent procedures, all other aspects of the study were equivalent. It seems likely, therefore, that the US consent procedures were directly responsible for at least a few thousand unnecessary deaths, in the pursuit of "informed consent" that many doctors would consider inhumane.

Random versus haphazard treatment: avoidance of double standards

The consent procedures used in the USA for ISIS-2 and those used for many trials in this country would not generally be considered appropriate outside a clinical trial. In routine practice, however, treatment is quite often chosen haphazardly (rather than randomly) and, at least in the case of SK, inappropriately, since almost all doctors around the world were not using SK at all before ISIS-2. Comparisons of practice between different countries—with wide variations in the use of certain treatments—underline the haphazard nature of many treatment decisions. And, if treatments that are used widely in some countries but hardly at all in others (e.g. intravenous nitrates in acute MI) do have worthwhile effects, then the sooner this is reliably established the sooner that unnecessary deaths will be avoided. Similarly, if such treatments have no worthwhile effects (or even cause harm, e.g. prophylactic antiarrhythmics in MI, which have been used widely in the USA) then it is important to demonstrate this quickly and clearly. Placing obstacles in the way of properly randomized evaluation of current "haphazard" treatment is, therefore, not appropriate.

ISIS-2 results: general implications

Figure 1 shows the main ISIS-2 results: there are four survival curves because a "factorial" (2×2) design was used, in which aspirin was given to half of the active-SK group and to half of the placebo-SK group.

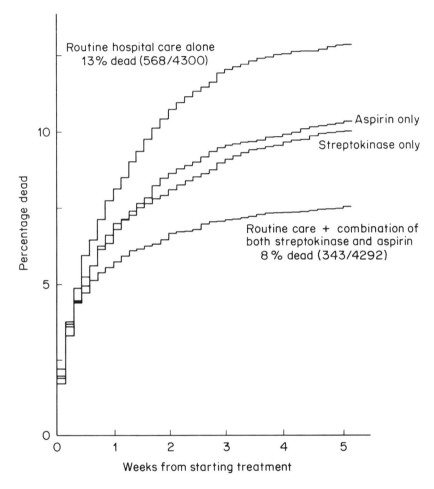

Figure 1. Lives saved in ISIS-2 among 17 187 heart attack patients who would not normally have received streptokinase or aspirin, divided at random into four similar groups who receive aspirin only, streptokinase only, both or neither. (Any doctor who believed that a particular patient should be given either treatment gave it, and did not include that patient in ISIS-2.)

ISIS-2 shows five things:

(1) Large, simple trials can save many lives.

(2) As long as trials are governed by the "uncertainty principle", there is an approximate parallelism between good science and good ethics, *so there is no pressure to be any more unethical than ordinary medical practice is.*

(3) Excessively detailed consent may severely damage recruitment, causing (directly or indirectly) many deaths.

(4) Excessively detailed consent may also be distressing and inhumane.

(5) Patients do not cease to be human when considered for trials, so the degree of informed consent that is humanly appropriate in routine medical treatment outside trials may not differ greatly from that which is humanly appropriate in a randomized comparison of different treatments that is governed by the uncertainty principle—or, to use Professor Baum's phrase, *"double standards" are not appropriate* [9].

These are the main considerations that underlie our request that the ethics of randomized treatment comparisons that are governed by the uncertainty principle should be considered separately from those of other research (just as the ethics of routine medical treatment outside trials is considered separately). Unless this is done, there may well develop a tendency to impose on trials, in the name of "ethics", procedures that may be progressively less and less humane for today's patients, and that may very seriously damage the interests of future patients, even to the point of directly and predictably causing large numbers of unnecessary deaths.

REFERENCES

1. Responsibility in investigations on human subjects. Report of the Medical Research Council for 1962–63: 21–25
2. Yusuf S, Collins R, Peto R (1984) Why do we need some large, simple randomized trials? Stat Med 3: 409–420
3. Early Breast Cancer Trialists' Collaborative Group (1990) Treatment of early breast cancer. Volume 1: Worldwide evidence 1985–1990. Oxford University Press
4. Yusuf S, Collins R, Peto R et al (1985) Intravenous and intracoronary fibrinolytic therapy in acute myocardial infarction: overview of results on mortality, reinfarction and side-effects from 33 randomized controlled trials. Eur Heart J 6: 556–585
5. GISSI Collaborative Group (1986) Effectiveness of intravenous thrombolytic treatment in acute myocardial infarction. Lancet i: 397–402
6. ISIS-2 Collaborative Group (1988) Randomised trial of intravenous streptokinase, oral aspirin, both, or neither among 17,187 cases of suspected acute myocardial infarction: ISIS-2. Lancet ii: 349–360
7. ISIS-2 Collaborative Group (1985) Second International Study of Infarct Survival: UK protocol (personal communication ISIS, Oxford)
8. ISIS-2 Collaborative Group (1985) Second International Study of Infarct Survival: US protocol (personal communication ISIS, Oxford)
9. Baum M (1986) Do we need informed consent? Lancet ii: 911–912

APPENDIX 1: EXAMPLE OF POSSIBLE CONSENT FORM (IF REQUIRED) FROM UK PROTOCOL FOR ISIS-2

As already noted, the degree and timing of consent is entirely a matter for individual doctors to decide for individual patients in the light of local requirements and advice from any relevant ethical committees. In those cases where written consent is deemed necessary, the following example, adapted as appropriate, may be helpful.

Statement to be read by, or to, patient or relative, suggesting use of research medication

We'd like to explain to you some of the research we're doing, and then ask if you would want to help with it.

Every day, all over the country, lots of people come into hospital who have just had—or nearly had—a heart attack. In this hospital, we use all the *standard* treatments for this, and then we invite patients to join in a study to find out if, in addition, blood-thinning treatments are useful. The idea of blood-thinning is that dissolving or preventing a blood clot in the heart may make a heart attack less severe, or even prevent one from developing. But, blood-thinning can, very occasionally, give people a really serious allergy or bleed. What we—and the hundreds of other doctors working with us—all hope is that these treatments will do much more *good* than harm.

This is what the research project involves. In addition to all the standard treatments, you'd get *two* research medicines. The *first* is given as one pill a day for a month, and the *second* is given immediately into the tube in your arm, and takes about an hour. The research medicines would be either active blood-thinning treatments or inactive ones. Neither we nor you would know whether your treatments were active or not—this information is kept on a secret code list at another hospital. There wouldn't be any extra tests; we'd just send off the important details of how you'd been in hospital (to be used, in confidence, for medical research purposes only).

Have you got any questions before you choose whether to sign up for this research project? Various technical details are available, if you'd like them, *first*.

AFTER A READING OF THE ABOVE STATEMENTS, I HAVE NO IMMEDIATE QUESTIONS UNANSWERED, AND I AM WILLING FOR THE ABOVE-MENTIONED RESEARCH MEDICINES TO BE GIVEN, ON THE UNDERSTANDING THAT THEY CAN BE STOPPED AT ANY TIME IF I WISH.

Signed _____ Patient/Responsible relative

NB: Some technical details are available (see below).

Technical details of treatments

We're specially interested in two different types of blood-thinning treatment, one of which is just ordinary aspirin.

Streptokinase: (to dissolve clots)	One and a half megaunits of "Streptase" (or matching placebo) infused over about an hour in about a tenth of a litre of normal saline.

Aspirin: (to prevent clots)	One tablet of 160 mg/day for a month (or matching placebo), with a special enteric coating to avoid irritation to the stomach.

Technical details of possible side-effects and benefits from streptokinase

Previous studies in Britain and Italy of this streptokinase dosage suggest that reversible allergic reactions (e.g. shivers, faintness, etc.) and reversible bruises or bleeds (e.g. in the mouth, nose, skin, urinary tract or gut) may temporarily affect about 10% of all patients, but that fatal or permanently damaging reactions are extremely rare[*] perhaps no more than one or two per thousand patients treated. Against this, the hope is that at least 15 or 20 deaths from heart disease can be avoided.[†]

Technical details of possible side-effects and benefits from active aspirin

Any side-effects should be less than with standard aspirin tablets, first because our study is of only about *half* an ordinary aspirin a day (160 mg), and second because our aspirin has an "enteric" coat to protect the gullet and stomach from irritation. Correspondingly, however, any benefits from aspirin may also be somewhat smaller than those from streptokinase.[‡]

Technical details of possible side-effects and benefits from inactive medications

The inactive preparations should produce no material risk or nuisance, for no extra skin puncture is involved, and all standard treatment is still given. However, they also offer no benefits.

---

[*]The type of allergic reaction recently described and reviewed (*JAMA*, 1984, 252: 1314) had no long-term consequences, and the preparation we now have is purer and, hence, much less likely to cause an allergic reaction, than some of the old preparations.
[†]Benefits about twice as large as this were suggested in a survey of earlier studies of streptokinase (*N Engl J Med* 1982, 307: 1180).
[‡]*Lancet* editorial, 1980, i: 1172.

Technical details of effects on patient's rights

None. Patients can, if they wish, withdraw at any time; of course, if they believe they have been negligently managed, the normal means of legal redress are unaffected.

Technical details of finance

The physicians at this hospital are not making any money out of collaborating in this study. Only the actual costs of the study (e.g. postage, telephones, medications, etc.) are paid for by the drug suppliers (Behringwerke/Hoechst streptokinase, and Sterling aspirin), and because both drugs are old ones that are out of patent, other suppliers can manufacture them freely if they work. Our aim in this study is not to make money for anybody, but just to find out what's best for patients.

APPENDIX 2: CONSENT DETAILS FROM US PROTOCOL FOR ISIS-2

All research projects involving human subjects in the United States must be approved by the Institutional Review Board (IRB) at the hospital where the project will be carried out, prior to the beginning of the study. To assist participating CCUs in obtaining IRB approval of ISIS-2, the US Coordinating Center has prepared a sample IRB Application and Patient Consent Form in accordance with the guidelines of the Brigham and Women's Hospital Committee for the Protection of Human Subjects, who have reviewed and approved these materials. These guidelines incorporate the requirements of both the US Department of Health and Human Services and the Food and Drug Administration.

Six areas are addressed in the Patient Consent Form:

(1) the purpose of the trial;
(2) trial procedures;
(3) associated risks and discomforts;
(4) possible benefits of participation;
(5) alternatives to trial treatment;
(6) standard paragraphs addressing issues such as the preservation of confidentiality, patients' rights, compensation for injury, etc.

These materials are provided as samples only; they may well require modification to conform with the policies at your institution. The exact form of the application required may differ from institution to institution. More importantly, hospital policies on the issues raised in the standard paragraphs are likely to vary. Participating centers should be careful to state the specific policies of their institution regarding these issues.

Again, formal written approval of the IRB for this study must be obtained before any participants can be recruited into the trial. We will require a copy of the approval for each participating hospital before randomization at that unit can begin. Signed Patient Consent Forms should be obtained and kept on file for all patients enrolled at your institution.

If you have any questions regarding your hospital's policies for the protection of human subjects, you should contact a representative of your IRB. You should also feel free to contact the staff of the US Coordinating Center to discuss either the application or the sample Patient Consent Form.

SAMPLE PATIENT CONSENT FORM

Purpose

Your attending physician believes you may have had or are having a heart attack. We are therefore asking you to participate in a research study investigating the usefulness of two experimental drug treatments that can be given along with standard therapy for patients having or suspected of having heart attacks. These drugs are streptokinase administered intravenously (i.e., through a tube inserted into a vein) and coated aspirin administered orally.

Most often, heart attacks are caused by a blood clot in the coronary arteries that prevents blood flow to the heart muscle, thereby causing permanent damage to the heart. Previous research has demonstrated that intravenous streptokinase, administered promptly after the onset of symptoms over a one-hour period, can often dissolve such a clot and thus restore blood flow, which may limit the amount of damage to the heart. However, after the effects of the streptokinase wear off, a new clot can form in the coronary arteries, which can once again prevent blood flow to the heart. For this reason, treatment with aspirin, which interferes with blood clot formation, may prove beneficial.

There have been few controlled studies of intravenous streptokinase or aspirin for the treatment of patients having heart attacks. Therefore such use of these drugs is considered investigational and the FDA does not allow them to be marketed for this purpose. In order to determine the benefits and risks of these drug treatments, they need to be assessed in a large-scale trial such as this one, which has participants from 14 countries and over 500 collaborating hospitals.

Procedure

If you participate, in addition to receiving whatever standard treatments for heart attacks you and your doctor may determine, you will immediately be assigned, at random, to one of the four possible treatment groups. The treatments are as follows: streptokinase or its placebo (an identical-appearing substance which contains no active ingredients) will be given through the intravenous tubing already in place. In addition, a tablet containing 160 mg of coated aspirin (about half the amount contained in a standard adult aspirin) or an aspirin placebo, will be taken right away and then once daily for a month. Thus, you might receive streptokinase or aspirin or both of these active treatments or neither active treatment (only placebos). For purposes of the research, neither you nor anyone else at the hospital will know whether you are receiving active or placebo medications. However, that information will be on file at the trial coordinating center and can be made available to your physician if needed for your care and treatment.

While the medication is being prepared, a blood sample (about one tablespoon) will be withdrawn through the intravenous tube. This blood will be analyzed to attempt to determine what factors put people at risk for heart attacks. Then you will be given the first tablet of aspirin or placebo, which you should chew in order to achieve a more immediate effect. After taking this tablet, you will be given the infusion of streptokinase or placebo, which will take about an hour and will not be repeated. Thereafter, the tablet of aspirin or placebo will be taken once daily and should be swallowed whole. Any tablets remaining at the time of your discharge from the hospital should be taken daily until you have completed the prescribed course.

In several days, when you feel up to it, we will also ask you to complete a brief questionnaire about your general health. When you are discharged from the hospital, important details of your hospital course will be recorded for purposes of the study and sent to the study coordinating center. Approximately one year after your discharge from the hospital, you will be sent a brief form with a few follow-up questions, which you will be asked to return to the coordinating center.

No additional charge will be made for the study medications or for the blood test mentioned above. The total length of your planned involvement in the study will be one month, until your supply of study pills runs out.

Risks and discomforts

Previous studies with the dosage of streptokinase that will be used in this research suggest that allergic reactions such as fevers, chills or rash and temporary bruising or bleeding in the mouth, nose, skin, urinary tract or arms may occur in about 10% of patients. All these effects subside after treatment is stopped. In addition, serious but usually transient heart rhythm disturbances may sometimes occur when the clot in the coronary arteries dissolves and blood flow is restored, and in this event immediate treatment will be given. The major risks from the use of streptokinase are the possibility of bleeding from the stomach or intestinal tract, stroke, and possibly death. However, it appears that such reactions are rare, with permanently damaging or fatal reactions affecting only perhaps 1–2 patients per thousand who receive intravenous streptokinase.*

Standard aspirin can cause indigestion or other stomach upset, and it increases the tendency to bleed, particularly in the stomach or intestinal tract. The risks and discomforts from the aspirin you might receive in this study are expected to be less than those that may occur with the use of standard aspirin. This is because the dose to be used will be only half the amount contained in a standard adult aspirin tablet, and because the study tablets are coated with a preparation designed to reduce irritation to the esophagus and stomach. (The protective coating will not be effective for the first aspirin dose, since chewing that tablet destroys the coating.) Some people may find chewing the first aspirin/placebo tablet distasteful.

While the combination of streptokinase and aspirin might, in theory, be expected to worsen bleeding tendencies caused by either drug alone, we know of no evidence of increased instances of bleeding in patients receiving streptokinase and aspirin as compared with patients receiving streptokinase alone.

---

*This conclusion derives from unpublished data on the first few hundred patients randomized in the British pilot study for ISIS-2 (R. Collins, personal communication) and on the first few thousand patients in the randomized Italian "GISSI" trial of intravenous streptokinase (G. Tognoni, personal communication).

There is also the possibility of allergic reactions to aspirin or streptokinase, such as fever, chills or rash. If you have had previous allergic reactions to either aspirin or streptokinase you should tell us, and you should not participate in the study. If you have any questions about whether your particular medical condition or your standard treatment may affect these risks or discomforts, you should discuss this with your doctor.

No risk or discomfort is anticipated from the blood drawing, which will be done through an intravenous tube already in place.

Benefits

The potential benefits for those who receive the streptokinase, or aspirin, or both, are that one or both of these treatments may limit the amount of damage caused by the heart attack, prevent an early recurrence of heart attack, and/or prolong life. In addition, regardless of your treatment assignment, your participation in the study will contribute to medical knowledge resulting in the selection of better methods of treatment for and better understanding of the causes of heart attacks.

Alternative procedures

The main alternative to the study procedures is the standard medical treatment for your condition as determined by you and your physician. Standard treatment may include various heart and pain medications, oxygen, and monitoring of your physical status so that emergency medical care can be given if needed. Most standard treatments can be given along with the study agents, at the discretion of your doctor.

There is another relatively new mode of therapy, intracoronary administration of streptokinase, which requires emergency threading of a tube through blood vessels leading to the heart and to the blocked coronary artery. If you and your doctor determine that your treatment will include intracoronary streptokinase, then you should not participate in the study. [Whether you choose to include these statements regarding intracoronary streptokinase will depend upon the availability of this method of treatment at your institution.]

Standard paragraphs

In the event that at any point during this project, you feel that you have not been adequately informed as to the risks, benefits, or alternative procedures, or feel under excessive duress to continue this treatment against your wishes, or wish to report or discuss any injury you believe may be related to the research, a representative of the Human Subjects Committee [or Institutional Review Board] is available to speak with you.

Confidential information contained in your medical record may not be furnished to anyone unaffiliated with the hospital or the study without your written consent, except as required by law or regulation.

There is a possibility that your medical record, including identifying information, may be inspected and/or photocopied by the Food and Drug Administration or other Federal or state government agencies in the ordinary course of carrying out their governmental functions. If your record is used or disseminated for government purposes, it will be done under conditions that will protect your privacy to the fullest extent possible consistent with laws relating to public disclosure of information and the law enforcement responsibilities of the agency.

In the event that you should be injured during the course of this study, [insert your institution's policy regarding the availability of medical treatments and/or compensation if injury occurs, and if available, what they consist of or where further information may be obtained].

A signed copy of this consent form will be made available to you.

Participation in this study is voluntary, and you are free to refuse to participate or to withdraw your consent and to discontinue participation at any time. Such refusal or discontinuance will not affect your regular treatments or medical care in any way.

I have fully explained the procedures, identifying those which are investigational, and have explained their purpose. I have asked whether or not any questions have arisen regarding the procedures and have answered these questions to the best of my ability.

Date _____ Responsible Investigator _____

I have been fully informed as to the procedures to be followed, including those which are investigational, and have been given a description of the attendant discomforts, risks and benefits to be expected and the appropriate alternate procedures. In signing this consent form, I agree to this method of treatment and I understand that I am free to refuse to participate or to withdraw my consent and discontinue my participation in this study at any time. I understand also that if I have any questions at any time, they will be answered.

Date _____ Patient _____

or GUARDIAN/NEXT OF KIN _____

ABOUT THE AUTHORS

Rory Collins qualified in medicine at St Thomas's Hospital Medical School, University of London, in 1981 and obtained BSc in statistics from George Washington University, Washington DC in 1977 and MSc in statistics from the University of Oxford in 1983. In 1981 he obtained an appointment as a research assistant to Richard Peto in the Imperial Cancer Research Fund/Medical Research Council Clinical Trial Service Unit, Oxford University, and to Professor Peter Sleight in the Department of Cardiovascular Medicine, John Radcliffe Hospital, Oxford, primarily to co-ordinate large-scale clinical trials of the acute treatment of heart attacks. In 1985 he was appointed co-director of the MRC/ICRF Clinical Trial Service Unit, with Richard Peto as director, and in the following year was elected to the Staines Medical Research Fellowship of Exeter College, Oxford University, and was awarded a British Heart Foundation Senior Research Fellowship.

Dr Collins' work has been in the establishment of really large-scale randomized controlled trials of the treatment of heart attacks, of other vascular disease, and of cancer, while also being closely involved in developing approaches to the combination of results from related randomized controlled trials ("systematic overviews" or "meta-analyses") that allow the more reliable assessment of treatment effects.

Sir Richard Doll qualified in medicine at St Thomas's Hospital Medical School, University of London in 1937 and obtained MD Lond. in 1945, DSc Lond. in 1958, and DM Oxford in 1969. After qualifying he worked for two years as a hospital intern and for six years in the Royal Army Medical Corps before turning to research. In 1946 he obtained an appointment as a research assistant to Sir Francis Avery Jones at the Central Middlesex Hospital and two years later joined the Medical Research Council's Statistical Unit under Sir Austin Bradford Hill. In 1961 he succeeded Sir Austin as director of the unit and continued in that post until his appointment as Regius Professor of Medicine in the University of Oxford in 1969. In 1979 he was appointed to head Green College, a new foundation in Oxford that had been established to take a special interest in clinical medicine. In Oxford he also directed the Cancer Epidemiology and Clinical Trials Unit that had been established by the Imperial Cancer Research Fund and has continued to work with the Fund, since his retirement, as an honorary member of the Cancer Studies Unit under Mr Richard Peto.

Sir Richard's work has included studies of the causes and treatment of peptic ulcers, the causes of lung cancer and leukaemia, the occupational hazards of cancer, and the effects of smoking, exposure to ionizing radiations, and the use of oral contraceptives.

He was elected FRCP Lond. in 1957 and FRS in 1966, was knighted in 1971, and has received honorary degrees from the universities of Newcastle, Belfast, Reading, Newfoundland, Tasmania, New York, Harvard, London and Oxford. His awards include the United Nations Award for Cancer Research in 1962, the Gairdner Award, Toronto, in 1970, the General Motors prize in 1979, the BMA's Gold Medal in 1983, the Royal Society's Royal Medal in 1986 and the Helmut Horten Foundation Award in 1991.

Richard Peto obtained BA in natural sciences from the University of Cambridge in 1966 and MSc in statistics from the University of London in 1967. In 1967 he obtained an appointment as a research assistant to Dr (later Sir) Richard Doll in the Medical Research Council Statistical Research Unit in London and then the Department of the Regius Professor of Medicine at the University of Oxford. In 1975 he was appointed as University Reader in Cancer Studies, University of Oxford, and he then set up the Imperial Cancer Research Fund Clinical Trial Service Unit to facilitate multicentre collaborative trials.

Richard Peto's work has included studies of the causes of cancer, the effects of smoking, and the establishment of really large-scale clinical trials in a variety of diseases, as well as being instrumental in developing statistical approaches to the combination of results from related randomized controlled trials ("systematic overviews" or "meta-analyses") that allow the more reliable assessment of treatment effects.

He was elected FRS in 1989, and was made an Honorary Member of the Royal College of Physicians in London in 1987 and of the Swedish Society of Internal Medicine in 1988. His awards include the Guy Silver Medal from the Royal Statistical Society in 1986 and the Helmut Horten Foundation Award in 1991.

5 Informed Consent and the Introduction of New Cancer Treatments

JEFFREY S. TOBIAS

Quite apart from the clinical problems in confirming whether a new cancer treatment is genuinely superior to established approaches [1, 2], the ethical and moral difficulties relating to the introduction of a novel treatment raise fundamental issues [3]. The conflict between compassionate but impartial treatment of the individual, coupled with the natural desire of all clinical oncologists to move the field forward, has attracted increased attention [4] and seems certain to remain contentious for the foreseeable future. Much of the debate has revolved around the concept of "informed consent" yet neither lawyers, ethicists nor medical scientists have to date agreed precisely what this term actually means (see Chapters 1 and 2). It is generally held to imply a full declaration of treatment options to any patient who has been invited to become a participant in a clinical study, and is of course of particular relevance in randomized controlled prospective clinical studies. Together with the full description of any treatments there should be an explanation of the possible side-effects of the new or standard treatments. It is also widely assumed that whenever the study is controlled by random allocation, this fact should be laid before the patient. Inherent in this explanation is of course the additional implication that the patient must also be made aware of the shortcomings of current treatment, and the essential need for clinical research to establish superior methods. Among the many difficulties concerning informed consent is the fundamental question of how full an explanation can reasonably be regarded as sufficient to help the patient to become "informed". In the USA it has become customary to provide a lengthy written document for the patient to read, which outlines not only the trial under consideration but also, necessarily, a frank exposition of the sometimes poor results achieved by current conventional treatment, together with an often startling account of possible side-effects relating to the new treatment under study. Such written explanations have often been regarded—quite rightly in my view— as more likely to be protective of the doctor than the patient, and are often couched in jargon of such legal precision that medical anxieties about a possible lawsuit for negligence seem surely to provide the subtext. On

Introducing New Treatments for Cancer: Practical, Ethical and Legal Problems. Edited by C. J. Williams
© 1992 John Wiley & Sons Ltd

the other hand, one might reasonably ask how else the patient can become truly informed, if unable to take away with him a carefully written document to study and to consider calmly. Alternative approaches such as a conversational explanation via the doctor are clearly open to misconception, failure of comprehension by the patient, or over-anxiety to conform with the doctor's enthusiastic advice to become a participant in a study which the patient does not fully understand (see Chapter 5).

ALTERNATIVE APPROACHES IN HELPING PATIENTS DECIDE

If a patient is about to enter (or be asked to enter) a prospectively randomized controlled study, the alternatives open to the doctor are full disclosure, partial disclosure or no disclosure at all. There is little doubt that in many studies performed before the 1970s, when informed consent became such a major ethical issue, many randomized studies were performed both in the UK, the USA and elsewhere, without any disclosure whatsoever to the participating patients. Indeed, the whole issue was brought to light, at least in Britain, following an inquest in 1982 at which it was discovered that an elderly patient had died as a result of neutropenic sepsis following administration of the cytotoxic agent 5-fluorouracil as an infusion into the liver (see Chapter 16 for further discussion) [5]. The coroner decided that such treatment was not normally regarded as standard for the bowel cancer from which she was suffering, and it became apparent that she had been a participant in a prospectively randomized clinical study in which half the patients were receiving adjuvant cytotoxic treatment, and half were not. The consultant in charge of her case explained that the ethical committee to whom he had referred the trial protocol had not regarded disclosure as a vital element and, perhaps predictably, many ethicists and newspaper reports expressed outrage at this state of affairs. Although no legal proceedings were brought, it was widely regarded at the time that failure of disclosure that the patient might be undergoing a non-standard form of treatment was no longer acceptable in the Britain of the 1980s. Indeed, the legal correspondent of *The Lancet* commented [5]:

> I find the concept of secret random control trials wholly unacceptable, and the reason offered to justify them both unconvincing and unsatisfactory.

The case certainly aroused considerable public interest, making clear for perhaps the first time the large number of clinical studies (par-ticularly in cancer medicine) that were presently being undertaken. Since this medico-legal *cause celebre*, the public has clearly become increasingly interested in cancer trials, and indeed a second case, in which a leading breast cancer surgeon was pilloried by the press for apparently failing to disclose information, was even more widely discussed [6, 7]. The fact that this particular issue related not to formal cancer treatment but to a controlled study assessing the possible benefit of counselling and adjuvant breast cancer treatment, at a time when these approaches were not widely available, received rather little attention to the irritation of many research clinicians in oncology.

Despite these difficulties there are of course many advantages for the patient in not being aware that he or she is a participant in a clinically controlled study of a new cancer treatment. First of all, the patient is spared the anxiety of knowing for certain that the treatment on offer is not yet established as proven. Many patients, indeed probably the majority, have a fear of clinical "experiments" without the understanding that in a sense, any treatment whatever, however well established, is experimental in that the doctor cannot be certain that it will work. Furthermore, the patient is spared the inevitable anxiety of knowing that a new approach is being offered since the standard treatment does not always work sufficiently well in the particular type of cancer from which he or she is suffering. It may seem surprising to sophisticated, well-informed professional people that many patients are prepared to trust fully in their doctor and in the efficacy of the treatment, with the misguided but sometimes happy result that their last few months of life are a good deal calmer than might otherwise be the case. Although this view might be regarded as unreasonably paternalistic, the medical profession must realize that many patients do not wish to have too full an explanation of every detail of their condition and its likely implications or outcome. Such denial is a well-known coping mechanism which can serve patients well and should be respected by the doctor—though not, on the other hand, blithely used as justification for a blanket withholding of information from all patients. This delicate balance between information and discretion can never be straightforward, yet any disclosure to the patient that treatment for his cancer may be contingent on a random decision will necessarily remove this option for them.

Partial disclosure is a more complex and more sophisticated concept, and was first described by Zelen and others [8] as a means of overcoming the difficulties inherent in both full disclosure, with its complete and frank discussion of treatment options, possible failures and potential side-effects; and the increasingly unacceptable non-disclosure described above. The fundamental approach was to regard the new form of treatment in any randomized study as essentially experimental, but the control arm, which generally consisted of standard management not normally regarded in this same light, as "established". The argument then progressed to include all patients in the former group as requiring a full explanation of the clinical trial, including of course the fact of randomization and the position of the patient within the "experimental" arm of the study, whereas patients who were about to receive established treatment would not require any explanation on the grounds that the treatment would be precisely similar to what would normally be offered at major institutions if the patient were not participating in a clinical study (see Chapter 15 for a full discussion of this topic). This at least would spare all these patients the uncertainties and anxieties which, it was argued, they simply did not need to know about, whilst respecting the rights and the needs of patients in the "experimental" arm who were made well aware of the fact that a clinical study was in progress and that they had been selected by random allocation for the newer treatment. When first described, this approach was warmly welcomed by many as an excellent compromise. It was already clear that many important clinical studies were foundering for lack of recruitment, largely as a result of patients' or physicians' dislike or disinclination to accept the rigours of a clinical study which demanded lengthy explanation and possibly a franker account of the inherent difficulties of treatment than the doctor would normally be prepared to offer. On the other hand, any patient about to become the recipient of a novel treatment would do so only in the knowledge that the new medication or therapeutic proposal was not yet fully established, and could reasonably be refused if the patient so wished.

For the technique to work at all, clearly it was necessary for patients to be randomized before any explanation or informed consent procedure was offered, and a full discussion of the study could then be provided for all patients receiving the new treatment. This essential precondition has led to both moral and statistical objections to the method. Many ethicists argue that any patient has an undeniable right to self-determination, making it essential to offer a full description of a randomized study to all those participating within it, even those in whom the allocated treatment proves to be "standard", i.e. the established treatment which they would have received anyway. It is certainly difficult to counter the view that patients who are allocated to the standard treatment arm have as much right as the other group to know about any potentially beneficial treatment on offer, even if they choose to participate in the study in full knowledge that they might not be allocated to it. Furthermore, from the statistical point of view any such study would clearly be weakened if many patients in the "experimental" arm chose after full explanation to refuse the new treatment and opt instead for the standard treatment. Clearly they would have to be included, for statistical purposes, as having received the new treatment (see Chapter 15) though of course, in actual treatment terms, they had not received it. Any possible small benefit in the newer treatment would therefore be more difficult to demonstrate, particularly if a substantial number of patients declined the new treatment on offer.

Partial disclosure, or disclosure of the facts of the randomized study only to some (usually half) of the participants, is clearly an ethical minefield which makes it unattractive to many clinical researchers. Yet there are of course many advantages, often overlooked. Partial disclosure works as a means of respecting the right of patients not to be allocated novel treatments which are not yet fully established (and might never be) whilst at the same time ensuring reasonable recruitment for clinical studies since, at the very least, the group undergoing standard treatment are highly unlikely to reject it because they are unaware that they are participating in any clinical study at all. Furthermore, as previously pointed out, these latter patients are spared the anxiety of knowing that further improvements or refinements in their treatment are urgently needed. Although many regard the principle of self-determination as paramount, one could perhaps also argue that partial disclosure, with the alleviation of anxiety and uncertainty in patients who are to receive standard treatment, is itself a substantial gain for the individual and also for any group of patients with the same illness since valuable academic information might well flow from the study being undertaken.

My personal feeling is that these advantages should rightly be regarded as considerable, and that in certain circumstances partial disclosure is not unreasonable. Consider for example the case of a promising, unproven, potentially valuable but highly toxic form of treatment, not previously available but currently under investigation in a group of cancer patients, the majority of whom might well be young women below the age of 50. The intense study and public interest relating to adjuvant combination chemotherapy for advanced carcinoma of the cervix is a good illustration of this paradigm. It seems clear that valuable responses, both objective and subjective in terms of pain and symptom relief, are frequently seen in the majority of patients who would otherwise be suitable only for treatment by radical irradiation [9]. Although radiotherapy can be curative in advanced carcinoma of the cervix, the long-term results of treatment are poor, particularly in the later stages, and most patients do not survive to five years. There is some evidence that the disease is even more likely to be lethal in younger women. Despite the high response rate to combination chemotherapy described in several studies, there is as yet no clear-cut long-term survival benefit, and it may well prove impossible to improve the overall outlook with presently available agents, despite a high response rate and tolerable treatment-related side-effects. In view of the encouraging early results there is no dispute that studies of combination chemotherapy used as an adjuvant with radiotherapy are essential. This is particularly important since there could be a small long-term survival advantage of the kind recently recognized in breast cancer, by a systematic overview of all randomized trials of adjuvant therapy, most of which failed to show a significant survival benefit individually (see Chapter 29) [10]. Despite this wide agreement, all our studies in cervical cancer have so far been dogged by limited recruitment even though the numbers of potential patients in the UK, USA and Europe are considerable. Clearly, no type of study apart from a randomized controlled clinical trial is likely to provide results sufficiently reliable to be trustworthy, yet the necessity for informed consent in this type of study does provide an additional disincentive to many researchers. Is it reasonable to dwell on the very poor results of standard treatment, particularly in patients with advanced disease who might well be under the age of 40 years, with young families? Is it proper to point out that there is a promising new treatment only to find that the patient, having agreed to enter the study, is allocated to "radiotherapy alone" and thus denied what she might regard as a most valuable addition to her treatment? Increasingly it is patients like this who have been allocated to what they consider "the wrong treatment" who prove most difficult to reassure; the physician finds himself furiously back-peddling, playing down the possible advantages of the new treatment, and perhaps over-emphasizing the likely side-effects [11]. At best, this is an extremely distressing situation for the patient and a most uncomfortable one for the physician. The mutual trust between them, so critical for the patient's future, may have been permanently dented.

Full disclosure is, at least at first sight, clearly the only answer! Both the patient and the doctor can be entirely frank about the advantages, disadvantages and dangers of the clinical trial, and a no-holds-barred discussion can take place which will allow the patient to decide for him or herself whether or not this clinical trial is acceptable. The problems, however, are considerable. Many physicians, myself included, find the explanation of randomization a difficult one, since it seems to the well-informed clinician so simple, straightforward, unbiased and academically attractive, yet to the patient randomization is a blunt and brutal tool. Can we really expect our patients to understand that, for example, the choice between breast preservation and mastectomy should be decided in this way? Only ten years ago this was a critically important question before it became clear—thanks to a randomized controlled study run by the National Surgical Adjuvant Breast Project (NSABP) in the USA—that the two treatments were probably identical, from the point of view of overall survival [12]. Can we reasonably expect a patient to agree to highly toxic chemotherapy, with the attendant hair loss, nausea and myelosuppression on what seems like the whim of the computer or trialist? In truth, randomization is a highly sophisticated concept which most patients as individuals, and indeed the public at large, are largely unable to accept, mostly in consequence of the long-established model that patients and doctors hold of each other, namely that the doctor is there to make decisions, the patient to accept them. If the partnership is unequal, this perhaps is an inevitable consequence; the doctor should be able to provide all the answers, and not express uncertainty, above all where the patient's life might be at stake. This traditional view is quite at odds with the need to advance our understanding by randomization in clinical trials. It is all very well to extol the advantages of patient self-determination, yet we most certainly should respect the patient's right of denial, if that is his chosen approach, or of simply preferring to behave as the trusting patient and allowing his chosen physician to take the right decisions for him [13]. This latter point was clearly demonstrated by the late Franz Ingelfinger, formerly editor of the *New England Journal of Medicine*, who himself died of a carcinoma of the oesophagus—having ironically been in the forefront of clinical gastroenterology throughout his career. As he pointed out:

> I received from physician friends throughout the country a barrage of well-intentioned but contradictory advice . . . as a result not only I but my wife, my son and daughter-in-law (all doctors), and other family members became increasingly confused and emotionally distraught. Finally when the pangs of indecision had become nearly intolerable, one wise physician friend said "What you need is a doctor". He was telling me to forget the information I already had and the information I was receiving from many quarters, and to seek instead a person who would dominate, who would tell me what to do, who would in a paternalistic manner assume responsibility for my care. When this excellent advice was followed, my family and I sensed immediate and immense relief. The incapacity of enervating worry was dispelled, and I could return to my usual anxieties such as deciding on the fate of manuscripts.

Here was a highly professional, well-informed and thoroughly capable physician who, at the time of the greatest crisis in his life simply wanted a good doctor to tell him what to do. Again, one would not insist that this willing reliance on the traditional paternalist view of the physician's role is acceptable to all, but the point surely is that it is highly valued by many, and not to be dispensed with lightly. Other highly gifted physicians have argued persuasively against the insistence on full disclosure as an essential prelude to a physician's selection of treatment from a number of alternatives [14]. Brewin, for instance, has pointed out that for some patients, even the use of the word "cancer" is unwise, since their understanding of the term might be quite different from what is appropriate to their case:

> The idea that the mere fact of randomization always requires special informed consent—with all its disadvantages and potential for causing misconception and anxiety—is surely illogical. A doctor in his normal practice, giving treatment without randomization, is trusted to choose from several options, even though there may be no way that he can be sure which is best. Why should we not also trust a doctor who submits such options to randomization, while taking full responsibility for the suitability of each? Are the two situations really so different?

From the academic point of view, full disclosure does of course carry an additional major penalty in the form of slower recruitment. Many patients find themselves so bewildered by the description of possible outcomes, and by the nature of the doctor's uncertainty, that they decline to enter. The more critical the question, the more likely this is to be true since, quite clearly, the treatment alternatives are likely to be very different and perceived by the patient as too important to leave to the randomization process.

THE ROLE OF THE NON-TRIALIST, AND A WAY FORWARD

Earlier I made the point that all treatments are in a sense clinical experiments, since the outcome can rarely if ever be certain. In cancer medicine, this is particularly poignant since even the most established of treatments are frequently unsuccessful. For instance, in non-small-cell carcinoma of the bronchus, all would agree that in the young, fit patient with an operable peripheral tumour, without evidence of distant or mediastinal node involvement, thoracotomy and tumour resection is the treatment of choice. Yet none would disagree that even using the most efficient and selective technological criteria to exclude all unsuitable patients, the long-term results are highly unsatisfactory, the majority of patients developing local or distant recurrence with fatal consequences. In patients with small operable carcinomas of the breast, it is even more widely accepted that our attempts to define a curable group have not allowed us to predict with any certainty that a particular individual is indeed likely to be cured by the initial treatment. Despite these self-evident facts, cancer physicians and surgeons who choose *not* to involve themselves in the demanding strictures of clinical trials are rarely if ever accused of complacency or callousness by their patients, the ethical–moral lobby or by the national press, even though there is a suggestion that their treatment results are less good than those of clinicians participating in trials (see Chapter 9)! It is as if a double standard has subtly been operating, with a strict code of conduct for those concerned with clinical cancer studies—often to the point of sensationalist "exposure" and undesirable, often misinformed scrutiny—whereas physicians who purport to know all the answers, and have no academic interest in contributing to further knowledge, are let off far more lightly [15]. Only by increased public awareness and education would it be possible to alter this difficult state of affairs. Treatments which do not fall into the general category of "clinical trials" are of no direct interest to ethics committees which nowadays, in most large centres, occupy an influential and powerful position, generally providing both advice and caution and, increasingly frequently, composed not only of doctors but also nursing staff and lay members. The role of research ethics committees (Chapter 6) in the delicate balance between academic research and the patient's rights has been widely discussed [16–18], and I will not explore this further. However, the concept of a national ethics committee (Chapter 7) to consider the merits of large multicentre national trials has already gained considerable acceptance since, inter alia, such committees would once and for all do away with the rather absurd present situation whereby the same large multicentre study might be regarded as entirely acceptable to the ethics committee of one centre, though deemed unsatisfactory by another.

In my own view, the way forward is conceptually simple yet extremely difficult to implement. Only by better public education and understanding of our current failures in cancer treatment can we develop a sufficiently frank exchange with patients to be able to offer them more candid explanations and thereby develop a more open partnership than has been traditionally possible [19, 20]. In the past decade, fewer than 10% of patients with cancer in the UK were admitted into clinical studies, though in some areas, particularly acute leukaemia, the figure was far higher. In other parts of the world, notably Scandinavia, clinical researchers have been more successful, particularly in certain areas such as breast cancer which have been of special interest to a small number of prominent and respected clinicians. British patients have in the past been too compliant, too malleable and too trusting. Perhaps we are now seeing the inevitable backlash from an over-dependence on an unrealistically paternalist attitude on the part of physicians. Perhaps our relative failure of commitment to clinical studies portrays no more than the disappointing inertia of a naturally cautious professional group. Whilst medical conservatism has served us well on occasion it may lead to too great a scepticism for new treatments. For instance, the use of adjuvant chemotherapy in node-positive pre-menopausal breast cancer patients, which we now know to be of real value and capable of saving lives, is still by no means thoroughly accepted and used in this country.

"Patient power" has become a favoured catch-phrase, yet in my own view a proper relationship between patient and doctor is more likely to emerge when doctors learn to accept that patients not only have rights but also brains as well, and can no longer be dealt with in a dismissive and off-hand way. On the other hand, patients too must recognize that asking for more information, and fuller participation in decision making, will inevitably bring more responsibilities and anxieties. Whether or not the physician chooses to discuss all aspects of the clinical trial with full disclosure in every case will always remain contentious; what is clearly established, however, is the critical importance of prospectively randomized clinical studies, which have already made substantial contributions to our current practice and will clearly continue to do so for the foreseeable future.

REFERENCES

1. Sacks HS, Berrier J, Reitman D (1987) Meta-analyses of randomized controlled trials. N Engl J Med 316: 450–455
2. Laupacis A, Sackett DL, Roberts RS (1988) An assessment of the consequences of treatment. N Engl J Med 318: 1728–1733

3. Cancer Research Campaign Working Party in Breast Conservation (1983) Informed consent: ethical, legal and medical implications for doctors and patients who participate in randomised clinical trials. Br Med J 286: 1117–1121
4. Tobias JS, Tattersall MHN (1985) Doing the best for the cancer patient. Lancet i: 35–38
5. Brahams D (1982) Death of a patient who was unwitting subject of randomised controlled trial of cancer treatment. Lancet i: 1028–1029
6. Anonymous (1988) Research without consent continued in the UK. Bull Inst Med Ethics 40: 13–15
7. Raphael A (1988) How doctor's secret trials abused me. Observer 9 October
8. Zelen M (1979) A new design for randomised clinical trials. N Engl J Med 300: 1242–1245
9. Tobias JS, Buxton J, Blackledge G et al (1989) Neoadjuvant therapy in cervical cancer. Proc ECCO 5, London, Abstract 0–1068
10. Early Breast Cancer Trialists' Collaborative Group (1988) Effects of adjuvant tamoxifen and of cytotoxic therapy on mortality in early breast cancer. N Engl J Med 319: 1681–1692
11. Tobias JS (1988) Informed consent and controlled trials. Lancet ii: 1194
12. Fisher B, Bauer M, Margolese R et al (1985) Five year results of a randomised clinical trial comparing total mastectomy and segmental mastectomy with or without radiation in the treatment of breast cancer. N Engl J Med 312: 665–671
13. Inglefinger FJ (1980) Arrogance. N Engl J Med 303: 1507–1511
14. Brewin TB (1982) Consent to randomised treatment. Lancet ii: 919–922
15. Baum M, Zilkha K, Houghton J (1989) Ethics of clinical research: lessons for the future. Br Med J 299: 251–253
16. Warnock M (1988) A national ethics committee. Br Med J 297: 1626–1627
17. Lock S (1990) Monitoring research ethical committees. Br Med J 300: 61–62
18. Royal College of Physicians (1990) Guidelines on the practice of ethics committees in medical research involving human subjects, 2nd edition. London
19. Brahams D (1988) Randomised trials and informed consent. Lancet ii: 1033–1034
20. Tobias JS (1990) Problems with informed consent. Br J Hosp Med (in press)

ABOUT THE AUTHOR

Dr Jeffrey Tobias is Consultant in Radiotherapy and Oncology at University College Hospital, London. His particular clinical interests are in the management of breast cancer, gynaecological cancers and cancer of the head and neck. He is particularly concerned with the ethical problems relating to new treatments for cancer and with clinical trial methodology and analysis. He is currently Chairman of the UKCCCR (United Kingdom Co-ordinating Committee in Cancer Research) head and neck cancer trial group.

Dr Tobias qualified from Cambridge University and St Bartholomew's Hospital in 1971 and is a Fellow of the Royal College of Radiologists and of the Royal College of Physicians. His junior posts were spent at St Bartholomew's Hospital and the Hammersmith Hospital, London, and he was a Clinical Fellow in cancer medicine at Harvard University, Boston,

Massachusetts, from 1974 to 1975. He was trained in radiotherapy at the Royal Marsden Hospital. In addition to over 100 scientific papers, he is joint author of three books on cancer, the most recent in collaboration with Dr Williams, the editor of the present volume. Other interests include medico-legal aspects of clinical practice, and the integration of terminal/ supportive care into the general practice of Oncology.

6 Issues in Informed Consent

MARTIN H. N. TATTERSALL and R. JOHN SIMES

When seeking consent from patients for medical treatments, the amount and kind of information which should be given, and the kind of consent which should be obtained, are the subject of considerable debate (see Chapter 4). Much of the discussion has focused on the contrasting requirements of consent for treatment outside controlled studies versus participation in randomized trials comparing different standard treatments. Baum [1] has highlighted the double standards which exist in this setting, and Brewin [2] has raised the issues of ordinary versus special consent. Brewin has argued that the mere fact of randomization in allocating treatment raises no "special" consent issues when the treatments being compared are "standard". He has proposed that doctors participating in randomized treatment trials should not be thought of as research workers "but simply as a clinician with an ethical duty to his patients not to go on giving them treatments without doing everything possible to assess their true worth".

The Declaration of Helsinki [3] states as a basic principle that "in any research on human beings, each potential subject must be *adequately* informed of the aims, methods, anticipated benefits and potential hazards of the study". Other bodies which have issued guidelines for consent also do not distinguish between the consent requirements when the treatment being given is standard, as part of a randomized trial comparing different standard treatment, versus when the treatment is novel or a phase I trial [4]. It is our view that different issues are raised in the latter circumstances and that the ethical issues require special consideration particularly in regard to "seeking and obtaining" consent. In this chapter we review ethical issues in regard to consent to treatment in general, and we discuss consent to participate in randomized controlled trials comparing different standard treatments. Finally we consider the special case of seeking and obtaining consent to novel therapies.

INFORMED CONSENT (HOW MUCH?)

The rationale for informed consent is to safeguard the autonomy and integrity of the individual and to ensure the patient plays an active role in

Introducing New Treatments for Cancer: Practical, Ethical and Legal Problems. Edited by C. J. Williams
© 1992 John Wiley & Sons Ltd

decisions about his care. The doctrine of informed consent contains four requirements:

(1) that the patient should be capable of giving consent;
(2) that the consent should be freely given;
(3) that patients should be given all information material to the decisions to agree;
(4) that patients should understand the information.

The amount of information that should be disclosed varies between countries. Discretion is allowed in the UK and Australia particularly when there is thought to be some conflict between the potential harm of additional information and allowing the patient to make a totally autonomous decision. The focus on how much information to disclose due to regulations rather than active communication between patient and doctors has been argued to be detrimental to ensuring patients optimal care.

The inability of patients to comprehend detailed information given during informed consent has been a sharp practical argument as to the limitations of the concept. Several studies have demonstrated patients' inability to understand important details relevant to their consent. This is particularly so when the studies relied on consent forms to communicate information.

Although full comprehension may not be attainable, some studies have demonstrated means to increase the level of patient understanding. The policy of allowing patients to keep the consent forms overnight has been shown to increase understanding. Furthermore, some controlled studies have demonstrated better understanding in patients given more information.

The concern that detailed disclosure of information may unnecessarily distress patients has led many to argue against unsolicited risk disclosure. This concern is not supported by some clinical studies and in fact disclosure of operative risks has been associated with reduced postoperative anxiety and improved postoperative pain control. Informed consent has also led to more realistic expectations of disease and treatment. However, other studies have shown harm associated with more information with side-effects experienced as a psychosomatic disorder or associated increased anxiety.

A number of investigations have demonstrated that patients do wish to be informed about their treatment or diagnostic procedures. Other studies have indicated that some patients do not wish to be informed of additional risks or details. Practising indiscriminate informed consent may also be "an ethically unjustifiable form of medical paternalism".

Several authors have emphasized the importance of preserving a good doctor–patient relationship and expressed concern that detailed informed consent may interfere with the relationship. This is one reason given for physicians' reluctance to participate in a randomized trial of breast cancer surgery. However, there is little empirical data that detailed disclosure of information does interfere with the doctor–patient relationship.

Several recent studies have shown that most patients want to play an active role in their treatment decisions but were usually content to let the doctors take the responsibility for the actual decisions [5]. A recent randomized trial has shown that patients can be taught to take a more active role in their treatment and that this can have favourable impacts on their health.

Further light on how much information should be given in trials comparing standard treatments in a randomized setting is given by examining the results of a consent trial which we reported some years ago.

THE CONSENT STUDY

STUDY OUTLINE

This trial, first reported in 1986 [6], compared two approaches to seeking consent for clinical trials of different standard cancer therapies: an individual approach at the discretion of each doctor; and a policy of total disclosure of all relevant information given both verbally and in writing. The basic design of the study is outlined in Figure 1. The major objectives of the study were to compare the effect of these two consent procedures on patients' understanding of their illness and treatment, on their willingness to participate in clinical trials, on anxiety levels and on the patients' perception of the doctor–patient relationship. These outcomes were assessed by means of a questionnaire designed and pre-tested for this study given soon after the consent interview and about three to four weeks later. Information was

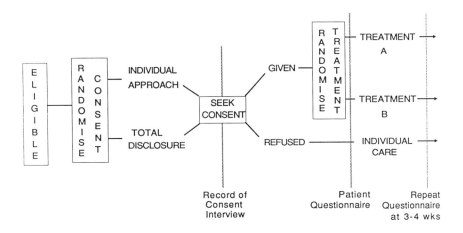

Figure 1. Informed consent study design

also collected on patients' attitudes towards informed consent issues and towards participation in medical decision.

MAIN RESULTS

Fifty-seven patients, eligible for 11 different cancer trials, were randomized to one or other consent procedure. Patients receiving total disclosure were generally given more information, particularly on uncommon side-effects of treatment and on the research nature of the trials, su⌐h as treatment randomization. These patients usually received the consent form to read overnight before giving consent. Patients receiving the individual approach had a variable amount of information given based on the doctor's judgment and the patient's wishes, with consent being obtained verbally. All patients were given the opportunity to ask further questions, which were answered honestly.

The main effects of total disclosure compared with the individual approach are summarized in Table 1. Those receiving total disclosure were more knowledgeable of their illness and treatment ($p=0.0001$) and about the research aspects of the cancer treatment ($p=0.03$). However, these patients were less willing to participate in the trial of cancer treatment and had a higher anxiety score ($p=0.02$). The patients' perception of the doctor–patient relationship was not significantly different between the two consent procedures for any of the three summary measures: confidence in the doctors; personal doctor–patient relationship; and individualized care. Differences found at the time of the initial questionnaire were no longer apparent three to four weeks later on the repeat questionnaire.

The results of this trial suggest there are trade-offs in the amount of information patients are given before consenting to cancer trials. More detailed information, given indiscriminantly, resulted in a more

Table 1. Major outcomes of informed consent trial: initial questionnaire (scores expressed as mean $\pm$ SEM)

	Individual approach ($n=29$)	Total disclosure ($n=26$)	p-value[a]
Willingness to participate	88±3	65±7	0.01
Patient confidence	73±3	73±3	0.90
Personal doctor–patient relationship	76±2	77±3	0.87
Individualized care	71±3	66±3	0.17
Knowledge: treatment side-effects	56±3	82±4	0.0001
Knowledge: research aspects	59±4	73±5	0.03
Anxiety	42±2	49±2	0.02
All outcomes			0.0001

[a]p-values are two-sided based two-sample t-test for individual outcomes. A test for all outcomes together (Hotelling's T^2 statistic) was significant at $p=0.0001$.

knowledgeable yet more reluctant and anxious patient. This raises the issue as to whether the amount and kind of information given to each patient should be tailored to the individual circumstances. This concept is supported by a further exploratory analysis of the trial data.

CLUSTER ANALYSIS

In order to see whether different patients might be approached differently when seeking consent, patients were first divided into three well-defined

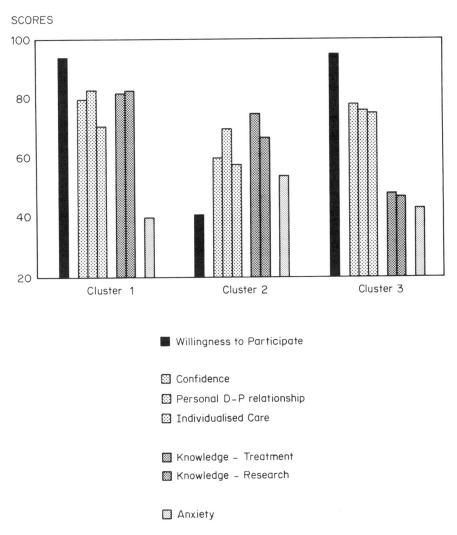

Figure 2. Informed consent study cluster profiles

groups of similar outcomes using the method of K-means clustering [7]. This method groups together those patients with more similar scores. The clusters were defined according to the similarity of patients in terms of the seven major outcomes of the trial: knowledge of the treatment; knowledge of research aspects; willingness to participate; anxiety; and the three measures of doctor–patient relationship (confidence; personal; individualized care).

The cluster profiles of the three relatively distinct groups are illustrated in Figure 2. Cluster 1 contained patients with greater knowledge, a positive doctor–patient relationship, greater willingness to participate and less anxiety. Cluster 3 also contained largely patients with a positive doctor–patient relationship, less anxiety and greater willingness to participate. However, these patients had much less knowledge of the treatment or the trial. By contrast, patients from cluster 2 had a less positive doctor–patient relationship, were more reluctant to participate in trials and were considerably more anxious. This group was also more knowledgeable (similar to cluster 1).

Table 2 shows that clusters 1 and 2 received significantly more information during the consent interview and that these two groups contained significantly more patients allocated to the total disclosure procedure ($p = 0.003$). Patients from cluster 3 were almost all allocated to the individual approach. Hence for some patients (cluster 1) more detailed information appears to be beneficial with greater knowledge, a positive doctor–patient relationship and reduced anxiety levels. However, for patients in cluster 2, the more detailed information may be harmful with a less positive doctor–patient relationship and increased anxiety levels. If some patients are less able to handle detailed disclosure of information this would be a strong argument against the indiscriminate policy of total disclosure and emphasize the need for tailoring the consent process to individual needs and wishes.

Table 2. Relation of clusters to consent interview

	Clusters		
	1	2	3
Consent procedure[a]			
individual	7	6	16
total disclosure	12	11	3
Consent interview[b]			
% areas covered	85 (4)	91 (3)	76 (4)
% side effects mentioned	74 (7)	81 (7)	57 (8)

[a]Number of patients in each cluster.
[b]Results expressed as mean (SE) for each cluster.

PATIENT ATTITUDES

Opinions regarding informed consent of the 55 patients who answered the initial questionnaire are summarized in Table 3. For normal cancer treatment most patients felt they should be given any information their doctor considered important, plus be told about anything they ask. However, for experimental treatment most felt they should be told everything. Few patients (16%) felt their doctor alone should decide how much information they are given and married patients in particular wanted to be involved in this decision ($p < 0.05$). Virtually all patients (98%) preferred to be *involved*

Table 3. Patient attitudes regarding informed consent ($n = 55$) (expressed as number (%))

Question 1: How much information should patients like yourself be given about their illness and treatment?

	Normally	For experimental treatment
(a) Should be told only what their doctor thinks is important for them to know?	1 (2)	1 (2)
(b) Should be told only about things they ask?	0 (0)	0 (0)
(c) Should be told about anything they ask and also anything their doctor thinks is important for them to know?	29 (53)	20 (36)
(d) Should be told everything unless they ask not to be told it all.	12 (22)	14 (25)
(e) Everyone should be told everything regardless.	13 (24)	20 (36)

Question 2: Who should decide how much you are told about your illness and treatment?

(a) Your doctor	9 (16)
(b) Yourself	12 (22)
(c) You and your doctor	14 (25)
(d) You and your family	1 (2)
(e) Your doctor and your family	0 (0)
(f) You, your doctor and your family	19 (35)

Question 3: Do you think there should be any laws which have a say or influence in how much information you are given?

(a) Definitely yes	8 (15)
(b) Yes	7 (13)
(c) Not sure	11 (20)
(d) No	8 (15)
(e) Definitely no	21 (38)

in decisions about their medical care and treatment but most patients (85%) preferred to leave the *actual decisions* to their doctors. The opinions regarding the influence of the law on informed consent procedures were diverse but with approximately one-half of the patients feeling the law should not have any say. An opinion for the law to have a say in such matters was expressed particularly by the younger patient (less than 55 years) compared with older patient ($p < 0.05$). Both informed consent groups expressed similar opinions on these issues.

In general, patients were well satisfied with the information they had received *regardless* of the informed consent procedure used. In both groups, most patients felt they had a good understanding of their illness and treatment programme, had plenty of opportunity to ask questions and felt more confident as a result of the information they received. Almost all patients from both groups (95%) felt they had been given about the right amount of information to help them decide what to do. This illustrates the importance of controlled studies in consent and not accepting measures of patient satisfaction for a particular consent procedure as sufficient argument for its use.

It is interesting that patients drew a distinction between experimental therapies where most felt they should be told everything versus standard cancer treatment where most patients felt they should be given any information their doctor considered important.

ETHICAL ISSUES IN TRIALS OF NEW THERAPIES

The clinical trial allows appropriate scientific appraisal of new treatments to ensure that patients are offered the best treatments. Without the use of clinical trials, standard treatment may be suboptimal and some treatments may be ineffective or even harmful. However, to evaluate each new therapy, it must be tested at a time when it is not known if it is better or worse than standard therapy, and inevitably this means that patients participating in a clinical trial are being exposed to unknown risks of the new therapy. This creates a potential dilemma particularly when "standard best therapy" has not been given. Most ethical guidelines for clinical research recommend that clinical trials are justifiable only if the foreseeable risks are reasonable in terms of the anticipated benefits to the patient and the community. A recent review [8] of 211 reports of phase I cytotoxic studies published between 1972 and 1987 reported objective tumour response in 4.5% of 6639 patients and toxic deaths in 0.5% (see Chapter 12). This review, while providing some reassuring information about fatal toxicity in the exploration of novel cancer chemotherapies, indicates the infrequency of tumour response in these patient trials, and notes that only 9% of the patients had received no prior treatment, and 75.3% had received prior chemotherapy. In an editorial about this article, Sessa and Cavalli [9] question whether all of the early clinical trials are justified, and consider whether phase I trials should be limited to only those compounds for which a "conclusive rationale can be previously demonstrated".

A proper selection of patients for phase I clinical trials, and a correct procedure for seeking and obtaining informed consent, are seen by Sessa and Cavalli to be mandatory. Not every patient who fits into the eligibility criteria of a phase I protocol is psychologically capable of handling the type of information which is required for informed consent. No guidelines have been presented relating to this aspect of patient selection, but Sessa and Cavalli recommend that the following categories of patients are the best candidates for phase I trials: strong believers in chemotherapy; those who would like to contribute to future knowledge and help other cancer patients; and those who want to please their relatives by maintaining a combative spirit.

There has been recent discussion about the evaluation of new drugs in previously untreated patients with chemosensitive advanced cancers such as extensive-stage small-cell lung cancer. Some clinicians believe that conducting phase I and II studies in previously untreated small-cell lung cancer patients is unethical while others have suggested that it is the only way to give new drugs "the fairest possible test for their development". Ettinger [10], in an editorial reviewing two reports in the *Journal of Clinical Oncology* of the evaluation of new drugs in previously untreated patients with small-cell lung cancer, concludes that it is now reasonable to test new drugs in this group of patients. He advocates either a randomized design comparing novel therapy followed by standard treatment at time of progression versus standard treatment, or novel treatment followed by standard treatment on failure as a single treatment policy. He comments that the "ultimate success of such new drug studies will depend on these studies being well designed, the selection of appropriate patients and the availability of effective salvage therapies". While emphasizing the need for and importance of the informed consent of patients participating in such studies, Ettinger maintains that patients must know of both the risks and benefits of the treatment options. However, he does not state what the benefits may be.

Chalmers, in a meeting debating patient research and informed consent, highlighted the widespread lay assumption that a new treatment must have a high probability of being "better" than the older one. By the very nature of the screening of new therapies the chance of a new therapy being found superior than existing ones is probably small. Dr Anderson, at the same meeting, argued that the prejudices of today tend toward an over-enthusiasm for research and for new treatment methods, partly fuelled by career advancement of clinical investigators. False optimism can easily affect the judgment of both the doctor involved in research and his patients. The recent movement in the UK towards defining standard treatment approaches for particular tumour types and stages may help to clarify for patients when experimental therapies are reasonable options.

The presentation of information to patients eligible for phase I clinical trials has not been studied, nor are data available about the proportion of eligible patients invited to participate who decline. However, criticisms have been voiced that current consent documents read as if they were written more for the protection of the investigator and the institution than to help to provide helpful information for the patient. The difficulties raised by the dual role of physician and clinical investigator further complicate the utilization of written consent to investigational new cancer treatment. Penman et al [11] investigated the perception of the consent procedure for phase II and III cancer trials of 144 patients and 68 physicians. Patients recalled the consent procedure positively, and relied heavily on physicians' advice. They felt most clinicians wanted them to accept while 29% felt that their participation in the decision was not encouraged. The major reasons given for accepting were trust in the physician, belief that the treatment would help, and fear that the disease would get worse without it. Twenty-two per cent did not recall three weeks later the information given that treatment was investigational. Most patients expected large benefits from treatment, and only 4% expected little or no benefit. Forty-seven of the 144 patients gave as one of the reasons for accepting treatment "to be part of research", but only six of them included this reason as one of their top three reasons, and none gave it as first in importance.

It is self-evident that the method of presenting data about the possible outcome of differing treatment approaches, i.e. second or third-line therapy versus a new treatment, will have a significant impact on patient choice. McNeil et al [12] have investigated how variations in the way information is presented to patients influences their choices between treatment options. The same information can result in different patient preferences depending on whether treatment outcomes are presented as survival probabilities or duration, as chances of living or dying, and with treatment identified or not. They suggest that an awareness of these effects among clinicians and patients should "reduce bias and improve the quality of medical decision making".

Since cancer therapies are often not curative, the goals of treatment in cancer patients need to be carefully considered in the light of patient preferences. These decisions can be especially difficult in the debilitated or terminally ill when debating whether to try to prolong life or to allow the patient to die. These patients may also be those who are considered as candidates for phase I clinical trials. We feel that detailed information about the risks and likely benefits of experimental therapy should be provided, and whenever possible patients should be encouraged to discuss with their families whether or not they wish to be entered in trials of novel therapies.

CONCLUSIONS

When seeking consent for medical treatments the amount and kind of information which should be given are still the subject of considerable debate. Ethical guidelines stress the importance in clinical trials of adequately informing each patient of the anticipated benefits and potential hazards of study treatment. Inadequate distinction is made in most guidelines between ethical guidelines for trials of experimental or novel therapies and those trials comparing treatments in a randomized fashion that are already regarded as standard by many in the medical community.

For experimental therapies, owing to their low chance of success with a greater uncertainty about possible major adverse effects and owing to the greater potential conflict between individual versus community benefit, there is an additional responsibility on the doctor for ensuring the patient is adequately informed before seeking consent.

For standard therapies being given as part of a randomized trial, similar ethical principles should apply as for routine treatment. Whilst all patients should receive sufficient information so they can make an informed choice of treatment, it should be recognized that trade-offs may exist in giving detailed unsolicited information. A caring and sensitive consent process tailored to the individual's needs and wishes is recommended.

REFERENCES

1. Baum M (1986) Do we need informed consent? Lancet ii: 911–912
2. Brewin TB (1985) Truth, trust, paternalism. Lancet ii: 490–492
3. World Medical Association (1964) Declaration of Helsinki: recommendations guiding medical doctors in biomedical research involving human subjects. World Medical Association, Helsinki
4. National Health and Medical Research Council (1988) NHMRC statement on human experimentation and supplementary notes. NHMRC, Canberra
5. Lebacqz K, Levine RJ (1977) Respect for persons and informed consent to participate in cancer research. Clin Res 25: 101–107
6. Simes RJ, Tattersall MHN, Coates AS et al (1986) Randomised comparison of procedures for obtaining informed consent in clinical trial of treatment for cancer. Br Med J 293: 1065–1068
7. Wong MA (1982) A hybrid clustering method for identifying high-density clusters. J Am Stat Assoc 77: 841–847
8. Decoster G, Stein G, Holdener EE (1990) Responses and toxic deaths in phase I clinical trials. Ann Oncol 6: 175–181
9. Sessa C, Cavalli F (1990) Who benefits from phase I studies? Ann Oncol 1: 164–165
10. Ettinger DS (1990) Evaluation of new drugs in untreated patients with small-cell lung cancer: its time has come. J Clin Oncol 8: 374–377
11. Penman DT, Holland JC, Bahna GF et al (1984) Informed consent for investigational chemotherapy; patients' and physicians perceptions. J Clin Oncol 2: 849–855
12. McNiel BJ, Pauker SG, Fox HC, Tversky A (1982) On elicitation of preferences for alternative therapies. N Engl J Med 306: 1259–1262

ABOUT THE AUTHORS

Professor Martin Tattersall is a medical oncologist and biochemical pharmacologist trained at the Royal Postgraduate Medical School, London, the Institute of Cancer Research, Royal Marsden Hospital, and at the Harvard Medical School. He is Professor of Cancer Medicine at the University of Sydney, and head of clinical oncology at Royal Prince Alfred Hospital. His clinical research interests are in gynaecological and breast cancer management, and in ethical issues in clinical cancer research.

Dr John Simes is a medical oncologist and biostatistician trained at Royal Prince Alfred Hospital in medical oncology and at the Harvard School of Public Health in biostatistics. Recently he has taken up the position of Director of the NHMRC Clinical Trials Centre, a recently established national trials centre in Australia. Dr Simes' research interests include ethics of randomized trials and methods for translating the results of clinical trials into clinical decision making.

7 Research Ethics Committees in Britain

CLAIRE GILBERT FOSTER

Medical research develops apace, bringing with it not only remarkable new skills and techniques but also what appear as completely new ethical problems. There is a moral obligation for the research undertaken by members of the clinical community to be done in an ethical way. A sharp increase over the last decade of public interest in this area compounds the need not only for the research to be ethical but also for it to be seen to be ethical.

Although there has been a lurking concern about human experimentation since Nazi rule in Germany, anxiety in Britain did not begin to be vociferous until the 1960s. In 1962 the *British Medical Journal* (*BMJ*) published an editorial which stated:

> The publication in the *Twentieth Century* of an article by Dr M.H. Pappworth entitled "Human Guinea Pigs: A Warning" has provoked widespread comment in the national press. There has for some time been public uneasiness about investigations carried out in hospitals which have not always been obviously in the interest of the subject of the investigation. (27 October 1962: 1108–1109)

Mrs Hodgson, then Chairman of the Patient's Association, wrote in 1963:

> Clinical trials are obviously going on, and on a big scale. Patients are not told if they are receiving new or orthodox treatment. I maintain that they should be told. ("Now a voice for the patient", *The Times*, 17 June 1963)

An editorial in the *BMJ* in 1963 quotes this statement from Mrs Hodgson and speaks of her as having a voice to be reckoned with: "Mrs Hodgson, according to an article in *The Times* headed 'Now a Voice for the Patient', is moving forward with some determination." The editorial adds: "We agree with Mrs Hodgson" (6 July 1963).

Desmond Laurence's proposal in 1966 that medical research should be subject to ethical review, following the example of the USA, seemed to

Introducing New Treatments for Cancer: Practical, Ethical and Legal Problems. Edited by C. J. Williams
© 1992 John Wiley & Sons Ltd

provide a solution to the growing demand that research should be both ethical and seen to be ethical. He quotes the then Surgeon General of the USA, Dr William H. Stewart:

> We are assuming, essentially, that the medical school, hospital, or other research institution—by accepting the administration of public funds—accepts also a share of responsibility for their use. We are asking that the institution assure us that research proposals related to the use of human subjects are being systematically subjected to independent review, and we are urging that qualified individuals from outside the scientific area be involved in this review. (Quoted in Dr Laurence's letter to the President of the Royal College of Physicians, 1966)

Professor Laurence's suggestion was taken up by the Royal College of Physicians (RCP) and then by the Ministry of Health. In 1968 the Ministry sent a memorandum, which included a statement by the RCP, to regional hospital boards, hospital management committees and boards of governors. It indicated that hospital authorities should organize ethical review boards on an informal, advisory basis. But no legal requirement was placed upon authorities to establish ethics committees and no formal legal status was offered to these committees. Specific guidelines on their practices and methods were not given, as strict rules of conduct, it was thought, would not be readily adaptable to local needs.

The lack of specificity in the Ministry of Health's request reflects a tendency on its part to be coy about dictating to the medical profession its ethical imperatives. It also helps to explain the muddle now apparent in research ethics committees in Great Britain, which were left to work out their own methods and practices. Surveys conducted during the last decade indicate that committees are becoming part of the medical furniture; currently there is at least one research ethics committee in nearly every health district. The Department of Health (DoH) has now told all NHS institutions that they must establish a research ethics committee by February 1992 [1]. There are others attached to pharmaceutical companies and independent organizations of which we have evidence only by their members' attendance at educational conferences for ethics committees. These committees, which are independent of the National Health Service (NHS), are not included in the register compiled by the RCP. This has implications if the register is to be used as a mailing list for information about developments, new guidelines, etc.

The DoH has, until its recent publication *Local Research Ethics Committees* [1], left ethics committees alone. Surprisingly they were not even acknowledged when, in 1984, the DHSS sent a health notice out about the administration of radioactive substances to persons. This notice clarifies regulations about doctors and dentists administering radioactive substances and emphasizes that the regulations are concerned with "the protection of the patient or volunteer . . . rather than with the protection of the staff who are involved" (*Administration of Radioactive Substances to Persons*, 1984). Research ethics committees would need to know about this document yet it is not addressed to them, but rather to regional health authorities, district health authorities, special health authorities for the London postgraduate teaching hospitals, boards of governors and community health councils (CHCs). It would have been left to the bodies listed above to realize their local ethics committee would need to see the document. The survey carried out in 1989 on district research ethics committees showed that out of 28 committees only one mentioned this document in its literature for applicant researchers [2].

Guidance about the ethics of research and the practice of research ethics committees has been on offer from other quarters, however. The RCP in particular, having laid the foundation for establishing ethics committees, has produced a number of guidelines for ethics committees. The most important of these are the *Guidelines on the Practice of Ethics Committees in Medical Research* [3] and its updated version which was published in 1990 (Chapter 3). It has also produced two documents on the ethics of medical research, entitled *Research on Healthy Volunteers* [4] and *Research Involving Patients* [5]. Other documents produced by the RCP have an important bearing on the deliberations of ethics committees, such as *The Relationship between Physicians and the Pharmaceutical Industry* [6]. The World Medical Association's Helsinki Guidelines [7], the Association of British Pharmaceutical Industries' Guidelines [8], the British Medical Association's Guidelines [9], and a *Code of Practice* from the Human Fertilisation and Embryology Authority for human in vitro fertilization [10], all provide detailed, particular, or more general advice and guidance useful to those whose responsibility it is to assess the ethics of medical research.

However, these guidelines, according to the four surveys [2, 11–13] conducted over the last ten years, seem often to have been ignored. Exactly why this is so is not known, although bad communication, ideas about not needing help and lack of time or willpower will be among the reasons.

CURRENT AND POTENTIAL PROBLEMS

Ethical opinion is always debatable, and the paradigmatic ethics committee has not yet been created. There is room available, then, for some diversity amongst committees. But the confused situation we currently have is open to exploitation, and can easily become injurious to subjects of medical research, to medical research itself and to the reputation of the medical profession.

For the sake of the argument, and to illustrate the possibilities of the current situation, imagine a doctor who was asked by a pharmaceutical company to research a new drug on his patients, for a large fee. Desirous of the financial rewards and of the acclaim when the research was completed and the new drug appeared on the market, the doctor agreed. Caution told him he should gain ethical approval; ambition told him this was the way to gloss his research with respectability. He did his homework and found an ethics committee which did not ask about the sponsorship of the project, nor about the financial rewards the researcher himself may receive. The committee's application form merely asked whether he was to be gaining consent from his research subjects, and did not ask to see the letter of invitation or information sheet he may or may not have been providing for his subjects. The committee had no lay member and so was unlikely to be very aware of the patients' needs and wants.

The doctor can find out all this information about committees, because the written constitution and application form of any committee is public property, and there is no reason for a secretary or a chairman to withhold information about his or her committee over the telephone. He does not have to apply to his most local committee; any committee's approval will do.

Having found an ethics committee which would be unlikely to cause trouble, the doctor submitted his application and had it approved. Armed with "ethical approval", he went ahead with his research. The appearance was that his research was as ethical as any other research, because it had formal approval from an ethics committee. If the drug turned out to be a failure he was not required to publish negative results. If it was a success he would have no trouble publishing: he had ethical approval.

While the story is itself not true, all its parts come from real-life situations. It was in fact a pharmaceutical company, not a doctor, which researched ethics committees across the country to discover in which centres it would be easiest to have its protocol for a multicentre trial approved. The present author's survey [2] shows that many ethics committees do not ask about finance, that a number of ethics committees ask if informed consent is to be obtained, but do not ask how, and that some committees still have no lay member. Others have lay members who are entirely left out of the discussion and decision-making process, either because business is conducted by post and the lay member cannot understand the protocol, or because the preponderance of articulate medical membership overwhelms the lay membership. These observations were made at a meeting of lay members of ethics committees, organized by the College of Health and Riverside CHC in April 1989. Once the research has ethical approval, no other body is required to scrutinize it; it is entirely left to the researcher to ensure the research continues to be conducted in an ethical manner. In other words, if the ethics committee does not do its job properly, there is no official back-up. Research is currently being undertaken by Dr Phillipa Easterbrook in Oxford and Harvard Medical Schools to investigate the thesis that journals tend to favour publication of positive results (Chapter 25), so that trials which fail, or which produce negative results, are rarely exposed.

Another illustration shows the opposite possibility. In this case, the doctor was at the vanguard of developing a new therapy. The knowledge was quite new and radical, and the proposed therapy was technically complicated. He wished to put his research to the test and so formulated a research proposal. A grant-giving body, persuaded of the science of the research, agreed to fund his work pending ethical approval. Accordingly, the doctor presented his research application to his local ethics committee. This committee was thorough; its members were anxious to avoid the reputation of a rubber-stamp committee, and its ethical standards for approved research projects were high. One of its lay members was possessed of strong ethical opinions and a mission to protect any potential research subjects, be they healthy or patient volunteers. He was not afraid to speak, and had a lurking mistrust of the medical profession, members of which he believed would try to "get away with it" if he let them. The research application, now neatly inserted into the committee's exacting application form, was duly made, and came up at the next meeting of the committee. The committee was always very careful with its applications: none went through on the nod; chairman's approval was never given; each item was thoroughly discussed, no matter how long it took. The committee prided itself on its rigour, and prided itself that it never bowed to peer pressure. If a multicentre trial had already been approved in all but its own district, it would not give its own approval unless the protocol matched its ethical requirements. If the research looked like it was going to save humankind forever more from some dread disease, and yet failed to meet the committee's ethical requirements, it would not be swayed to approve it until it did.

This particular research proposal was for a new cancer therapy. None of the members of the committee was a trained oncologist (an ethics committee which had on it representatives from every medical speciality would be far too large to function) and the scientific basis of this research project was not properly understood. The committee was not convinced that the research needed to be done. The zealous lay member insisted that the procedures involved would be far too complex and invasive of the subjects to warrant the study's validity, and the project was rejected. This again is a story which though fictional as a whole is the sum of parts which have happened or could happen.

A third scenario is that of the multicentre trial. Epidemiologists and other specialists who have to conduct research over large areas, both geo-graphically and demographically, face real problems with gaining ethical approval. Currently, the most correct way to undertake this kind of multicentre trial is to apply for ethical approval from every local ethics committee whose district is to be involved in the research. A protocol which went to fifty committees, each of which had a different method and a different set of ethical criteria, would be so modified, after fifty examinations, that it would be unrecognizable from its original. Certainly, no protocol would be capable of pleasing every committee. In fact, many such researchers bypass local committees. There is an argument which suggests that their work is closer to audit than research and is therefore not obliged to be scrutinized by research ethics committees. This begs a different though related question to do with the fine line between research and therapy, and research and audit, which is beyond the scope of this essay.

The other kind of multicentre trial is that which is organized by a central body, such as the International Study on Infarct Survival (ISIS) trials being coordinated in Oxford, or large drugs trials organized by pharmaceutical companies. Here individual researchers based in particular localities will be asked to undertake the research on a certain quota of subjects in their areas. It will be up to them to approach their own local ethics committees for approval. Some committees, being more rigorous than others, may well turn down or substantially alter a protocol, where others will not. This can jeopardize the trial. It can also put the ethics of the trial under suspicion. Opportunists can exploit the situation by ensuring that only the less rigorous committees scrutinize their protocols.

PROPOSALS

The aim of research ethics committees is to ensure that medical research is ethical and seen to be ethical. The problem with the current situation of ethics committees is apparently simple. It is basically that there is a great diversity of committees and this has given rise to the difficulties now faced. Thus, in the extreme case, if all committees knew exactly what their remit was, and what standard of practice they had to meet, and this remit and standard were uniform across the country, such situations as those described in the three illustrations could not arise.

Unfortunately people are not built to be uniform; committees would not be decision-making bodies if outcomes were already determined, and fixed ethical criteria cannot always provide an appropriate framework for medical research. There are always exceptions. A simple example is that of the obtaining of so-called informed consent. The Nuremburg Code decrees that "the voluntary consent of the human subject is absolutely essential". This is a just and fair ethical principle, in theory. But by virtue of it, research on children, on mentally ill patients, on comatose or emergency patients is outlawed. Committees obliged to ensure this ethical criterion was met would be obliged to disapprove of all the above categories of medical research. It would, in any case, be a rubber-stamp committee and its members, persons with discriminating abilities, would not always agree with the rubber-stamping they had to do. Thus the solution to the problem is not as simple as the problem itself. Merely enforcing uniformity would create numerous hidden problems.

Two practical proposals have entered the debate about ethics committees in Britain. The first and most widely discussed and supported is that of setting up a national research ethics committee. The second is to create a national association of ethics committees. Either of these organizations would have certain functions to fulfil in order to bring local committees to the point where they were able to meet their purposes. These functions are: adequate publicity of guidelines and assurance that they were being followed; training or assistance to bring committees up to an acceptable standard; assistance with difficult scientific or ethical problems with particular research; and some sort of co-ordination of the scrutiny and approval of multicentre trials.

A NATIONAL RESEARCH ETHICS COMMITTEE

The proposal to create a national ethics committee has found support from many different sides. Early in 1987, responses from local ethics committees to the British Medical Association's proposal for such a committee were collated, and found to be 80% in favour. Discussion of the subject, in particular in the correspondence columns of the *BMJ* in 1990, has shown that different people wish for a national research ethics committee for different reasons. Some ethics committees wish to see a national committee set up to deal with multicentre trials, because of the aggravation caused when they, perhaps alone among all the other committees assessing the multicentre project, insist on certain changes to the protocol. Others whose concern is about inadequacy of practice, lack of communication between committees, their unregulated proliferation and the apparent lack of interest in or knowledge about current guidelines, wish to see a national ethics committee as a kind of overseer, with regulatory authority. Some hope for a national ethics committee as an advisory board for particularly difficult ethical questions faced by local committees. The same proposal is advocated by some researchers whose work is frustrated by ethics committees which, the researchers feel, do not understand their research. Finally, a committee which had a high public profile would fulfil the criterion noted above, that research should be seen to be ethical, for the committee would be highly visible.

There are difficulties, however, with this proposal. First, the committee would need to paradigmatic. Nobody knows what a paradigmatic ethics committee is like, but most people involved in such matters have an opinion, ranging from a committee entirely made up of lay members plus a token doctor, to no lay membership at all. Ideas about practice also differ, as mine and other surveys indicate. A committee consisting of the "great and the good" will be unconvincing. Selecting the most important people on offer, medical and lay, to sit on the committee will not create the best committee. Professor Baum has suggested, in a letter to the *BMJ* (10 February 1990), that lay membership should consist only of those with "scholarship in medical ethics"; others feel they should be chosen because they have high profiles. The RCP suggests they should be "persons of responsibility and standing". But the most important quality they can have, more than those mentioned above, is an ignorance of medical language, and a willingness to ask what things mean. A very useful function of lay members is to ensure that the letter of invitation to patients or volunteers from researchers will make sense to them. Words like "venous cannulation", "placebo", "serial blood samples" and "slit lamp", part of a doctor's vernacular, are meaningless to the man on the Clapham omnibus or the woman in the out-patients' clinic.

Second, whatever the constitution of the committee and however it decides it will function, it will need to be good enough to earn the trust of local committees. If it has a policing function, and the power to approve multicentre trials, and if local committees will be expected to refer difficult cases to the national committee, local committees will have to concur and accept the role of the national committee. I suspect this would be difficult no matter how excellent the national committee, for there are a number of committees which have devised their own methods and practices, who feel they do a good job, and enjoy their independence and direct responsibility for the research taking place in their districts.

Finally, there will be logistical and administrative problems. How is a large and unwieldy collection of local committees policed? How can a central committee know and understand each local area well enough to make decisions about research proposed to take place there, and about how the local committee should run itself?

It is worth looking at other countries which have national ethics committees or national research ethics committees to see how they fared. Denmark, in 1980–81, created a comprehensive two-level system with a "central scientific–ethical committee", and regional committees, for examining medical research projects. The central committee has one scientific and one lay member from each regional committee, and a chairman and a vice chairman appointed by the Danish Medical Research Council. Its current chairman has stated "until now the committee system has not rested on legislation, but a commission has recently been appointed to advise the government how to give a legal basis to the control of research". The central committee is also an appeals body.

In France an ethics committee was created in 1974 by the National Institute of Health and Medical Research. Its remit then was to examine research projects involving human subjects. In 1983 this committee became the National Consultative Ethics Committee for the Life Sciences and Health, and was established by law. Its mandate is much broader now. Its members are nominated from all the "major corps" of the nation; the majority are doctors but there are also jurists, social scientists, philosophers and representatives from different spiritual traditions. It is now responsible for formulating opinions on all the major ethical issues, and in this regard has published several reports.

In Germany there is a central governmental committee which meets to discuss issues rather than individual research projects. Switzerland established a central committee for medical ethics based on the Declaration of Helsinki and the "Guidelines for experimental research on man" of the Swiss Academy of Medical Sciences. It has several clearly defined tasks, which are: to reply to questions concerning medical ethics; to co-ordinate with local committees, promoting the exchange of information; to operate as a local committee for the hospitals which have none; to draw up recommendations on specific ethical problems; and to endeavour to build up trust between patients and the clinical community by improving contact between the public and the medical profession. Its membership is entirely medical apart from one teacher in the Faculty of Law at a Swiss University.

It should be noted that only the central committee in Denmark is concerned solely with research ethics. All the other national committees are concerned with medical ethics in general as well as research ethics. It should also be noted that the system of committees in Denmark was set up as a discrete event. The national committee was thus part of the system from its beginning and would be accepted as such by regional committees. In France, the National Committee was created before local committees, but in any case it has no responsibility for them. Germany's governmental committee likewise has little to do with local committees, chiefly because its function is different from theirs. The Swiss national committee also seems to have been established before committees had been created at a local level and has a responsibility to keep in contact with them. The Swiss model is the most comprehensive and useful, were we to seek one, but it is important to recognize how much work being a member of such a committee would involve.

A national research ethics committee which tried to fulfil all the functions that would be asked of it would be over-stretched. My fear would be that it would deal with the more obvious needs—multicentre trials and the really difficult, high-profile issues in medical research, such as embryology—and leave the policing altogether, thus dealing with one or two symptoms of the problem of local ethics committees and not with its cause. It would be assumed that all was well because a national ethics committee was up and running, while local committees continued to be as diverse and in some cases inadequate as they always were. In effect, a similar assumption to that made in the late 1960s would be made; then it was thought that simply advising hospitals and research institutions to create ethics committees would bring to an end all unethical research. Now it would be thought that a national committee would bring to an end all problems with the ethics committees set up without detailed advice in the 1960s.

A NATIONAL ASSOCIATION OF RESEARCH ETHICS COMMITTEES

The idea for a national association of ethics committees has been less widely canvassed. Significantly, the two persons who have suggested it in public are both chairmen of local ethics committees.

A national association might provide a more sophisticated and flexible method by which to better the practices of local ethics committees. Established as an enabling rather than a regulating body, it would admit to membership only those committees which agreed to meet a certain standard of practice (such as the one outlined in the DoH *Guidelines*). Thus membership would be voluntary, but membership would be a guarantee to outsiders that the committee functioned adequately. In time, credence would only be given to those committees which were members.

Training programmes for members of ethics committees are already available, run by different organizations (see below). An association might be instrumental in co-ordinating and disseminating information about these programmes. It would also be in a position to set up training programmes of its own. One approach might be that of "action research", which has been successfully used to evaluate and simultaneously to improve a ward sister training project at Guy's and Whipps Cross hospitals.

An association might be in a position to provide better administrative care for committees than would a national committee. It might, however, be less effective in the other two functions needed at the present time: assistance with the scrutinizing of multicentre trial proposals, and advice about difficult cases. But there is no reason why the association could not include a national research ethics advisory committee within its organization to meet these needs. It could, moreover, co-ordinate a floating membership of such a committee. Thus, for example, representatives from all or some of the local committees in whose districts a multicentre trial is proposed to take place could be co-opted to the national committee assessing that trial's protocol, thus enabling communication of decisions made at a national, central level to local areas where the effects of such decisions will be felt. Furthermore, the association could build up a store of people with different expertise, ready to be co-opted as and when necessary, on to this floating national committee, rather like the way that local committees, when faced with a proposal which needs the scrutiny of a specialist, should co-opt that specialist on to the committee while assessing those projects.

NO FURTHER ASSISTANCE

It may be the case that no further assistance should be organized, for there is already some considerable activity in Britain aimed at improving the practice of research ethics committees. It could be argued that there is no need to create a new organization when, eventually, all the current needs of committees will be met by different organizations already in existence. The RCP has held a meeting of chairmen of ethics committees and intends to continue to do so on a regular basis. It has compiled a register of ethics committees in Great Britain, not yet complete but the first of its kind. Its own Committee on Ethical Issues in Medicine is considering setting up a national research ethics committee to look at multicentre trials and to advise local committees on difficult protocols. The Association of Community Health Councils has produced an information pack for lay members of research ethics committees, which includes a booklist, addresses of organizations considering the role of ethics committees, information about training that is available and two articles—one about the experience of a lay member of an ethics committee, and the other about consent to participate in research. The Institute of Medical Ethics is considering producing a newsletter for ethics committees to facilitate communication and information exchange. The Centre for the Study of Philosophy and Health Care at University College Swansea is holding annual three-day training conferences for members of ethics committees. The Centre for Social Ethics and Policy, University of Manchester, held two one-day seminars in 1991 for members of ethics committees and intends to continue. The College of Health is considering a series of one-day seminars around England and Wales for lay members of ethics committees. The Centre of Medical Law and Ethics, King's College London, is planning "starter packs" for new members of ethics committees and training courses for committees around the country. Consumers for Ethics in Research (CERES) has held public meetings on the advantages and disadvantages of medical research. The Royal College of Obstetricians and Gynaecologists and the British Paediatric Association are drawing up a checklist for ethics committees of questions to ask about proposed research during pregnancy and following birth. Finally, the guidelines which the DoH has produced may serve their purpose and bring ethics committees into line.

CONCLUSION

It may well be the case that the needs ethics committees face will be met by different organizations. However, we should be aware that with the proliferation of individual offers of assistance to ethics committees, the worrying level of diversity that is the principal problem of ethics committees may well remain. Some kind of central organization is therefore advisable, and on balance that of a voluntary association of ethics committees seems to be the best solution at present.

REFERENCES

1. Department of Health (1991) Local Research Ethics Committees
2. Gilbert C, Fulford KWM, Parker C (1989) Diversity in the practice of district ethics committees. Br Med J 299: 1437–1439
3. Royal College of Physicians (1984) Guidelines on the practice of ethics committees in medical research. RCP, London (amended 1990)
4. Royal College of Physicians (1986) Research on healthy volunteers. RCP, London
5. Royal College of Physicians (1984) Research involving patients. RCP, London
6. Royal College of Physicians (1986) The relationship between physicians and the pharmaceutical industry. RCP, London
7. World Medical Association (1964) Declaration of Helsinki: recommendations guiding physicians in biomedical research involving human subjects. WMA, Helsinki (amended Tokyo 1975 and Venice 1983)
8. Association of British Pharmaceutical Industries (1983) Guidelines: clinical trials—compensation for medically induced injury. ABPI, London
9. British Medical Association, Royal College of General Practitioners, and Association of British Pharmaceutical Industries (1983) Code of practice for the clinical assessment of licensed medicinal products in general practice. Br Med J 286: 1295–1297
10. Human Fertilisation and Embryology Authority (1991) Code of Practice. HFEA, London
11. Thompson IE, French K, Melia KM, Boyd KM, Templeton AA, Potter B (1981) Research ethical committees in Scotland. Br Med J 282: 718–720
12. Nicholson RH (ed) (1986) Medical research on children: ethics, law and practice. Oxford Medical Publications
13. Neuberger J (1991) Ethics Committees in the United Kingdom. King's Fund

ABOUT THE AUTHOR

Claire Gilbert Foster, having completed an honours degree in theology at Balliol College, Oxford, has since worked as a research officer at the Ian Ramsey Centre for the study of ethics in science and medicine. Her research has specialized in the function and practice of research ethics committees in Britain. She has also undertaken research on the social responsibility work of the Church of England. She has helped set up the Oxford Practice Skills Course, a project which aims to teach medical students about medical ethics, communication skills and legal issues as an integral part of their clinical course at the Oxford Medical School. She is now a research fellow at the Centre of Medical Law and Ethics, King's College London, working on the research ethics committees project.

8 Research Ethics, Journals and Bioethics*

STEPHEN LOCK

In Britain for the past few years there has been a growing consensus of unease over medical ethics. In part this has reflected the demonstration that the surveillance of the ethical aspects of clinical research is so haphazard, with practice varying enormously throughout the country (see Chapter 7). In part also it is an acknowledgement that at present most medical ethics are retroactive (to use the current jargon), whereas what is also needed is guidance proactively—particularly on the dilemmas raised by the new techniques such as in vitro fertilization, surrogacy, gene therapy and so on. Hence the calls to put things on a more formal basis with some sort of national machinery for both supervision (a medical research ethics committee) and guidance (a medical bioethics committee).

Inevitably the next question to be asked is: one organization or two? My personal preference would be for one—or rather a central body serving two separate functions. Topics will inevitably overlap, the expense should be less with a single secretariat, and with two bodies the public and the media will find it difficult to know which does what (similar to the traditional confusion between the British Medical Association (BMA) and the General Medical Council). Against this is the argument that the central research ethics committee will contain predominantly medical and nursing members and be concerned with training and monitoring, while the national bioethics committee will probably have fewer than half its members from these two professions and include representatives from other disciplines such as philosophy, theology, law, social sciences and public affairs. In any case, I suspect that, given that creating a supervisory agency is agreed to be urgent and is the easier task of the two, the die has already been cast in favour of creating two separate organizations—while this volume already contains Claire Gilbert Foster's discussion of a central research ethics committee. So here I shall confine myself to a short discussion on the need for a national bioethics committee. But first I have been asked to precede this with a note about the role of

---

*Part of the last section of this chapter is based on an editorial in the *British Medical Journal*, 1990, 300: 1149–1150.

Introducing New Treatments for Cancer: Practical, Ethical and Legal Problems. Edited by C. J. Williams
© 1992 John Wiley & Sons Ltd

journals and the development of modern ethical concepts, given that historically it was in journals that the ideas were thrashed out and that, as one form of the "gatekeepers" of science, they were in a position to disseminate any codes and to enforce them.

Soon after the war the horrific details of the experiments on prisoners in the Nazi concentration camps emerged, and a vigorous debate ensued, in the journals and elsewhere. On the one hand, was the way in which such data had been obtained so repellent that editors should automatically deny publication to any paper based on these, whatever their originality, scientific reliability and clinical importance (the usual criteria for publication)? On the other hand, given that the work had already been done, should not some "good" come of it, and would not scientists learn how *not* to do research in man if the actual details of these programmes were put on record?

Such debates have recurred in the emotionally less fraught context of clinical research with a dubious ethical background—for example, where truly informed consent had not been obtained, still perhaps the most difficult conundrum editors are faced with. But 45 years ago most people felt that there was some sort of absolute bar to publishing the results of research in the concentration camps and it did not appear (though recently, and ironically, it has also been shown that scientifically the work was unsound, its results worthless, and possibly the methods also fraudulent). Thus the principal positive result was the development in 1946 of the Nuremburg Code, which spelt out the three requirements for human experimentation: truly voluntary consent by the subject, previous animal studies to clear the procedure of danger, and performance of the research under proper medical supervision.

During the remainder of the 1940s and early 1950s little was published about the ethics of clinical research, though a mounting feeling that decisions could not just be left to individual doctors was typified by debates at bodies such as the Royal Society of Medicine and the publication of a memorandum by the Medical Research Council. The last was described as inconclusive, however, and clearly something more than guidelines was needed. So in the late 1950s two doctors who were not only prominent in editing national journals but also in the then influential World Medical Association started wide discussions about an influential code for human experimentation. Both Hugh Clegg, then editor of the *British Medical Journal* (*BMJ*), and Tapani Kosonen, editor of the *Finnish Medical Journal*, had been disturbed by receiving papers for publication reporting non-therapeutic research on patients who had not been asked for full consent. Not only was there no comprehensive code they could cite to authors in support of their disquiet, but some articles published in other major journals could be criticized even more, given that they were based on research of even less acceptable standards.

The eventual Declaration of Helsinki appeared in 1964 and it is a tribute to Clegg and Kosonen that, with revisions, it is still the basis for theory and practice in this difficult subject. And its acceptance was helped around this time by the appearance of two books documenting some of the abuses and making suggestions for control: *Experimentation in Man* by H. K. Beecher, professor of research in anaesthesia at Harvard University, and *Human Guinea Pigs*, by Maurice Pappworth, a British physician. The response to all this was swift. In the same year, 1964, the MRC issued a statement of general guidance; in 1966 the US Public Health Service stated that it would not support projects unless they had first been reviewed by a committee of fellow professionals; in 1967 the Royal College of Physicians proposed that hospitals should establish informal review boards, and this idea was repeated by the Ministry of Health a year later.

Since then most medical authorities have set up ethics committees and further official guidance and suggestions have been issued from time to time. Nevertheless, compared with the USA, where ethical review is a federal legal requirement, done mostly by institutional review boards, sadly in Britain, where it is voluntary, the evidence has shown a "worrying degree of variation" in the practice of these committees. Hence the call for national standards, set and maintained by a national research ethics committee—a topic further discussed by Claire Gilbert Foster in the preceding chapter. So I will now turn to emphasizing the valuable role of medical journals in the evolution of thinking on this subject.

ROLE OF MEDICAL JOURNALS

Journals have been said to have four main functions: informing, instructing, commenting, and miscellaneous. Information is mostly the province of the original articles and news, and instruction that of the editorials and other didactic articles; comment may be either external, as letters to the editor in the correspondence column, or editorial, in leading articles; and miscellaneous includes news, medical politics, hypothesis, personal views, reviews of books and media programmes. In the past 40 years, moreover, the realization has grown up that the medical professions can no longer stand alone and that their interaction with society is something that concerns us all. Thus the miscellaneous function of medical journals has become increasingly important.

A good example of the part a journal can play arose out of the discussions on the definition of brain death. This was triggered by a television programme entitled "Are the patients really dead?" The programme was inaccurate; so are many programmes and surely the details could be put right in a review? Indeed they could, and were, in the *BMJ*'s Medicine and the Media column—but there was much more to it than that. Brain death is an exceptionally difficult concept, understood at the time of the programme by only a few specialists. Hence not only did the concept have to be explained to the public—who also had to be reassured, given that otherwise their vital co-operation in the transplant programme would have been lost—but its whole basis had to be got over to most doctors as well. Thus there were editorial discussions of principles, practice and ethics, and eventually a whole series of medical practice articles, *ABC of Brain Death*; the correspondence columns enabled professionals who felt that their patch had been trampled over to let off steam about the media, and for those in the media to debate the dilemma of balancing public interest against unjustified alarm.

Many of us concerned in the brain death debate over-reacted but in the end I think good came out of it, not least in the general message that doctors and other professionals have to take the public with them. And the same message applies to the more general recent ethical debates, particularly that of randomization in clinical trials such as multivitamins in pregnancy to prevent spina bifida or adjuvant chemotherapy after mastectomy. Such questions can be answered only after public debate, however tedious and inconvenient this may seem to the professionals at the time. To be sure, editors can do a lot. Self-evidently they have to be vigilant in checking that articles submitted for publication discuss the ethical implications besides recording that the clinical research has been approved by research ethics committee. But is the latter sufficient, particularly since some committees are much more lenient than others? Should the editor take it on himself, with or without expert help, to challenge an ethics committee's fiat? And if, as many might agree, the answer is yes, does this merely cover the obviously risky procedures, or a relative lack of explanation, or does it extend to the clinical details or the design of the study? (Some have contended, for instance, that a study that has inadequate statistical power to show a difference at its conclusion is unethical and should be rejected for publication.)

My own view is that the dilemma resembles that currently seen with medical misconduct. The editor has a responsibility to try to put things right in the first place (by expert peer review and so on) and to put the record straight if he has inadvertently published fraudulent work. But, lacking the detailed knowledge and the resources he is not a policeman; that is the role of the author's institution and the primary responsibility lies with the dean or similar official. Similarly the editor can make reasonable checks that work described in a paper has received ethical approval, but the prime details of this must rest with the local ethics committee. What is worrying is that so many of these have adopted a relaxed attitude, which is why we need a national committee not only to train and monitor standards but also to debate new and difficult issues and issue guidance about them.

NEW BIOETHICAL DILEMMAS

In some ways public anxieties about new developments in medical scientific research mirror those of 40 years ago about clinical research. There seems to be a feeling that the medical scientists' capacity to tread new paths has outstripped their ability to take account of all of their implications—and, anyway, even if an individual limits his own activities on ethical grounds, in the mad scramble for priority of achievement another scientist will not. Such debates have occurred over organ transplants in practice and over gene therapy in theory, but particularly over the issues raised by the new reproductive technology: in vitro fertilization, surrogacy and embryo research.

Several countries have a single body to which existing bioethical problems can be referred for assessement, and which can anticipate new ones. In 1988 Australia established a National Bioethics Consultative Council, with the aim of achieving a national uniform approach. It provides advice and undertakes studies on major new developments. Similarly, despite initial political difficulties in getting it established, there is now a flourishing National Ethics Council in Denmark, which is currently dealing with embryo research, preimplantation diagnosis, and gene therapy. Nevertheless, the most conspicuously successful of these bodies, the President's Commission in the USA, was discontinued by President Reagan; between 1980 and 1983 it had published ten high-quality reports, including those on stopping life-sustaining treatment and protecting human subjects of research. France has had a national bioethics committee since 1983, whose activity has been based on developing new statutes rather than codes of practice; given this philosophy and the large size of the committee (37 members, some representing various interests), not surprisingly progress has been limited. The same seems likely to be true for the Italian National Bioethics Committee, established in 1990, which has no fewer than 40 members, appointed to balance various political interests.

So far Britain has referred difficult and contentious issues piecemeal and as they arise to various bodies not primarily concerned with ethical matters, such as the Department of Health, the MRC, the medical royal colleges and the British Medical Association.

It has set up ad hoc committees to consider individual problems that could be ignored no longer—for example, the interim licensing authority on in vitro fertilization. And it has also consulted special interest groups including the pharmaceutical industry, religious bodies and consumer organizations. But Britain has lacked a national body to keep the issues under review and it was left to the MRC and the Royal College of Obstetricians and Gynaecologists to set up the interim licensing authority on in vitro fertilization.

The need to establish a national bioethics committee in Britain was first discussed in depth in 1989, by both the Ciba Foundation and Gresham College. But the major impetus came from a weekend meeting at Cumberland Lodge in April 1990 organized by the Nuffield Foundation, attended by experts in the disciplines—lawyers, theologians and philosophers, as well as doctors, including three peers, seven knights, five heads of Oxbridge colleges, and five Fellows of the Royal Society. There was substantial agreement about the need for a new committee and what shape it should take, and a consultation document was circulated widely.

The consultation document cites five arguments in favour of the committee: the need for a body to survey the whole field of bioethics; the need for anticipating or rapidly responding to new problems; the need for a national UK voice to play a greater part in European discussions; the need to coordinate discussions within Britain; and the need to highlight the issues in the public mind. The principal task of the committee would be guidance, rather than regulation, at least initially, as well as educating public opinion. So it would work by commissioning studies directly, a good example of an initial and imminent one being the problems raised by genetic screening. The committee would contain no fewer than 12 and preferably no more than 15 members, chosen for their individual qualities rather than as representatives, while a majority should be "lay"—that is, neither professional scientists nor clinicians—as should the chairman (who might well be an eminent lawyer). The authority of the new body, it is intended, will indeed arise out of the quality of its membership, the value of the work done, and its independent character.

However the details change as a result of the consultations and the initial experience, a priority will be to participate in the current European discussions. As I write, many of these are going on: a resolution has been passed recently about the need for a "Convention for the protection of the human person with regard to biomedical science", an ethics committee (described as "unnecessarily unsatisfactory") has been set up for the EC human genome and there is the likelihood of a similar committee for embryology. All these will assume particular importance in 1993, given that Britain will not then be able to opt out of European legislation. So I hope that our government will see the wisdom not only of supporting the idea of such a committee, but also of contributing to its funding and running costs while allowing it to remain independent.

NOTE ADDED IN PROOF

The rapidity of change in this topic is shown by two announcements in the summer of 1991, since this article was written. Firstly, the Nuffield Foundation has announced the formation of the Nuffield Council on Bioethics, whose remit will be largely on the lines discussed at the Cumberland Lodge conference. Secondly, the Department of Health has produced "Local Research Ethics Committees", a booklet giving advice on establishing these, the principles they should follow, and special considerations concerning particular groups. As always in the subject, doubts can be raised about both of these. My personal ones about the former include its composition, drawn principally from the "good and the great", and the highish average age of its members, which might give active research workers the impression that this body might find it difficult appreciating their day-to-day problems. The Department of Health document, which is still interim, goes a little further in its recommendations on detail—such as of the composition of the committee, its working procedures, keeping a register, and follow-up, but still ignores the central problem of ensuring uniform standards across the country.

ABOUT THE AUTHOR

Dr Stephen P. Lock was editor of the *British Medical Journal* (*BMJ*) from 1975 to 1991; he is now a senior associate fellow at the Research Unit of the Royal College of Physicians. Trained as a haematologist, he served on the staffs of London teaching hospitals before being appointed assistant editor of the *BMJ* in 1964. He became deputy editor in 1974. He was medical correspondent to the BBC Overseas Services from 1966 to 1974. Dr Lock's special interest is medical writing and biomedical communication, including evaluating scientific information, the role of peer review, the editing process, and the impact of new information technology. He has taught many courses in medical writing in Britain, Finland, Iraq, Kuwait, Canada and Australia. He is a founder and member of the International Committee of Medical Journal Editors (the Vancouver Group) and immediate past president of the European Association of Science Editors. His books include *Better Medical Writing*, the *Medical Risks of Life*, and *A Difficult Balance: Editorial Peer Review in Medicine*. Dr Lock is a graduate of Queens' College, Cambridge University, and the Medical College of St Bartholomew's Hospital. He has received many international honours, among them the Donders Medal (*Netherlands Journal of Medicine*), and the International Medal (Finnish Medical Society). He is an Honorary Fellow of the Royal College of Physicians of Ireland and Edinburgh, and an Honorary Fellow of the American College of Physicians. In 1991 the honour of the CBE was conferred upon him.

Section II

CLINICAL TRIALS

Notes on Section II

This section is mainly concerned with the nuts and bolts of carrying out clinical trials to test new anticancer treatments. There is inevitably, however, a considerable overlap with other sections. **Charles Stiller** (Chapter 9) reviews extensively data on the influence of inclusion of patients into clinical trials on treatment outcome. One possible perception on the part of patients and clinicians is that inclusion in a trial will restrict normal choice of best treatment and may result in worse care and poorer survival. This hypothesis presupposes that the clinician already *knows* what the best therapies are—a doubtful proposition at best. As a corollary to this question Charles Stiller also asks whether referral to a specialist centre improves outcome. Clearly, categorical answers to these two questions are impossible since there is considerable bias both in those selected to be included in clinical trials and for referral to specialist centres.

Because the data are largely anecdotal and rely on numerous single reports, this is one of the chapters that has much data in tabular form and which has been heavily referenced. His overall conclusion is that there is no evidence that patients included in clinical trials do worse than those treated outside of trials. Indeed, the reverse seems true. Similarly, treatment in a specialist centre is not associated with a worse outcome and there is some data to suggest that the outlook is improved. The encouraging message, for patients and clinical researchers, of this chapter is that inclusion in a clinical trial may be beneficial and is certainly not to the disadvantage of patients.

Much of current chemotherapy has been based on empirical principles. Drugs have usually been selected from screening systems and are tested in phase I and II studies (see below) in an uncritical manner. Dose is frequently based on surface area and schedules have paid no attention to pharmacokinetics. This has been allowed to happen for pragmatic reasons. There is a real need for new drugs in what is a group of rapidly fatal diseases. For this reason regulatory authorities have accepted a "lower standard" of data for drug approval than would be necessary for instance in the case of a new anti-arthritis drug—see Notes on Section III.

Phase I and II studies are already difficult enough to perform (see Chapters 10 and 11) using a simple dose escalation scheme based on surface area.

Introducing New Treatments for Cancer: Practical, Ethical and Legal Problems. Edited by C. J. Williams
© 1992 John Wiley & Sons Ltd

The introduction of complex pharmacological studies and development of dosing schedules based on these has been considered too cumbersome. However, there is reason to think that we are not using current drugs in an optimum fashion and that future drug development may be substandard if we continue in our current crude fashion. Most new non-anticancer drugs are tested initially (phase I) in human volunteers. However, cytotoxic drugs cannot be used in such a population since they usually have severe short and long-term side-effects. The patients that are included in these initial trials (see **George Blackledge and Frank Lawton**, Chapter 10) are often dying of their cancer and extensive pharmacological studies may be inappropriate because they become an additional burden to the patient. Data gained in such patients may also be less than reliable because they often have a variety of systems failure, making interpretation difficult. Despite these difficulties, a strong case can be made for considering a more systematic approach to ascertaining the most favourable dose and schedule of new (and old) drugs.

George Blackledge and Frank Lawton discuss some of the problems in identifying new drugs that might be useful in human cancers and the first steps in their clinical use. At present we have had to rely on in vitro and animal tumour models to select drugs likely to be active in human cancer. These, however, suffer from all manner of problems and are clearly inadequate for the task. The catch-22 that we are caught in is that new models are validated by testing known active drugs (identified by old tumour models) to see if they are recognized as useful by the new system. This process of course tends to only select new models that are similar to the old ones! What we need are models that detect active drugs, especially in solid tumours, that old models failed to detect—an open-ended research commitment that may be too risky and expensive. One alternative currently being tested by the National Cancer Institute is the use of human tumours in in vitro systems and in immune-suppressed animals.

Blackledge and Lawton go on to stress the problem of selection of suitable patients for phase I and II studies. It is clear that these are of paramount importance and that active drugs may be rejected by only testing them in very sick patients who have failed extensive pretreatment. For instance, 5-fluorouracil (an antimetabolite) was originally extensively tested in colon cancer: response rates varied from 0 to 89% depending on the trial. The true response rate is 20–25%, demonstrating how patient selection can give a false impression of drug activity.

It has been suggested that phase II studies can be done in patients who are receiving their first chemotherapy treatment provided that such treatment is essentially palliative in nature. For instance, there are a couple of trials of this type in breast cancer and extensive small-cell lung cancer: tumours which are often responsive to chemotherapy but where few if any patients are cured. Such patients could be treated initially with a phase II agent, being switched to standard therapy only on failure to respond or on relapse.

However, this radical approach *needs* to be verified by a controlled trial. Ideally, such a trial should randomize patients to the new drug followed by standard treatment on disease progression, or to standard therapy followed by the phase II drug on progression. As well as survival, symptom control and quality of life should be measured. Only if such studies show no detriment to patients receiving initial treatment with phase II drugs is it likely that new drugs will be tested in this way in previously untreated patients. Clearly such a trial has major ethical implications and would only be feasible in tumour types where there was *uncertainty* about whether delaying standard therapy was a bad thing to do (see Chapter 12 by Sally Stenning).

The more general chapter by Blackledge and Lawton is followed by an in-depth analysis of phase I trials of anticancer chemotherapy (**Eduard Holdener** and his colleagues, Chapter 11). It is reassuring to see that the rate of deaths attributable to the new drugs being tested was very low. However, despite *some* objective tumour responses there is no evidence that patients feel physically better or live longer because of the treatment. This point is underlined by Victor Tunkel (Chapter 2) in his discussion of whether this type of clinical research is non-therapeutic in nature. His legal and ethical standpoint on this is made clear in his chapter.

As discussed in subsequent chapters (**Sally Stenning**, Chapter 12; **Bob Souhami**, Chapter 13), there has been a major failure to realize that large numbers of patients are required in phase III studies designed to identify optimal treatment. Rather, we have concentrated on complex and restrictive treatment protocols together with extensive data collection. Such studies may be fine in single institutions, when the question is appropriate, but just do not work well in the sort of large-scale trials we now need. One of the problems in defining appropriate questions is the inability of clinicians to agree on the detail of the protocol. Thus in discussions on possible Medical Research Council trials in early ovarian cancer it was quickly obvious that surgeons had different opinions on what constituted optimal staging and surgical resection, pathologists could not agree on classification and grading, whilst oncologists wanted to vary the chemotherapy. However, all basically wanted to ask the same question because there was genuine *uncertainty* over the best treatment for some patients with early resected ovarian cancer. A pragmatic trial based on the "uncertainty principle" was therefore proposed (Chapter 12)—instead of clearly defining which patients were eligible for the trial, the clinician was asked to decide based on his own experience. Thus patients he was sure would not benefit from chemotherapy and those he was sure would benefit from such treatment were excluded: only those patients where he was *uncertain* whether such treatment was indicated were eligible for inclusion in the trial. They were randomized to immediate chemotherapy or chemotherapy delayed to disease progression.

Such a device can increase accrual by attracting clinicians who might not agree with the requirements of a restrictive protocol. In addition, it is ethically sound since each patient is dealt with by his physician as an individual and is only considered for the trial if the clinician has uncertainty about which approach is best. It is hoped that this principle of uncertainty will aid in the development of true large-scale studies.

These types of trials are the basis of Chapter 13, by Bob Souhami. In this he puts forward the hypothesis that chemosensitivity is a property of tumours and not of drugs and comments on the difficulty of developing suitable tumour models (see above). Souhami underlines the relative insensitivity of the majority of cancers to cytotoxic chemotherapy and the fact that new therapies are, at best, only going to improve survival modestly. If accepted (and there is at present no real argument against this conclusion), this leads to a number of important factors which must be taken into account when planning new trials.

So far there have been remarkably few attempts to ascertain what differences in treatment outcome are important to the patient and clinician (see Chapters 30 and 31). If treatment is essentially palliative improvement in outcome must be balanced against the toxicity and practicability of the treatment. If outcome differences are likely to be small, very large numbers are needed in trials if we are to come to firm conclusions about optimal treatment. Bob Souhami argues cogently for a pragmatic approach to such trials. Based on the uncertainty principle they should be free from rigid restrictions and should cause minimal extra work or upset to the clinician and patient. Only in this way can we attract the 95% of cancer patients who currently are treated outside of clinical trials. One criticism of such an approach is that it dilutes the "good" results achievable in expert centres. However, few such centres seem to be able to mount studies capable of answering important questions. Though it is feasible that a "loose" protocol used by many clinicians may result in less good results than those of a single institution, it seems highly likely that the difference will be a simple decrease in the differences between two treatments—the effect is quantitative and not qualitative (Chapter 12). Thus a trial showing a small (say 5–10%) difference is still likely to give a statistically significant result if the trial is very large—a result that is also significant to the community in that the data are from multiple doctors looking after a wide variety of patients and not a single institution caring for a carefully selected group of patients using a very strict treatment protocol. In other words, large-scale studies mirror the "real world".

The scope of such an enterprise is underlined by Bob Souhami's discussion of the need for national and international trials. Such large-scale collaboration is possible, as witnessed by the success of the ISIS studies in coronary artery disease, which has accrued tens of thousands of patients. If more detailed information on, say, quality of life is needed in such large studies this may be gathered by those with a special interest in this area or, if all clinicians agree, from a random sample of all patients randomized.

As has been discussed in Section I informed consent for clinical trials has been a necessary but problematic area for clinicians engaged in research on patients. **Max Parmar** (Chapter 14) tackles the suggestion first put forward by Zelen that randomization into a trial can take place *before* discussion of the trial with the patient. In this way the patient, knowing which treatment they *would* receive in this trial, may find it easier to make their mind up as to whether they wish to be included. However, as Parmar points out this has the disadvantage that some will refuse inclusion in the trial which results in the need for more patients in the study. Since the whole point of the device is to increase the number of patients accepting inclusion in the trial the crux of pre-randomization consent is whether the extra number of patients accepting the study exceeds the number of extra patients required because randomized patients have selected treatments other than that to which they were randomized in the trial. Parmar demonstrates that trials to present have been very mixed in this regard—some showing a real benefit by the extra patients accrued whilst in others the approach was counter-productive. In my own mind the double-consent randomization method discussed is much preferable to the single-consent design where patients receiving *standard* therapy are not told of the trial—a potentially dubious practice ethically. At present there seems no way of knowing whether this device (double-consent post-randomization) will yield the sought-after result or could be counter-productive in an individual proposed trial.

The ethical need to avoid continuing randomized trials in which treatments are detrimental to patients or when the new treatment is quickly found to be superior to standard therapy has led to the development of "stopping rules". **David Machin** (Chapter 15) reviews current thinking in this difficult area. Integral to this problem is the influence of interim analyses—frequent examination of data from randomized trials increases the chance that, due to normal fluctuations in results, a statistically significant difference will be seen. Because of this a variety of methods of handling interim analysis and more importantly sequential interim analysis have been developed. In general these have been conservative in their outlook, demanding a high degree of statistical significance, in order to avoid early discontinuation of a study. Clearly, if a treatment has excessive morbidity or mortality early stopping is scientifically and ethically justified. However, the situation is more complicated if the investigator thinks that there may be *some* benefit from the new treatment. Early stopping may result in a situation where there appears to be benefit from the treatment, but because the numbers entered in to the study are low problems arise. Since more events will occur after stopping the trial the degree of advantage may fall back and become non-significant statistically (even though there is a *true* advantage to the new treatment). Just as worrying, the final result may continue to show a significant advantage to the new therapy but because of low numbers the confidence limits are wide; for example, the treatment may show a 12% improvement in five-year survival with confidence limits of 2% to 25%. In this situation clinical judgment as to whether to apply the treatment is greatly open to previous prejudice—believers anticipating a worthwhile advantage approaching 25% and nihilists expecting a worthless difference of a few per cent. To a certain extent this is what has happened to the CALGB study in non-small-cell lung cancer discussed by Machin. This trial, which was stopped early because of significantly better survival in the new treatment group, has remained controversial—even those accepting the results have been heard to say in the same sentence that a confirmatory trial is necessary. If the original trial was large enough this would not be necessary; although by stopping early the trialists will have ensured that, if the results are right, the number of patients in the trial denied useful treatment is minimal, they will have less of an impact on the medical community as a whole. As a result more patients may be accrued into the control arm (with poorer results) of a second trial and fewer patients in the general community will be given the new treatment because some clinicians remain unconvinced. Thus, the outcome of early stopping may be very ethical for the study itself, but produces an overall situation where there is detriment to patients in further trials and in the community. Should the ethics only consider potential patients in a particular trial or the ethics of the result for the community at large? If the second option is accepted then trials should only be stopped early if the results are so clear cut that there are narrow confidence limits.

Graham Thorpe in Chapter 16 discusses an often neglected topic: experiments on the dying. This crosses over to a certain extent with Chapters 10 and 11 on phase I and II studies. However, only one or two per cent of such patients enter studies, leaving 98% or so of dying patients not being entered into studies.

Too little cancer research has been devoted to developing better ways of helping dying cancer patients; nearly all the effort has been directed at eradicating or controlling the tumour, often with little success. As Thorpe discusses, those working primarily with dying patients have been partly to blame as they have avoided research. He makes a strong case for including the patient and their family in the decision as to whether or not to join in a trial of palliative care. To date carers have often been paternalistic; although this may be appropriate for some very sick or distressed patients there must be many of the 130 000 patients who die of cancer in Britain each year who would be willing to help with research into better care. As Thorpe points out such trials will often need to include multiple centres; this will require those caring for dying patients to trust other centres, something which the present protective attitude has not always fostered.

9 Survival of Patients in Clinical Trials and at Specialist Centres

CHARLES STILLER

Cancer is a major cause of death in industrialized countries. In 1987 in England and Wales, for example, 16% of all deaths among persons aged 1–34 and 38% among those aged 35–64 had a malignant neoplasm as the underlying cause. Nevertheless, there have been many advances in treatment resulting in substantial improvements in survival rates. It is common knowledge that patients with different types of cancer have not shared equally in these advances. Within a given diagnostic group factors such as the age of the patient and the stage of the disease can be important determinants of prognosis. Other factors which are not characteristics of the patient or tumour may, however, also affect the probability of survival. In particular, there has been a continuing debate over the roles of entry to clinical trials, use of standardized treatment protocols and referral to specialist treatment centres. These interrelated topics were, for example, briefly surveyed in a recent editorial in the *British Medical Journal* [1]. The purpose of this chapter is to review and discuss the evidence in greater detail. Much of the research hitherto has been in relation to relatively rare cancers which occur mainly in children. This review will therefore be weighted towards childhood cancers, but the comparatively small amount of published material on adult cancers will also be considered.

SOURCES OF LITERATURE REVIEW

The issues reviewed in this chapter have been considered in a series of studies using data from the population-based National Registry of Childhood Tumours (NRCT), which covers the whole of Great Britain and is maintained at the Childhood Cancer Research Group (CCRG). Reports on other studies were drawn from the comprehensive collection of publications on childhood cancer epidemiology at the CCRG. It is extremely unlikely that any important, relevant publications relating to childhood cancer have been missed. For adult cancers, the principal English language general medical and oncological journals were searched for references to population-based cancer survival rates and accrual to clinical trials for at least the past decade. Publications from these sources, and other publications to which they

Introducing New Treatments for Cancer: Practical, Ethical and Legal Problems. Edited by C. J. Williams
© 1992 John Wiley & Sons Ltd

referred, were supplemented by other reports known to colleagues. It is possible that some reports may have been missed, but it seems very likely that the most substantial studies have all been included. Table 1 gives details of all the publications known to me which contain original data on survival of cancer patients related to inclusion in clinical trials, treatment at specialist centres and other measures of clinical experience such as numbers of patients treated at particular hospitals.

It is well known that the survival rates reported from clinical trials or from case series at single hospitals are often higher than those obtained from population-based series, and in many instances the difference might be at least partly accounted for by a tendency for more patients with favourable prognostic features to be treated in trials or at specialist centres. This possible bias can be allowed for in comparative studies of the type discussed here by taking into account major prognostic factors such as age and primary site in the statistical analyses. For acute lymphoblastic leukaemia (ALL), the white cell count is an important prognostic factor on which data are often available. For many solid tumours, stage is of overriding prognostic importance though this is hard to allow for without very detailed data, since investigations may well have differed between trial and non-trial patients and between those treated at different types of hospital. Greater weight should generally be attached to those studies where efforts have been made to reduce the effect of biased inclusion in trials or referral to major centres by allowing for other prognostic factors, as indicated in the following review.

CHILDHOOD LEUKAEMIA

Some of the earliest evidence is from a study by the Medical Research Council (MRC) Working Party on Leukaemia in Childhood of children with acute leukaemia diagnosed during 1963–1967 in England and Wales [2]. At this time the survival rate was extremely low. For ALL, which accounts for about one-quarter of all childhood cancers in Britain, the five-year survival rate nationally was under 5%, compared with an actuarial rate of 70% for children diagnosed during 1983–1985. Nevertheless, the development of effective chemotherapy had begun and this resulted in the start of the trend towards higher survival rates that has taken place over the past quarter of a century. In this study, children were ascertained from cancer registries, resulting in a population-based series which was felt to be nearly complete. The patients were divided into two groups: the "study group" who had been treated from the time of diagnosis by specialists associated with the Working Party, and those who received initial treatment elsewhere. Since age is an important prognostic factor in ALL the results were analysed for three age groups. In all three groups the children in the study group had substantially longer survival times; among children aged 2–8 years, who had the best prognosis,

Table 1. Published studies of survival of cancer patients in relation to inclusion in clinical trials, treatment at specialist centres and other measures of clinical experience

Ref.	Years of diagnosis	Location	No. of patients	Diagnostic groups	Factors studied
1. Childhood leukaemia					
[2]	1963–7	England and Wales	879	ALL	Specialist centres; trial protocol
[8]	1971	South-east England	75	All leukaemia	Specialist centres
[3]	1954–68	Manchester region, England	461	Acute leukaemia	Specialist centres
[11]	1971–4	FRG (patients on standard protocols only)	530	ALL	Number of patients per hospital
[10]	1970–5	Greater Delaware Valley, USA	327	ALL	Specialist centres; national protocol
[12]	1980–5	FRG	1 655	ALL	Inclusion in national trials
			321	AML	
[7]	1968–82	Northern region, England	306	ALL	Specialist centres
			67	AML	
[14]	1977–84	Great Britain	389	ANLL	Specialist centres
[5]	1971–84	Great Britain	4 697	ALL	Inclusion in national trials; number of patients per hospital
2. Other childhood cancers					
[15]	1962–8	Great Britain	268	Retinoblastoma	Specialist centres
[16]	1969–80	Great Britain	431	Retinoblastoma	Specialist centres
[20]	1950–72	New York, USA	127	Wilms' tumour	Specialist centres
[17]	1970–3	Great Britain	313	Wilms' tumour	Inclusion in national trials; Specialist centres
[22]	1968–79	Connecticut, USA	278	Brain tumours	Specialist centres
[18]	1971–7	Great Britain	368	Medulloblastoma	Number of patients per hospital

(continued)

Table 1. (continued)

Ref.	Years of diagnosis	Location	No. of patients	Diagnostic groups	Factors studied
[21]	1970–9	Greater Delaware Valley, USA	147	Wilms' tumour	Specialist centres
			76	Medulloblastoma	
			87	Rhabdomyosarcoma	
[12]	1980–5	FRG	313	Hodgkin's disease	Inclusion in national trials
			347	NHL	
			399	Neuroblastoma	
			361	Wilms' tumour	
			181	Medulloblastoma	
			182	Osteosarcoma	
			157	Ewing's sarcoma	
			380	Soft-tissue sarcoma	
			190	Germ-cell tumours	
[7]	1968–82	Northern region, England	47	Hodgkin's disease	Specialist centres
			63	NHL	
			213	Brain tumours (five subgroups)	
			38	Osteosarcoma	
[14]	1977–84	Great Britain	435	Hodgkin's disease	Specialist centres
			497	NHL	
			486	Neuroblastoma	
			483	Wilms' tumour	
			240	Osteosarcoma	
			234	Ewing's sarcoma	
			351	Rhabdomyosarcoma	
[23]	1980–7	FRG	210	Osteosarcoma	Inclusion in national trials

123

3. Adult cancers

Ref.	Years	Location	Cancer type	Number	Factor
[29]	1976–81	USA (patients in ECOG studies)	Breast	772	Type of hospital
			Gastrointestinal	1440	
			Head and neck	528	
			Myeloma	148	
			Lymphoma	610	
			Leukaemia	262	
			Lung	916	
			Melanoma	346	
			Gynaecological and genitourinary	690	
[32]	1957–76	West Midlands region, England	Oesophageal carcinoma	1089	Number of patients per surgeon
[31]	1963–82	South Thames regions, England	Osteosarcoma	407	Type of hospital
[27]	1980–5	Ireland	Testicular germ-cell tumours	246	Standard protocols; speciality of clinicians
[28]	1979–85	Finland	Multiple myeloma	1978	Entry to clinical trials
[30]	1970–81	Finland	Breast cancer	16 678	Specialist centres
			Prostate carcinoma	9 105	

Abbreviations: ALL, acute lymphoblastic leukaemia; AML, acute myeloid leukaemia; ANLL, acute non-lymphoblastic leukaemia; ECOG, Eastern Co-operative Oncology Group; NHL, non-Hodgkin's lymphoma.

the median survival time for the study group (72 weeks) was double that for others (36 weeks). The authors found no significant difference in survival between children treated in accordance with MRC trial protocols and those treated according to other regimens, and concluded that the improved survival rate for study group patients was due to the availability of special facilities and expertise. In a study of children in the Manchester region diagnosed during 1954–1968 those who were treated in large paediatric hospitals survived significantly longer, but the analysis did not distinguish between ALL and other types of leukaemia [3].

Since 1970, large numbers of children have been entered in the MRC United Kingdom Acute Lymphoblastic Leukaemia (UKALL) trials [4]. During 1971–1984 there were 4697 children treated for ALL and included in the population-based National Registry of Childhood Tumours (NRCT). In 1971–1973, 52% of children with ALL were treated at centres with at least six new patients per year, and the proportion had risen to 66% by 1980–1984 [5]. The increase in the proportion entered in the MRC trials over the same period, from 46% to 51%, is less impressive but in the early 1980s large numbers of children were also treated according to pilot protocols for future trials or in a locally organized trial at one very large centre. By the mid-1970s virtually all children were treated according to standardized protocols. Nevertheless, the survival rates for children in the NRCT who were actually included in the trials were consistently significantly higher than those for non-trial children, though survival improved for both groups [5]. Five-year survival rates were 51% for trial patients and 26% for those not in the trials among children diagnosed in 1971–1973. These rates increased to 72% and 64% respectively during 1980–1984. Survival rates overall were highest at the 12 major centres treating an average of at least six new patients per year. For children in the trials, there was no difference in survival between centres with different numbers of patients but among non-trial children there was a marked pattern of higher rates at centres with large numbers of patients. Age at diagnosis and white cell count—two important prognostic factors— were allowed for in all these analyses. The effects of inclusion in trials and size of treatment centre remained significant when children dying within three months of diagnosis were excluded, and thus it is unlikely that the difference in survival rates can be explained by more frequent failure to achieve. remission outside the trials or at minor centres. Although the 12 centres with the largest numbers of patients collectively had the highest survival rates, there was considerable variation between individual centres in this group. Some of this variation was probably due to random differences in the proportions of children with good prognostic features at individual centres. By far the highest survival rates—64% at five years and 60% (actuarial) at ten years from diagnosis during 1970–1981 com- pared with 47% and 39% nationally—were achieved, however, at one centre where there was believed to be an unusually high degree of emphasis on strict adherence to the treatment protocol for this period in Britain [6].

A study in northern England also showed higher survival rates for children treated at specialist centres [7]; children at specialist centres and other hospitals had similar distributions of age and white cell count. A similar result was found in south-east England by McCarthy [8] but in this very small study no account was taken of other prognostic factors. Neither study examined the effect of inclusion in trials. The great majority of the children in these two series would also have been in the much larger NRCT study.

A broadly similar pattern has been observed in other countries. In a series of 101 children with ALL diagnosed in 1972 in five population-based registries in the USA, 27% were treated at hospitals participating in multicentre trials but the great majority were treated using accepted treatment regimens [9]. In a study of 327 children in the Greater Delaware Valley Pediatric Tumor Registry during 1970–1975, patients who were treated according to a standardized protocol had a four-year survival rate of 60% compared with 19% for those who were not so treated [10]. Children in this study who were treated at specialist paediatric cancer centres had a significantly higher survival rate than those treated at other hospitals. At both types of hospital, children treated on protocols had a markedly higher survival rate, but at the cancer centres there were few non-protocol patients and they tended to have an unusual clinical presentation with a poor prognosis. Among children treated on protocols, there was relatively little difference in survival between categories of hospital. The effects observed in this study were particularly marked for children with a low white cell count or who were aged 1–9 years—both favourable prognostic features.

In a series of 530 children treated according to one of two standard protocols in the German Federal Republic during 1971–1974 there was no difference in survival rate between children at centres with more than six patients per year and those with six or fewer [11]. The two groups had similar distributions for the principal prognostic features. In the same country during the early 1980s children with ALL who were not included in trials had a lower survival rate but this group may well have been biased towards patients with unfavourable prognostic features, since 91% of all children were in the trials [12]. Degree of adherence to protocol was examined in a study of 212 patients treated according to standardized regimens at the Hospital for Sick Children, Toronto, during 1976–1981 [13]; children who relapsed had received significantly less methotrexate than those who did not during the first and second years of continuing therapy.

There are fewer relevant data on the other, rarer childhood leukaemias. In Britain during 1977–1984, children with acute non-lymphoblastic leukaemia who were treated at paediatric oncology centres and other teaching hospitals had a three-year survival rate of over 25%—significantly higher than the rate of under 10% for those who were treated elsewhere;

age at diagnosis was allowed for in this analysis [14]. There was no significant difference in survival between major centres and other hospitals for children with acute myeloid leukaemia (AML) in the northern region of England treated during 1968–1982 but this series included only 67 patients [7]. In the German Federal Republic during 1980–1985, children with AML who were in trials had an actuarial three-year survival rate of 55%, compared with 28% for non-trial children [12]. Other prognostic factors were not allowed for in the analysis of the effects of type of hospital or inclusion in trials in either of these latter studies.

OTHER CHILDHOOD CANCERS

Similar studies have been conducted for a range of other childhood cancers. Retinoblastoma has for many years had an excellent prognosis, with a long-term survival rate of over 80% in the early 1960s. Two population-based studies have been published based on NRCT data for 1962–1968 [15] and 1969–1980 [16]. About 40% of British children with retinoblastoma are treated at two hospitals in London—one of them a specialist eye hospital—which together act as a national referral centre. Some children are treated at other specialist eye hospitals and the remainder at other, non-specialist hospitals. Survival rates were analysed allowing for the prognostic factors of tumour laterality and stage. In both study periods there was a significant trend towards higher survival rates at the national centre, lower rates at other eye hospitals and the lowest rates elsewhere.

For no childhood cancer other than retinoblastoma has a single centre come to treat such a high proportion of all patients. There has, however, been a continuing trend towards more centralized care and this has been accompanied by increased participation in multicentre clinical trials and studies.

The earliest British national trial for a paediatric solid tumour was the first MRC trial for Wilms' tumour (nephroblastoma), in which patients were entered from 1970 to 1974. An analysis of NRCT data for this period showed that from the start of the trial until the end of 1973, 57% of eligible children were included in the trial [17]. Survival rates were higher for children in the trial than for those who were eligible but not included—a highly significant difference when age and stage were allowed for. Survival rates were also higher for patients who had surgery at specialist teaching or children's hospitals, but there was no relationship between survival and the number of children treated at a radiotherapy centre.

Data from the NRCT have also been analysed for children with medullo-blastoma diagnosed during 1971–1977 [18]. There was no variation in survival rates between neurosurgical centres or between radiotherapy centres when these hospitals were classified according to the number of children treated for this tumour.

Data are not available on trends in centralization of treatment or entry to trials for other childhood cancers before 1977. In that year, the United Kingdom Children's Cancer Study Group (UKCCSG) was formed by a number of consultants specializing in paediatric oncology. Since then, membership of the UKCCSG has increased until almost every health region in England and Wales contains a paediatric oncology centre whose senior clinical staff are members of the group. There are also three centres in Scotland and one each in Northern Ireland and the Irish Republic. The proportion of children with cancer in Britain who were initially referred to paediatric oncology centres increased from under half in 1977 to around 70% by 1984 [14]. There were, however, substantial regional variations in referral rates. Children aged 12 and over were less likely to be referred to centres. Referral rates also varied widely with diagnostic group: over three-quarters of children with leukaemia and some embryonal tumours were referred to paediatric oncology centres, compared with around one-third of those with brain tumours. Since its formation, the UKCCSG has organized clinical trials and studies for children with Hodgkin's disease, non-Hodgkin's lymphoma (NHL), central nervous system (CNS) tumours, Wilms' tumour, Ewing's sarcoma and malignant germ-cell tumours. Members have also participated in national trials for acute leukaemia and international studies for CNS tumours, neuroblastoma, osteosarcoma and rhabdomyosarcoma. The proportions of all eligible patients included in these trials have not generally been published, but in many instances must be high. The first UKCCSG Wilms' tumour study included 78% of all eligible patients in Britain during 1980–1985 [19].

For seven different solid tumours, three-year survival rates for patients treated at paediatric oncology centres during 1977–1984 have been compared with those at other hospitals [14]. Age at diagnosis was allowed for in these analyses. For non-Hodgkin's lymphoma, Ewing's sarcoma and rhabdo-myosarcoma survival rates were significantly higher at paediatric oncology centres throughout the study period. There was overall a marked improve-ment in survival between 1977–1980 and 1981–1984 for NHL but the rates at other hospitals in the latter period only reached those attained at the paediatric centres four years earlier. Survival rates for children with osteosarcoma were low everywhere during 1977–1980 but in 1981–1984 the rates at paediatric oncology centres increased dramatically whereas there was no sign of improvement elsewhere. There was no significant difference in survival rates between treatment centre types for neuroblastoma but paediatric centres appeared to have a considerably higher proportion of patients with advanced tumours which have a poor prognosis. Survival rates were high everywhere for Hodgkin's disease and Wilms' tumour. During 1980–1982, however, several children with Wilms' tumour treated at other hospitals were apparently overtreated, mostly by receiving more radio-therapy than would have been prescribed had they been included in the UKCCSG clinical studies [19].

Among children in the northern region of England with several types of cancer diagnosed during 1968–1982 no significant effects were found of hospital treatment on survival but the numbers of patients in each diagnostic group were small and other prognostic factors were not allowed for [7].

As with leukaemia, data from the USA for childhood solid tumours present a broadly similar picture. In New York State from 1960 to 1972 children resident in and around Buffalo were more likely to be treated at hospitals which had larger numbers of Wilms' tumour patients, and these children also had a survival rate substantially higher than those from less populous, predominantly rural counties [20]; no other prognostic factors were allowed for. In the Greater Delaware Valley during 1970–1979, children with Wilms' tumour treated at specialist cancer centres and at other hospitals had similar survival rates, but the level of follow-up for late sequelae was better in cancer centres [21]. The Greater Delaware Valley study also investigated children with rhabdomyosarcoma and medulloblastoma. For both of these diagnostic groups cancer centre patients had a significantly higher three-year disease-free survival rate, although the rhabdomyosarcoma patients at cancer centres included a higher proportion with less favourable histology or tumour stage. In Connecticut, children with brain tumours diagnosed between 1968 and 1979 were studied [22]. For medulloblastoma and brain stem glioma, children treated at university cancer centres had higher survival rates, but no variation was found in survival with type of hospital for astrocytoma or ependymoma. No other prognostic factors were studied.

In the German Federal Republic survival rates for children in trials have been compared with those for non-trial children in a range of diagnostic groups using data from the population-based Co-operative Register of Childhood Malig-nancies [12]. Among children with NHL, medulloblastoma, Ewing's sarcoma and malignant germ-cell tumours, survival rates were higher for those included in clinical trials. For medulloblastoma, Wilms' tumour, osteosarcoma and soft-tissue sarcoma (mainly rhabdomyosarcoma), survival rates for trial and non-trial patients were very similar, though more recently published data point to a higher survival rate for children with osteosarcoma who were included in a trial [23]. Although no other comparisons of survival rates have been published for trial and non-trial patients in most of these diagnostic groups, the results should be interpreted with caution as allowance was not made for other prognostic factors and in many cases follow-up was very short.

ADULT CANCERS

Compared with childhood cancer, there is very little published research on the relationship between entry to trials, referral and survival for adult cancers, despite the fact that over 99% of cancer patients in developed countries are adults.

Much of what has been published relates to testicular germ-cell tumours. The prognosis for these tumours is now generally very good, largely thanks to advances in chemotherapy. One stage of the continuing debate on who should treat cancer opened with the reporting from a general oncology unit of a two-year survival rate of 80% for all patients with non-seminomatous tumours diagnosed in the early 1980s, while 67% of those with adverse prognostic features were alive and well between two and five years after diagnosis [24]. Even better results, however, were then reported from a centre specializing in the treatment of testicular teratoma, with corresponding survival rates of 90% for all patients and 86% for those in the less favourable group [25]. Regrettably, no formal comparative analysis has been published of the effects of inclusion in trials or treatment at specialist centres on survival rates for testicular tumours in Britain. Within one multicentre study, however, there was a marked trend for improvement in two-year survival rates from 68% to 89% over a six-year period [26]. The trend was still significant when allowance was made for changes in treatment and in the proportion of patients with good prognostic factors, suggesting strongly that part of the improvement in survival resulted from increasing clinical experience.

A registry-based analysis has been published from the Irish Testicular Tumour Registry [27]. In this study of 246 patients diagnosed over a six-year period, survival rates were significantly higher if the patient was under the management of a urologist, particularly if this was at the hospital of first presentation. No difference was found in a corresponding analysis of whether an oncologist managed the patient. Those under the combined care of a urologist and an oncologist had a higher survival rate but this failed to attain statistical significance. Entry to clinical trials was not analysed as such, but patients receiving unorthodox chemotherapy or reduced dosage of standard regimens had a markedly lower survival rate. The results are somewhat difficult to interpret, however, as a great many other comparisons were done of factors, including initial investigations and methods and frequency of follow-up, which would clearly be highly correlated with one another. The reasons for the use of non-standard chemotherapy were not specified, though tumour stage was allowed for in the statistical analysis.

The only population-based study of entry to trials and survival rates which has been published for an adult cancer relates to multiple myeloma in Finland [28]. In this study, the records of the national cancer registry were used to compare survival rates for different geographical areas, categorized according to whether it was local policy to enter patients with multiple myeloma in a clinical trial. During 1979–1985, 71% of the 569 patients aged under 71 were residents of trial areas, and 79% of the patients from these areas were actually included in the trials. Patients resident in the trial areas had a significantly higher five-year survival rate (38%) than those from the non-trial areas (28%). In the 20 years before the trials started, survival rates in both sets of areas were very similar to those in the non-trial areas during the study period. The sex ratios and mean ages of patients from the two types of area were very similar. The authors concluded that while the basic treatment may not have differed greatly between the two groups, there was a greater level of uniformity in the trial areas, where treatment was according to a defined protocol, and that the use of systematic treatment schedules produced the improved survival rate.

Within multicentre trials in the USA sponsored by the Eastern Cooperative Oncology Group (ECOG), survival times have been compared for patients treated at major centres and at local community hospitals [29]. No significant differences in survival by type of hospital were found for any of the nine major diagnostic groups in this study and this result was unchanged when adjustments were made for the performance status of patients at diagnosis.

In a more recent population-based study from the Finnish Cancer Registry, Karjalainen [30] examined survival rates for breast and prostate carcinoma, comparing patients living near to specialist treatment centres with those from other districts. Women with breast cancer who were residents of areas containing a university hospital and radiotherapy centre had a higher survival rate than those who lived elsewhere. Among men with prostate cancer there was no difference in survival rates between residents of the two types of area.

A study of patients aged under 65 with osteosarcoma diagnosed during 1963–1982 in the South Thames regions of England showed little variation in survival between major centres (teaching hospitals, and others where chemotherapy was used) and elsewhere when a model was fitted which also included calendar period of diagnosis, age, sex and type of treatment [31], but the improved results in younger patients at major centres probably occurred too recently to have been evident.

The effect of surgical experience on survival rates was studied in a series of over 1000 residents of the West Midlands region of England who had a resection for oesophageal carcinoma during 1957–1976 [32]. The operative mortality rate, defined as the proportion who died within 30 days of surgery, was 22% for patients whose operations were performed by surgeons who averaged at least six resections per year—significantly lower than the 39% mortality among those whose surgeons did at most three resections per year. Among patients who survived for 30 days, the five-year survival rates were similar for the two groups. There were no significant differences between the two groups in the distributions of various clinical features which could affect the prognosis.

There appear to be no other published comparisons of survival rates for adults with cancer who were or were not included in clinical trials. Rather more information is available on the proportions of adults in several diagnostic groups who have been included in trials. In the UK in 1978, a wide-ranging survey of then current randomized trials was carried out by Tate *et al.* [33], who estimated the proportion of patients entered in such studies in several diagnostic groups. Of the groups studied, only lymphoid leukaemia (for which an unusually high proportion of patients are children) had more than a quarter of all patients included in trials. The entry rates to trials for myeloid leukaemia and Hodgkin's disease were 14% and 17% respectively. No other diagnostic group in the survey had more than 10% of patients in trials. For breast cancer, despite the fact that 28 different trials were in progress, only 8% of patients were included in any of them. The entry rates for cancers of bone, brain and ovary were 6%, 4% and 4% respectively, and only 1% of patients with lung cancer were included in a trial.

At one district general hospital in 1980 there were over 1000 patients with malignant disease, with treatment given by a wide range of staff in many different departments [34]. The majority of women with ovarian tumours were entered in controlled trials, but no patients with any other type of cancer were included in trials.

In a more recent national survey of breast cancer treatment, only 37% of surgeons who gave adjuvant systemic therapy to more than half of their patients entered most of them in clinical trials [35].

In the USA also, low proportions of cancer patients are included in trials. A recent survey [36] investigated accrual of patients to Co-operative Group studies sponsored by the National Cancer Institute during 1988. Ten diagnostic groups were studied. The accrual rates to phase II and III studies were 3.7% for multiple myeloma, 3.3% for breast cancer and 2.8% for cancer of the cervix uteri. No other diagnostic group had a rate of more than 2%. Percentage accrual rates were not reported for leukaemias, lymphomas or germ-cell tumours but they would clearly have been somewhat higher, as in Britain. In 1985, 7.6% of potentially eligible American patients with brain tumours were treated in investigative clinical protocols, a proportion no higher than it had been five years earlier [37].

DISCUSSION

The way in which cancer treatment should be organized to maximize both the benefit to current patients and the rate of increase of knowledge has been under discussion for over half a century. Twelve years after its establishment, the Radium Commission [38] recommended that a cancer organization, which might consist of several hospitals, should serve a population of about a million so that at least 1000 cases should be treated in a year and each member of the medical team should see a large enough number of cases to become expert. At that time it was also already recognized that comparison of the effectiveness of different treatments should be made in trials with adequate numbers of patients to detect statistically any clinically important differences in survival rates [39].

More recently, in a number of studies the outcome for patients entered in clinical trials has been compared with that for patients who were not entered, as reviewed above. Some studies have also considered survival in relation to treatment at specialist centres and other hospitals. These investigations have only covered a tiny fraction of all cancers and have been largely concerned with rare diseases occurring predominantly in childhood.

In some studies a significantly higher survival rate was found for patients treated in trials or at specialist centres. In others, no difference in survival was found between trial and non-trial patients or between those treated at specialist centres and those treated elsewhere. In no published study, however, has entry to a clinical trial or treatment at a major centre been shown to result in a lower survival rate.

When patients are entered in clinical trials or treated according to standardized protocols, the evidence from several studies of childhood leukaemia and from the American ECOG is that the size of treatment centre has little or no effect on survival rates. Quality of participation of small centres in co-operative trials can sometimes be a problem. In a study of institutions participating in trials organized by the European Organization for Research on Treatment of Cancer, centres entering small numbers of patients were found to have a significantly lower percentage of valid patients [40]. In the ECOG study, however, no relationship was found between size of centre and percentage of patients who were ineligible; the rate of protocol violation at the small community hospitals was also similar to that at the major centres.

In addition to higher survival rates in some diagnostic groups, there are several other advantages for patients who are treated in clinical trials or at specialist centres. These can include the use of less treatment without compromising the probability of survival and improved follow-up for late effects, as found in the studies of Wilms' tumour discussed above. Patients with other tumours, for instance testicular germ-cell tumours, who are dispersed among many small centres with relatively little experience of the disease and not included in any multicentre study might receive treatment which is no longer the most effective and is itself associated with excess mortality [41, 42]; relatively unusual complications may also be missed.

Rosenberg [43] while reviewing the considerable progress which has been made in treating Hodgkin's disease, noted apprehensively that an increasing proportion of American patients were treated in small community hospitals and correspondingly fewer at major centres. This trend, with the small hospitals presumably not participating in co-operative trials, would lead to more departures from established modes of treatment and an increased error rate in diagnosis, staging and detection of complications; it would become harder to conduct clinical trials to improve survival still further and to reduce treatment-related morbidity.

In the USA, the National Cancer Institute has initiated measures to increase the number of patients in clinical trials but these have been directed mainly at clinicians already involved in research [44]. It has been suggested that more needs to be done to present clinical trials as the treatment of choice to patients if this initiative is to be successful [45]. Even when a major centre is participating in a trial, exclusions and refusal of consent can result in a low proportion of patients initially regarded as eligible being finally included in the trial [46].

For the great majority of types of cancer included in the studies reviewed here, it is clear that greater clinical experience and standardization of treatment, whether in the context of clinical trials or specialist treatment centres or both, is of direct benefit to patients. There is no evidence that inclusion in properly conducted trials results in poorer survival rates. For patients who are included in trials, treatment at large centres does not necessarily confer any substantial further advantage. As clinicians with an interest in oncology become more numerous, district general hospitals can increasingly provide a comprehensive service to cancer patients [47] and can participate in clinical trials in collaboration with regional centres. For the rarest cancers, however, including most of those occurring in childhood, it seems likely that patients should when possible be treated at specialist centres with a concentration of experience and facilities.

Finally, it should be stressed that while it may be reasonable to draw inferences from studies of rare tumours, there is little information on the effect of inclusion in trials on survival rates and other measures of outcome for most of the common cancers. In particular, elderly people are rarely included in trials although they account for a large proportion of all cancers [48]. While the more aggressive regimens used for younger patients may not be appropriate, the most suitable treatment for older people with cancer can only be discovered by research. No published studies so far have focused on the possible benefits to the oldest members of the study population of inclusion in trials or treatment at specialist centres. The ethics of excluding patients on grounds of age from clinical trials for diseases other than cancer have also recently been questioned [49].

Within clinical trials for cancer there has been an increasing tendency to examine quality of life of patients as well as their survival rates, but as yet there have apparently been no studies comparing the quality of life for patients who are included in trials and for those who are not included.

To elucidate the relationship between entry to trials, referral patterns and survival for the great majority of cancers, further research is needed, and population-based cancer registries have a vital role to play as the source of unbiased, reasonably complete series of patients.

ACKNOWLEDGMENTS

I wish to thank many colleagues for helpful discussions and reading earlier drafts, especially Dr I. Chalmers, Dr G. J. Draper and Professor K. Sikora.

I am very grateful to Mrs E. M. Roberts for secretarial assistance. The Childhood Cancer Research Group is supported by the Department of Health and the Scottish Home and Health Department.

REFERENCES

1. Stiller CA (1989) Survival of patients with cancer. Br Med J 299: 1058–1059
2. MRC (1971) Report to the Council from the Committee on Leukaemia and the Working Party on Leukaemia in Childhood. Duration of survival in children with acute leukaemia. Br Med J 4: 7–9
3. Marsden HB, Steward JK (1976) Leukaemia. In: Marsden HB, Steward JK (eds) Tumours in children, 2nd edn. Recent Results in Cancer Research, 13. Springer, Berlin
4. MRC (1986) Report to the Council by the Working Party on Leukaemia in Childhood. Improvement in survival for children with acute lymphoblastic leukaemia. Lancet i: 408–411
5. Stiller CA, Draper GJ (1989) Treatment centre size, entry to trials and survival in acute lymphoblastic leukaemia. Arch Dis Child 64: 657–661
6. Eden OB, Stiller CA, Gerrard MP (1988) Improved survival for childhood acute lymphoblastic leukaemia: possible effect of protocol compliance. Pediatr Hematol Oncol 5: 83–91
7. Craft AW, Amineddine HA, Scott JES, Wagget J (1987) The northern region children's malignant disease registry 1968–82: incidence and survival. Br J Cancer 56: 853–858
8. McCarthy M (1975) Medical care of childhood leukaemia. Lancet i: 1128–1130
9. Green SB, Myers MH, Fink DJ (1977) A population-based study of referral, diagnostic and treatment patterns for childhood acute lymphocytic leukaemia. Am J Epidemiol 106: 53–60
10. Meadows AT, Kramer S, Hopson R et al (1983) Survival in childhood acute lymphocytic leukaemia: effect of protocol and place of treatment. Cancer Invest 1: 49–55
11. Lampert F (1977) Kombinations-Chemotherapie und Hirnschadelbestrahlung bei 530 Kindern mit akuter lymphoblastischer Leukamie. Dtsch Med Wschr 102: 917–921
12. Kaatsch P, Michaelis J (1986) Jahresbericht 1985 uber die kooperative Dokumentation von Malignomen in Kindesalter. (West German Children's Tumour Registry annual report for 1985). University of Mainz, Institute for Medical Statistics and Documentation
13. Peeters M, Koren G, Jakubovicz D, Zipursky A (1988) Physician compliance and relapse rate of acute lymphoblastic leukaemia in children. Clin Pharmacol Ther 43: 228–232
14. Stiller CA (1988) Centralisation of treatment and survival rates for cancer. Arch Dis Child 63: 23–30
15. Lennox EL, Draper GJ, Sanders BM (1975) Retinoblastoma: a study of natural history and prognosis of 268 cases. Br Med J 3: 731–734
16. Sanders BM, Draper GJ, Kingston JE (1988) Retinoblastoma in Britain 1969–1980: incidence, treatment and survival. Br J Ophthalmol 72: 576–583
17. Lennox EL, Stiller CA, Morris Jones PH, Kinnier Wilson LM (1979) Nephroblastoma: treatment during 1970–73 and the effect on survival of inclusion in the first MRC trial. Br Med J 2: 567–569

18. Stiller CA, Lennox EL (1983) Childhood medulloblastoma in Britain 1971–77: analysis of treatment and survival. Br J Cancer 48: 835–841
19. Pritchard J, Stiller CA, Lennox EL (1989) Over-treatment of children with Wilms' tumour outside paediatric oncology centres. Br Med J 299: 835–836
20. Griffel M (1977) Wilms' tumor in New York State: Epidemiology and survivorship. Cancer 40: 3140–3145
21. Kramer S, Meadows AT, Pastore G et al (1984) Influence of place of treatment on diagnosis, treatment and survival in three pediatric solid tumors. J Clin Oncol 2: 917–923
22. Duffner K, Cohen ME, Flannery JT (1982) Referral patterns of childhood brain tumours in the state of Connecticut. Cancer 50: 1636–1640
23. Michaelis J (1988) Osteosarcoma. Lancet i: 1174
24. Naysmith A, Berry RJ (1985) Treatment of testicular teratoma in general oncology departments. Lancet i: 646
25. Bagshawe KD, Begent RHJ, Newlands ES, Rustin GJS (1985) What sort of oncology team should treat testicular teratoma? Lancet i: 930
26. MRC (1985) Report from the Medical Research Council Working Party on Testicular Tumours. Prognostic factors in advanced non-seminomatous germ-cell testicular tumours: results of a multi-centre study. Lancet i: 8–11
27. Thornhill JA, Walsh A, Conroy RM, Fennelly JJ, Kelly DG, Fitzpatrick JM (1988) Physician-dependent prognostic variables in the management of testicular cancer. Br J Urol 61: 244–249
28. Karjalainen S, Palva I (1989) Do treatment protocols improve end results? A study of survival of patients with multiple myeloma in Finland. Br Med J 299: 1069–1072
29. Begg CB, Carbone PP, Elson PJ, Zelen M (1982) Participation of community hospitals in clinical trials: analysis of five years of experience in the Eastern Cooperative Oncology Group. N Engl J Med 306: 1076–1080
30. Karjalainen S (1990) Geographical variation in cancer patient survival in Finland: chance, confounding or effect of treatment? J Epidemiol Community Health 44: 210–214
31. Gill M, McCarthy M, Murrells T, Silcocks P (1988) Chemotherapy for the primary treatment of osteosarcoma: population effectiveness over 20 years. Lancet i: 689–692
32. Matthews HR, Powell DJ, McConkey CC (1986) Effect of surgical experience on the results of resection for oesophageal carcinoma. Br J Surg 73: 621–623
33. Tate HC, Rawlinson JB, Freedman LS (1979) Randomised comparative studies in the treatment of cancer in the United Kingdom: room for improvement? Lancet ii: 623–625
34. Woll PH (1987) Who treats cancer? JRCP Lond 21: 61–66
35. Gazet J-C, Ramsbury RM, Ford HT, Powles TJ, Coombes RC (1985) Survey of treatment of primary breast cancer in Great Britain. Br Med J 290: 1793–1795
36. Friedman MA, Cain DF (1990) National Cancer Institute sponsored cooperative clinical trials. Cancer 65: 2376–2382
37. Mahaley MS, Mettlin C, Natarajan N, Laws ER, Peace BB (1989) National survey of patterns of care for brain-tumour patients. J Neurosurg 71: 826–836
38. Radium Commission (1942) Organization for cancer treatment. Br Med J ii: 48–50
39. Ellis F (1943) Planning in the treatment of cancer. Br Med J i: 570
40. Sylvester RJ, Pinedo HM, de Pauw M et al (1981) Quality of institutional participation in multicentre clinical trials. N Engl J Med 305: 852–855
41. Oliver RTD (1986) Rare cancers and specialist centres. Br Med J 292: 641–642
42. Ellis M, Sikora K (1986) Mortality in patients with testicular cancer: report of the Anglia and Trent testicular tumour groups. Br Med J 292: 672–674

43. Rosenberg SA (1986) Hodgkin's disease: no stage beyond cure. Hosp Pract 21: 91–108
44. Wittes RE, Friedman MA (1988) Accrual to clinical trials. J Nat Cancer Inst 80: 884–885
45. Gelber RD, Goldhirsch A (1988) Can a clinical trial be the treatment of choice for patients with cancer? J Nat Cancer Inst 80: 886–887
46. Jack WJL, Chetty U, Rodger A (1990) Recruitment to a prospective breast conservation trial: why are so few patients randomised? Br Med J 301: 83–85
47. McIllmurray MB, Gorst DW, Holdcroft PE (1986) A comprehensive service for patients with cancer in a district general hospital. Br Med J 292: 669–671
48. Fentiman IS, Tirelli U, Monfardini S et al (1990) Cancer in the elderly: why so badly treated? Lancet 335: 1020–1022
49. Chalmers TC (1990) Ethical implications of rejecting patients for clinical trials. JAMA 263: 865

ABOUT THE AUTHOR

Charles Stiller was awarded the degree of MSc in applied statistics at the University of Oxford in 1976. He is now a statistician and epidemiologist with the Childhood Cancer Research Group (CCRG), Department of Paediatrics, and Lecturer in Statistics at New College, Oxford. At the CCRG he has scientific responsibility for the National Registry of Childhood Tumours. This is a population-based registry covering the whole of mainland Britain. It ascertains around 1300 new cases per year and forms the basis of most of the research at the CCRG and of a wide range of collaborative projects. A number of these projects are carried out in cooperation with the United Kingdom Children's Cancer Study Group, of which Mr Stiller is also a member. He is an author of several publications on various aspects of survival of children with cancer, including the influence of referral patterns and entry to clinical trials. His other main research interest is in geographical variations in cancer incidence, and he was joint editor of a recent monograph on the international incidence of childhood cancer, which was published by the International Agency for Research on Cancer.

10 The Ethics and Practical Problems of Phase I and II Studies

GEORGE BLACKLEDGE and FRANK LAWTON

In theory the principle and practice of carrying out effective phase I and phase II studies of novel cancer therapies is easy. The phase I study establishes the dose that can be used in humans and the phase II study establishes whether that dose has the desired effect. Subsequent studies in the form of randomized phase III trials will determine whether that observed effect is worthwhile in comparison with established treatment.

Such simplistic statements do not unfortunately reflect the considerable problems and dilemmas that face the researcher in many phase I and II studies. This chapter attempts to identify and address some of these dilemmas.

WHERE IS THE STARTING POINT?

There is a need for new and better cancer treatments. The life-time risk of developing cancer for a person in the Western world is 30% and there is a 20% chance of dying from cancer. Only around one-third of patients who develop cancer stand a chance of being cured and whilst in many of the incurable cancers useful palliation and extension of life can be obtained, premature death is usually inevitable. The situation is far from perfect.

Metastatic disease remains one of the major problems in cancer treatment and is one of the most common reasons for the failure of local therapies such as surgery and radiotherapy. More effective systemic approaches are therefore needed. There are now over 40 different chemotherapy agents with demonstrated activity against cancer and over ten hormone therapies. A number of cytokines have been developed which have anticancer activity. With the exception of a few rare malignancies none of these compounds or combinations of them are completely effective against cancer. A process of developing, identifying and testing new compounds is therefore continually needed.

Introducing New Treatments for Cancer: Practical, Ethical and Legal Problems. Edited by C. J. Williams
© 1992 John Wiley & Sons Ltd

CHOOSING AGENTS FOR HUMAN TESTING

There are a number of methods by which new agents can be identified. One is through logical design, building on an observed difference between the specific cancer cell and normal or, alternatively, upon the chance observation of the action of a specific group of compounds. Agents such as the first effective anticancer treatment mechlorethamine, cisplatin and interferon were developed in this way. Experimental data suggested so strongly a potential role for these agents that they were introduced into the clinic after relatively little animal testing.

Screening of potential drugs using a panel of cancer cell cultures has been carried out by the National Cancer Institute for some years. Although tens of thousands of compounds have been tested the approach has identified relatively few useful agents. There are a number of probable reasons for this. First, a screening programme must make certain assumptions about the drugs for which it is screening, and whilst the cell cultures in which cytotoxicity is looked for cover a spectrum of cancers they have been chosen on the basis of the perceived activity of established drugs. A screening programme therefore is likely to be good at identifying further examples of those established agents. The test systems, however, are generally unsophisticated and may therefore be unable to detect novel compounds which may depend on metabolism in the human body or alter the way in which the body responds to the cancer. This flaw in screening systems is acknowledged and there are now a number of attempts to increase the sophistication of screening systems to detect the unexpected effect of an anticancer agent rather than to anticipate a conventional effect such as alkylating agent activity. Regardless of how effective any laboratory test system appears to be it is up to the clinical researcher finally to decide whether a new compound is worth testing in human beings.

WHAT IS THE MAXIMUM TOLERATED DOSE FOR AN ANTICANCER TREATMENT?

Most conventional anticancer agents have a narrow therapeutic ratio with significant toxicity either occurring within the effective therapeutic range or just above the therapeutic range. In addition to this some aspects of toxicity such as bone marrow toxicity may be an integral part of the action of the drug itself. Since the malignant process may be regarded as a function of altered gene expression many anticancer agents will affect DNA or RNA and there is therefore the potential for mutagenicity or carcinogenicity as a direct result of the desire for effect of the anticancer agent. These factors severely limit the volunteers on whom anticancer agents can be tested. The concept of testing on normal volunteers for most drugs is well established but the risks of short-term and long-term damage mean that normal volunteers cannot be used for anticancer testing. It is now regarded as ethically acceptable to use patients suffering from cancer in whom all conventional therapy has been tried and failed, but who are expected to live long enough for an adequate assessment of the toxicity of the compound being tested (see Chapters 1 and 2). This has led to phase I agents being tested in a highly selected subpopulation of patients with cancer. This population is unlikely to be typical of the population as a whole and any observations made in this subpopulation must be regarded with some caution, and not necessarily directly applicable to the patient population in whom the compound may eventually be used.

The characteristics of the subpopulation will be:

(1) Patients with a diagnosis of malignancy.
(2) Patients who cannot be cured by conventional methods.
(3) Most patients will have received some form of conventional treatment.
(4) The patients will have progressing, but not at that point life-threatening, disease.
(5) The patients will be highly motivated and will therefore not represent a typical psychological cross-section.
(6) Because of the presence of untreatable cancer there may be incipient organ failure (in particular liver and kidneys).
(7) There may have been damage to specific organs because of previous treatment, thus rendering the likelihood of toxicity in these areas far greater.

It can be seen from the above that this is not an ideal population in which to test a new agent. A recent overview of phase I studies [1] has suggested that there is little chance that patients entering phase I studies for cancer treatment will have a response (Chapter 11). The large majority of patients gain no benefit whatsoever and there is therefore an ethical dilemma in counselling and discussing phase I studies with these patients. In general terms they should be aware that they are volunteers and that the treatment they are receiving is highly unlikely to be of any benefit to themselves (see Chapters 1 and 2 for fuller discussion of ethical and legal points).

HOW IS THE MAXIMUM TOLERATED DOSE ESTABLISHED?

The existence of a narrow therapeutic ratio for most cytotoxic agents has meant that a relatively simple dose escalation schedule can be used in phase I studies for agents which are anticipated to have conventional toxicity. The Fibonacci escalation or modified Fibonacci escalation has worked well for agents in whom the primary dose limiting toxicity is expected to be myelotoxicity. Since this is the most common acute toxicity for most classes of cytotoxic drugs this approach has worked reasonably well. Problems arise with this approach when either the myelotoxicity is of unpredictable intensity or duration or when the toxicity is non-myelotoxic or non-dose related. For many new compounds this is the case. Additionally the administration of a bolus dose of chemotherapy is an inappropriate method of assessment for agents which are phase specific and for which the area under the curve is more important than the peak dose. For agents such as these, which include many of the antimetabolites, there remain unresolved problems decades after their introduction about the appropriate dose and scheduling to use. The conventional phase I study cannot answer these questions and it is only through a process of continued experimentation in man together with appropriate pharmacokinetics and observation of tumour response that such questions can be answered.

Another dilemma in phase I studies has recently emerged with the development of biological response modifiers. With these, conventional dose escalations cannot be used unless direct cytotoxic anticancer effect is anticipated. Many of these agents, however, have a putative mode of action through direct or indirect stimulation of the host's own immune system or through an anticancer effect which may not be related to dose but rather to total exposure time, scheduling and mode of administration. Evaluation of these agents is a complex task and one which has not yet been fully resolved.

PHASE II EVALUATION

The standard methods of phase II evaluation have been developed over several decades. They involve treating a group of patients with the same cancer who are refractory to conventional therapy. Usually around 14–20 patients will be treated if the compound has no activity. More will be treated if activity is seen, to gain some estimate of the level of activity.

Phase II studies do not attempt to prove that a new treatment is genuinely useful; they are merely a guide to the potential value of a new agent, which should then be tested in a randomized trial against whatever therapy is regarded as standard in a particular disease.

Although it might be perceived that the primary determinant of a positive phase II study is the activity of the drug being tested, there are now considerable data to suggest that other factors may influence the outcome. These are discussed below with special emphasis on epithelial ovarian cancer.

PROGNOSTIC FACTORS

In epithelial ovarian cancer prognostic factors associated with survival are well established and include, among others, tumour grade, residual tumour bulk and performance status [2]. Factors which may influence response to therapy, however, are less well defined. Most clinicians make some estimate of a patient's chance of response when being treated in a phase II or salvage setting, basing this on such factors as the patient's age and general medical condition, the type and duration of previous treatment and the duration of the previous response if it occurred. Few responses, for example, would be anticipated in a group of patients with ovarian cancer who have received cisplatin previously and who failed to respond. It may be argued that a population containing a large proportion of such patients is inappropriate for inclusion in a phase II study, yet it is likely that these patients, who have failed first-line therapy, are the first to be entered into a new phase II study, since "conventional" second-line treatment, after failure of cisplatin, will probably be ineffective.

A number of patient characteristics may affect the activity of a drug or, just as importantly, may influence the dose that the clinician is prepared to administer. Based on data gained from phase I studies, phase II investigations should be performed with adequate doses of the drug because of dose–response considerations. In many patients this may be difficult to achieve. Some of the factors which may influence patient, drug or dose selection in phase II studies are discussed below.

PATIENT AGE AND PERFORMANCE STATUS

Data are few as to whether the elderly suffer excess toxicity from cytotoxic regimens compared with younger patients, but it has been shown that they are more likely to be treated with less aggressive regimens and are more likely to have dose modifications [3]. Performance status and age may influence whether or not the patient is even considered for such a study.

INITIAL EXPECTATIONS IN A PHASE II STUDY WITH REGARD TO PREVIOUS TOXICITY

During the early part of a study while clinicians are developing experience with a new drug or drug regimen, patient recruitment may be influenced by two conflicting factors. Until the toxicity of the regimen has been defined, low doses may be employed, but until the activity has been confirmed clinicians may be tempted to treat only patients with little chance of prolonged benefit, relying on established second-line drugs rather than the new regimen. Previous toxicity suffered by a patient may influence the clinician as well as the patient who is to be entered into a study, which may produce side-effects that have already been experienced. The importance of these toxicities may differ, however, between clinician and patient. For example, a patient may worry about alopecia whilst a clinician will be more conscious of the potential for further bone marrow suppression. Once experience has been gained with the drug, clinicians may be more likely to enter patients who, it is felt, will tolerate full-dose therapy and who, by chance, may have other favourable prognostic factors for response.

PREVIOUS RESPONSE TO TREATMENT

Response to first-line therapy may have two important effects on subsequent responses in phase II studies. The first concerns the fact that a previous response to cytotoxic treatment will encourage both the clinician and the patient to "have another go". A patient who gains a long-term remission to first-line therapy and who has been off-treatment for a long period of time is a better candidate to receive full-dose phase II therapy and is therefore more likely to respond to an active regimen than is a patient with a poor response of short duration or one who has poor marrow, biochemical or renal function following heavy pretreatment. In addition, a patient who has had a good-quality response previously may be more likely to be entered into subsequent phase II studies. An important aspect when reporting the population under treatment in a phase II study is to define how the patients were selected.

In general, data relating to previous response, response duration and time "off-treatment" are not given in phase II studies. Most clinicians are aware of the influence of these factors, yet studies examining the effect of these factors on response have rarely been undertaken. It was this clinical problem that encouraged us to address the question of the influence of other factors on response apart from the activity of the drug under investigation [4]. A univariate analysis of five phase II studies of 93 patients with ovarian cancer showed that a number of factors were of significance in predicting the eventual response to treatment. These included the interval from the time of last treatment to the time of starting phase II treatment, the presenting stage of disease, the type of chemotherapy under investigation and the quality of the previous response to treatment. In a multivariate analysis only interval and International Federation of Obstetrics and Gynaecology (FIGO) stage were important, and a discriminant analysis using these factors predicted 89% of patients who did not respond to treatment and 75% of those who did. In the five studies, the response rate for those patients who progressed on first-line therapy or who relapsed within three to six months was less than 10%, compared with greater than 75% for patients who had a remission duration of greater than 15 months (Table 1). Since all the regimens tested had activity this factor alone could dramatically influence the likelihood of detecting a new active compound. Realistically it implies that many factors in different diseases could influence the chances of

Table 1. Response rate using interval from previous
treatment to phase II therapy only

Interval (months)	Total no.	No. responding	% responding
<3	39	4	10
4–6	11	1	9
7–9	11	4	36
10–12	6	1	17
13–15	4	2	50
16–18	4	3	75
19–21	1	1	100
>21	16	15	94

response for a new agent. It may not be possible to identify all these, but certainly the number of patients entered into phase II studies should, perhaps, be revised upwards to take account of such factors.

INTRAPERITONEAL REGIMENS

A number of studies have demonstrated that patients with small-volume disease with tumour masses of only up to 1 cm in diameter are the only ones likely to benefit from intraperitoneal drug administration [5,6]. This can affect potential recruitment to such a study, because physicians, knowing that the chance of obtaining a response in patients with bulkier disease is small, are unlikely to enter them in the study in the first place. Patients with small-volume disease, however, are difficult to assess for response, because clinically there will be nothing to measure. Such patients will be eligible for toxicity analysis, but unless they have evidence of disease progression while on treatment will require surgical assessment of response. Laparoscopic examination of the peritoneal cavity may be less morbid than second-look laparotomy, but response assessed using this method may be artificially elevated because of the high false-negative rate of the procedure. Even responses documented with a full surgical re-exploration should be regarded with care since up to 50% of patients with no evidence of disease at second-look laparotomy develop recurrent disease within 15 months. Nevertheless, patients with a macroscopically negative second-look operation are the ones most likely to benefit from further therapy especially if it is given as consolidation treatment immediately after surgery rather than at the time of relapse. Any relapses after this can then be regarded as treatment failures. Likewise tumour markers and imaging techniques are insufficiently specific or sensitive enough to be used to document response in patients with small-volume disease. The desire or ability of a patient to undergo a surgical restaging may affect her initial chances of being recruited into a phase II intraperitoneal study. In the authors' experience up to 20% of patients, otherwise eligible for phase II intraperitoneal studies, are unlikely to be included because of the anticipated difficulties of drug administration or assessment of response.

A further complicating factor regarding intraperitoneal regimens is that drugs inactive at standard systemic concentrations show activity at concentrations achievable after intraperitoneal administration and that second responses can be gained in patients with cancer resistant to a drug given intravenously, when the same drug is given by the intraperitoneal route [7].

RE-EXPOSURE TO CYTOTOXIC THERAPY

It is apparent also that some patients can be re-exposed to a particular intravenous regimen with good response. A recent report from the Royal Marsden Hospital has demonstrated that patients with relapsed ovarian cancer originally treated with cisplatin or carboplatin can be either successfully retreated with the same drug or crossed over to treatment with the other [8]. There was no significant difference in the response rate gained with these two actions. However, 17% of patients who relapsed within 18 months of primary therapy responded to the second regimen, compared with 53% of patients who relapsed after 18 months ($p=0.006$). In addition, the median survival from second treatment for patients who had a short first remission was 221 days, compared with 486 days for those who enjoyed a longer remission.

ASSESSING AGENTS WITH MINIMAL ACTIVITY

A review of some of the reports of anti-oestrogen therapy in ovarian cancer highlights many of the problems discussed above. In four studies the overall response rate was only 6.5% and, in addition, three of the four responses were contained within one of the reports. It may be assumed from this that hormone therapy has little place in the management of patients with ovarian cancer, but a detailed examination of the papers emphasizes the influence of the confounding factors detailed above. For example, nine of the 13 patients in the paper by Schwartz et al. were progressing on cisplatin therapy and five had evidence of small bowel obstruction when they began hormone treatment [9]. In addition all had been pretreated with at least two other regimens before recruitment to the study. The patients in the paper by Shirey et al. [10] had been heavily pretreated with 9–44 months of chemotherapy before entering the study in question and 43% of them had also been treated with radiotherapy. Data on the quality and duration of previous response to treatment in these patients was not given in the paper. Only five of the

22 patients in the report by Slevin et al. had any progression-free interval off-therapy before starting tamoxifen therapy [11]. Only the paper by Myers et al., where all three patients responded, has suggested any durable activity for hormone therapy in ovarian cancer [12]. However, a review of the detailed histories given in the paper shows again that in two cases it may have been patient characteristics rather than activity of the drug which accounted for this result. In one patient, treated with surgery only, there was a 16-year disease-free interval before she had evidence of recurrent cancer with liver and pulmonary metastases. She had a mixed response to a number of regimens over the next three and a half years before being treated with and responding to hormone therapy for 18 months. Another patient had initial debulking surgery, but it was five years later after responses to both melphalan and cisplatin that she developed chest metastases and an almost complete response to tamoxifen. These patients are untypical of the usual ovarian cancer population, and may therefore have either a second malignancy which responded to treatment or some other factor predisposing to endocrine response.

Similar controversy has occurred with the results of phase II studies of mitoxantrone in ovarian cancer. The response rate in the study by Lawton et al. was 12/46 (26%) but two other studies suggested minimal activity [13–15]. The patient populations, however, were quite different and this may explain the disparate results. For instance over 80% of the patients in the other studies had been previously treated with doxorubicin, compared with 11% of patients in the Lawton study, and 80% of patients in the study by Hilgers et al. were receiving mitoxantrone as third-line therapy or greater. Patients in the Lawton study had only received one prior regimen. In addition the dose of mitoxantrone used in the other two studies was 10–12 mg/m^2, whilst in the Lawton study patients started treatment at a dose of 12 mg/m^2 and escalation to 16 mg/m^2 or greater was possible in 14 patients.

These examples also demonstrate that patients with slow-growing cancers, presumably containing few chemotherapy-resistant clones, are also likely to be good candidates to demonstrate a response to a particular investigational regimen. Often, such patients have clinically apparent cancers which, however, are asymptomatic and may remain so for many months. The decision to treat in these circumstances may be influenced more by the need to test a new regimen rather than a worsening of the patient's condition.

In general, heavily pretreated patients are poor candidates for entry into new studies because the cumulative toxicity of their previous treatment precludes full-dose or full-duration phase II treatment. However, a subset of this population, namely those who have had a number of previous responses of good quality and duration—so-called "multiple responders"— should be recognized as having potential to respond again to the particular regimen under investigation. Of the 31 patients who had a response to treatment in the analysis of five phase II studies discussed above, five (16%) had at least a partial response to two prior regimens.

ANALYSIS OF PHASE II STUDIES

From the above discussion, in only one disease, it is clear that there are many factors which might influence the assessment of a new drug. These may be obvious, such as the number of previous treatments, or time to relapse, but there may be other, more subtle influences on patient selection for studies, such as not selecting patients in whom assessing response is difficult.

The phase II study, in a patient population which has failed conventional therapy, remains a reasonable approach to identifying active new agents. In soft-tissue sarcoma, a relatively chemoresistant disease, only three agents have significant activity as first-line therapy. All three showed responses in patients failing first-line therapy, in comparison with almost all the other chemotherapy agents which had negative phase II results in this setting [16]. It is therefore probably appropriate to continue evaluating new agents in this way, but it is important that potential confounding factors and prognostically important patient characteristics are documented in detail so that comparison can be made with other studies [17]. In this way, ethical and scientifically useful studies can be carried out, and the results made available to others.

REFERENCES

1. Decoster G, Stein G, Holdener E (1990) Responses and toxic deaths in phase I clinical trials. Ann Oncol 1: 175–182
2. Swenerton K, Hislop TG, Spinelli J, Le Riche JC, Yang N, Boyes DA (1985) Ovarian carcinoma: a multivariate analysis of prognostic factors Obstet Gynecol 65: 264–270
3. Walsh SJ, Begg CB, Carbone PP (1989) Cancer chemotherapy in the elderly. Semin Oncol 16: 66–75
4. Blackledge G, Lawton FG, Redman C, Kelly K (1989) Response of patients in phase II studies of chemotherapy in ovarian cancer: implications for patient treatment and the design of phase II studies. Br J Cancer 59: 650–653
5. Howell SB, Zimm S, Markman M, Abramson IS, Cleary S, Lucas WE, Weiss RJ (1987) Long term survival of advanced refractory ovarian carcinoma patients with small volume disease treated with intraperitoneal chemotherapy. J Clin Oncol 10: 1607–1612
6. Piver MS, Lele SB, Marchetti DL, Baker TR, Emrich LJ, Hartman AB (1988) Surgically documented response to intraperitoneal cisplatin, cytarabine and bleomycin after intravenous cisplatin-based chemotherapy in advanced ovarian adenocarcinoma. J Clin Oncol 6: 1679–1684
7. Hacker NF, Berek JS, Pretorius RG, Zuckerman J, Eisenkop S, Lagasse LD (1987) Intraperitoneal cis-platinum as salvage therapy for refractory epithelial ovarian cancer. Obstet Gynecol 70: 759–764

8. Gore ME, Fryatt I, Wiltshaw E, Dawson T (1990) Treatment of relapsed carcinoma of the ovary with cisplatin or carboplatin following initial treatment with these compounds. Gynecol Oncol 36: 207–211

9. Schwartz PE, Keating G, MacLusky N, Naftolin F, Eisenfeld A (1982) Tamoxifen therapy for advanced ovarian cancer. Obstet Gynecol 59: 583–588

10. Shirey DR, Kavanagh JJ Jr, Gerhenson DM, Freedman RS, Copeland LJ, Jones LA (1985) Tamoxifen therapy of epithelial ovarian cancer. Obstet Gynecol 66: 575–578

11. Slevin ML, Harvey VJ, Osborne RJ, Shepherd JH, Williams CJ, Mead GM (1989) A phase II study of tamoxifen in ovarian cancer. Eur J Cancer Clin Oncol 22: 309–312

12. Myers AM, Moore GE, Major FJ (1981) Advanced ovarian carcinoma: response to antiestrogen therapy. Cancer 48: 2368–2370

13. Lawton FG, Blackledge G, Mould JJ, Latief T, Watson R, Chetiyawardana AD (1987) Phase II study of mitoxantrone in epithelial ovarian cancer. Cancer Treat Rep 71: 627–630

14. Hilgers RD, Rivkin SE, von Hoff DD, Alberts DS (1984) Mitoxantrone in epithelial carcinoma of the ovary: a Southwest Oncology Group study. Am J Clin Oncol 7: 499–501

15. Muss HB, Asbury R, Bundy B, Ehrlch CE, Graham J (1984) Mitoxantrone (NSC-301739) in patients with advanced ovarian cancer: a phase II study of the Gynecologic Oncology Group. Am J Clin Oncol 7: 737–739

16. Blackledge G, van Oosterom A, Mouridsen H, Steward WP, Buesa J, Thomas D, Sylvester R, Rouesse J (1990) Doxorubicin in relapsed soft tissue sarcoma: justification of phase II evaluation of new drugs in this disease: an EORTC soft tissue and bone sarcoma group study. Eur J Cancer 26: 139–141

17. Buyse M, Staquet R, Sylvester R (eds) (1987) Cancer clinical trials: methods and practice. Oxford University Press

ABOUT THE AUTHORS

Dr George Blackledge was trained at Cambridge and St Bartholomew's Hospital, London. He did oncology training at the Christie Hospital, Manchester, and from 1982 to 1990 was Senior Lecturer then Reader in Medical Oncology at the University of Birmingham. During this time he was responsible for phase I and phase II trials in a wide variety of malignancies. Since 1990 he has been responsible for Clinical Research in Oncology at ICI Pharmaceuticals Group.

Mr Frank Lawton MD MRCOG is Consultant Gynaecologist at King's College Hospital. He received specialist training in gynaecological cancer in Manchester, Birmingham and Sydney. His main interests include combined modality therapy in ovarian cancer, gynaecological cancer screening and the management of the geriatric population with genital tract cancers.

11 Ethical Aspects of Phase I Studies in Cancer Patients

EDUARD E. HOLDENER, GENEVIEVE DECOSTER and
CAROL M. LIM

Spero, ergo sum,	*The one who hopes is ahead*
Sum, ergo spero	*of facts*
Wolfgang Hildesheimer, 1986	*Siegfried Lenz, 1986*

It is often stated that cancer patients who enter phase I trials have nothing to lose. However, it may be more important that they still have something to hope for. Although the likelihood of achieving an objective tumor response to an experimental drug at this stage of drug development is rather low [1,2], a chance always remains for the individual patient (see Appendix for summary of results of our review of phase I trials). Phase I clinical trials in cancer patients continue to be of pivotal importance in the development of a new drug since they represent the transition from the pre-clinical, experimental stage to the evaluation of clinical efficacy in man.

AVAILABILITY OF PRE-CLINICAL DATA AND DOSE FINDING

The first ethical question which arises in phase I trials in cancer is that often little pre-clinical toxicology and very limited efficacy data are available before the drug is used in man. The goal of phase I studies used to be to define the maximum tolerated dose (MTD) of a new cytotoxic agent. This may be less relevant than the search for the optimum biological dose for many of the recombinant proteins recently evaluated in cancer patients [3]. It is therefore mandatory to collect all necessary pre-clinical information on toxicology and efficacy from in vitro studies as well as in vivo animal studies, in order to minimize potential hazards and to optimize the safety of studies in man [4]. The limitations of the positive predictive value of these pre-clinical systems are well known but they may at least lead to the identification of ineffective drugs and thus prevent unnecessary treatment [5–9].

In our own review of phase I trials [1] we found that in only 76% of published papers was animal toxicology discussed, in 36% mention was

Introducing New Treatments for Cancer: Practical, Ethical and Legal Problems. Edited by C. J. Williams
© 1992 John Wiley & Sons Ltd

made of some preliminary toxicity data in man, but in 15% of the publications there was no reference to animal or to human toxicology.

Using classical dose escalation schemes [10], an average of 25 patients [1] is necessary to define the MTD of a new cytotoxic drug. In an attempt to reduce this number even further, thereby protecting patients from either ineffective and/or toxic treatment, new strategies employing pharmaco-kinetically guided dose escalation are currently being employed [11–13]. The moral benefits of intra-person dose escalation seem to outweigh those of inter-person escalation [14, 15], whereby all patients start treatment at a "non-toxic" entry dose and all eventually benefit from an optimum dose with the highest chance of being efficacious. A possible limiting factor of this approach, however, is the potential of cumulative toxicity. Specific study designs, in which the use of pre-clinical toxicity data is maximized, may help to reduce this risk.

CHOICE OF PATIENTS

A second ethical dilemma which arises in phase I studies is the choice of end-stage cancer patients as the target population for a drug of unknown benefit and potentially damaging effects [16]. The patient must also have exhausted all other therapeutic modalities that offer the possibility of success before being entered into phase I studies. In our review of the phase I literature [1], 82% of studies included patients who had been exposed to previous therapies such as chemotherapy and radiotherapy.

It has been argued by Oates that studies to determine whether a drug is effective and, if so, at which dose, should first be done on the patient population for whom the drug is intended [17]. If the drug is not effective, there is no need for normal subjects to be exposed to the risks of phase I studies which focus particularly on bioavailability and metabolism of the drug. Another reason to involve cancer patients in phase I trials in the field of cancer chemotherapy is that most of the drugs employed are very toxic [18]. It is therefore important that patients who are asked to participate in tests of new anticancer drugs are not misled about the likelihood of any therapeutic benefit they might derive [19].

Recently there have been an increasing number of exceptions from the trend to use cancer patients in phase I studies, such as in the early development of certain cytokines (e.g. interferons, hematopoietic growth factors) and other classes of compounds (e.g. retinoids), where phase I studies have also been done in healthy volunteers [20, 21]. One of the major objections to this approach is that healthy volunteers are not necessarily representative of the patient population and that any extrapolation of results from healthy volunteers to cancer patients may be dangerously misleading [22]. The metabolism of drugs may be changed by disease and drug interactions may modify effects which may necessitate phase I studies in both normal and patient subjects. The chief ethical objection to the use of normal subjects in any type of phase I study is that an unfavourable harm/benefit ratio exists for the individual subject. There is no possibility whatsoever of any direct health-related benefit so the harm/benefit ratio is always infinite.

When patients were questioned on whether or not they would consent to take part in clinical trials the most frequent reasons cited for agreement were advances in medical or scientific knowledge and potential benefit to others [23]. Nearly 80% of the patients questioned believed that contributing to scientific knowledge and helping future patients was extremely important and could make an important contribution to society. An interesting aspect of this survey was that there was no difference in the distribution of answers to the various questions between cancer patients, cardiology patients and the general public. Although clinical trials were generally viewed as important, ethical and as a means of obtaining superior medical care, there was, nevertheless, a minority of respondents who disapproved of patients serving as research subjects and who failed to attribute extreme importance to clinical investigations.

INFORMED CONSENT

According to The President's Commission [24] "although the informed consent doctrine has substantial foundations in law, it is essentially an ethical imperative". In our review of 211 publications covering 6639 patients who took part in phase I cancer trials [1], information on whether informed consent was obtained from the patients was inconsistently reported and it was rarely stated whether the consent, when given, was written, oral or witnessed. Considering the importance of this aspect of clinical research and the extensive information needed by a patient before he or she can consent to take part in a phase I study, including formal invitation to the study, statement of the objectives of the research, the basis for patient selection, an explanation of procedures, a detailed description of any discomfort or risks, and disclosure of alternative treatments that might be advantageous, it is somewhat surprising to see the inconsistency in the reporting of this matter [25].

There is evidence that today patients are more likely to participate in phase I trials as there has been a dramatic shift in physicians' stated policies of disclosure of the diagnosis of cancer to patients. In 1961, 88% of the physicians surveyed had a policy of non-disclosure of a diagnosis of cancer to the patient, whereas in 1979, 98% of those surveyed had a policy of telling the patient [26].

The informed consent doctrine requires that a patient consents to the medical procedures that are to be performed in a non-biased and informed manner. The ideal of shared decision making underlying this doctrine is that of the patient deciding, in collaboration with a physician, what type of health care, if any, will best cover his or her needs [27]. The fundamental values served by the practice of informed consent are promoting and protecting the patients' well-being while respecting their rights to determine, at least in part, the treatment which they believe will best ensure this. As is well known and as physicians are frequently quick to point out, however, the complexity of many treatment programs, together with the stress of illness, with its attendant fear, anxiety, dependency and regression—not to mention the physical effects of the illness itself—mean that a patient's normal decision-making abilities are often significantly diminished (see Chapters 5 and 6). It is therefore even more crucial that the information and recommendation given to a patient regarding participation in a phase I study is highly objective and "well balanced" between the principles of *benefit and no harm* to the patient on the one hand and the *autonomy* of the patient and *responsibility* of the physician on the other hand [28].

CANCER PATIENTS AND CLINICAL RESEARCH

Clinical research is by definition combined with professional medical care [29] but is coupled with higher degrees of uncertainty and unpredictability with respect to the safety and efficacy of the test drug than are present in established medical care procedures. This is particularly true in trials of potentially very toxic drugs in phase I clinical oncology. Since the risks of medical research seem to be small in comparison with the rates of accidental injury in the general population [30], there is a strong argument that patients should participate in studies which evaluate the risks and benefits of the practices to which they will be subjected. This justification is, however, insufficient for therapies which are on the frontiers of our knowledge, especially those which have the far-off goal of eventual cure and those which involve more than minimal risk. Support of and personal involvement in research of the latter type is a noble choice rather than a moral obligation. Pursuit of progress must take place within limits established by other values, including that of individual autonomy [31].

It is widely agreed that the prospective review of research protocols, and the institutional review board as a means of accomplishing this review, are effective in that they lead to the avoidance of excessively risky research and better enable the patient to consent to participation in the research [31]. Our own survey [1] showed that ethical review was rarely mentioned in European studies performed before 1980 whereas it was recorded more frequently in US studies. Today the process of ethical review has become an increasingly required process internationally and is carried out worldwide.

In contrast to consent at the institutional level, thereby allowing the research to be performed, informed consent from the patient, whereby he or she agrees to take part in the particular research, requires that the patient understands the circumstances, decides in the absence of control by others and intentionally authorizes a professional to proceed with the proposed medical research program.

CONCLUSIONS

The ethical aspects of phase I clinical trials are no different from those which apply to other patient populations or normal volunteers although, as was stated at the beginning of this chapter, the patient may have little to hope for. The three fundamental ethical principles recognized as being particularly relevant to the ethics of research involving human subjects, i.e. *respect for the individual*, *benefit* and *justice*, are just as relevant in a population of cancer patients as they are in the general public as a whole [32].

REFERENCES

1. Decoster G, Stein G, Holdener EE (1990) Responses and toxic deaths in phase I clinical trials. Ann Oncol 1: 175–181
2. Estey E, Hoth D, Simon R et al (1986) Therapeutic response in phase I trials of antineoplastic agents. Cancer Treat Rep 70: 71–80
3. Parkinson DR (1990) Endogenous substances as drugs: issues related to the application of cytokines in cancer therapy. Drug Safety 5: 75–83
4. Darry G, Dion S (1986) The ethical approach to phase I clinical trials in oncology. Drug Exptl Clin Res 12: 21–22
5. Ogawa M, Bergsagel DE, McCulloch EA (1973) Chemotherapy of mouse myeloma: quantitative cell culture predictive of response in vivo. Blood 41: 7–15
6. Moon TE, Salmon SE, White CS et al (1981) Quantitative association between the in vitro human tumor stem cell assay and clinical response to cancer chemotherapy. Cancer Chemother Pharmacol 6: 211–218
7. Salmon SE (1980) Applications of the human tumor stem cell assay to new drug evaluation and screening. In: Salmon SE (ed) Cloning of human tumor stem cells. Liss, New York, pp 291–312
8. Shoemaker RH, Wolpert-DeFilippes MK, Makuch RW et al (1983) Use of the human tumor clonogenic assay for new drug screening. Proc Am Assoc Cancer Res 24: 311
9. Von Hoff DD, Casper J, Bradley E et al (1981) Association between human tumor colony-forming assay results and response of an individual patient's tumor to chemotherapy. Am J Med 70: 1027–1032
10. Carter SK, Selawry O, Slavik M (1975) Phase I clinical trials. Natl Cancer Inst Monograph 45: 75–81

11. Collins JM, Grieshaber CK, Chabner BA (1990) Pharmacologically guided phase I clinical trials based upon preclinical drug development. J Natl Cancer Inst 82: 1321–1326
12. EORTC pharmacokinetics and metabolism group (1987) Pharmacokinetically guided dose-escalation in phase I clinical trials: commentary and proposed guidelines. Eur J Cancer Clin Oncol 23: 1083–1087
13. Gianni L, Vigano L, Surbone A et al (1990) Pharmacology and clinical toxicity of 4-deoxydoxorubicin: an example of successful application of pharmacokinetics to dose escalation in phase I trials. J Natl Cancer Inst 82: 469–477
14. Sass HM (1990) Ethical considerations in phase I clinical trials. Onkologie 13: 85–88
15. Arpaillange P, Dion S, Mathé G (1986) Proposals for ethical standards in therapeutic trials with humans. Drugs Exptl Clin Res 12: 11–19
16. Markman M (1986) The ethical dilemma of phase I clinical trials. CA-A Cancer J Clinicians 36: 367–1369
17. Oates JA (1972) A scientific rationale for choosing patients rather than normal subjects for phase I studies. Clin Pharmacol Ther 13: 808–811
18. Lipsett MB (1982) On the nature and ethics of phase I clinical trials of cancer chemotherapies. JAMA 248: 941–942
19 The President's Commission for the study of ethical problems in medicine and biomedical and behavioral research (1983) US Government Printing Office, Washington pp 41–43
20 Barouki FM, Witter FR, Griffin DE et al (1987) Time course of interferon levels, antiviral state, $2'5'$-oligoadenylate synthetase and side effects in healthy men. J Interferon Res 7: 29–39
21. Decoster G, Rich W, Brown C (in press) Adverse effects of G-CSF. In: Morstyn G, Dexter M (eds) G-CSF in clinical applications. Marcel Dekker, New York
22. Azarnoff DL (1972) Physiologic factors in selecting human volunteers for drug studies. Clin Pharmacol Ther 13: 771–778
23. Cassileth BR, Lusk EJ, Miller DS et al (1982) Attitudes toward clinical trials among patients and the public. JAMA 248: 968–970
24. The President's Commission for the study of ethical problems in medicine and biomedical research (1982) The ethical and legal implication of informed consent in the patient–practitioner relationship. US Government Printing Office, Washington
25. Levine RJ (1988) Informed consent in ethics and regulation of clinical research. In: Levine RJ (ed) Yale University Press, New Haven pp 96–153
26. Novack DH, Plumer R, Smith RL et al (1979) Changes in physician's attitudes toward telling the cancer patient. JAMA 241: 897–900
27. Buchanan AE, Brock DW (1989) Competence and incompetence. In: Buchanan AE, Brock DW (eds) Deciding for others: the ethics of surrogate decision making. Cambridge University Press, pp 17–86
28. Sass HM (1990) Ethical considerations in phase I clinical trials. Onkologie 13: 85–88
29. WHO (1976) Biomedical research: a revised code of ethics. WHO Chronicles 30: 360–362
30. Cordon PV, Dommel FW Jr, Trumble R (1976) Injuries to research subjects: a survey of investigators. N Engl J Med 295: 650–654
31. Capron AM (1989) Human experimentation. In: Veatch RM (ed) Medical ethics. Jones & Barthell, Boston, pp 125–172
32 Levine RJ (1988) Ethics and regulation of clinical research. Yale University Press, New Haven, pp 11–18

APPENDIX: SUMMARY OF RESULTS OF AN OVERVIEW OF PUBLISHED PHASE I TRIALS*

Table 1. Responses and toxic deaths per class of agents

Class	Agent	No. of studies	Total no. of patients	No. of CR+PR	No. of toxic deaths
Antimetabolites	sparfosic acid	5	201	3	0
	carmofur	1	111	3	0
	CB3717	1	99	7	2
	tiazofurin	5	96	1	3
	tegafur	4	94	8	1
	pyrazofurin	2	91	1	0
	azacitidine	4	90	8	2
	IMPY	3	83	1	0
	triciribine	3	77	0	1
	L-alanosine	2	71	0	1
	fludarabine	3	52	1	0
	diglicoaldehyde	1	40	2	0
	thioguanine	1	36	0	0
	doxifluridine	1	30	0	0
	flurocitabine	1	24	3	2
	trimetrexate	1	22	0	0
	ancitabine	1	19	0	0
	FMAU	1	17	0	0
	floxuridine	1	15	0	0
	cytarabine	1	14	2	0
	N6 benzyladenosine	1	14	0	0
	21 agents	*43*	*1296*	*40 (3.1%)*	*12 (0.9%)*
Alkylating	chlorozotocin	5	156	8	0
	pentamethylmelamine	4	128	0	1
	PCNU	3	125	10	0
	ICRF-187	4	121	3	0
	diaziquone	4	115	0	0
	anaxirone	3	111	5	1
	dianhydrogalactitol	3	109	6	0
	nimustine	1	109	0	0
	porfiromycin	1	103	5	1
	teroxirone	3	91	0	1
	semustine	2	82	9	0
	ifosfamide	2	62	3	0
	razoxane	2	53	1	0
	spiromustine	1	38	3	0
	mitozolomide	1	37	3	0
	chromomycin A3	1	26	0	0
	improsulfan HCI	1	25	5	0
	hycanthone mesylate	1	15	0	0

(continued overleaf)

*Reprinted with permission from Decoster et al., *Annals of Oncology*, 1990, 1: 175–181.

Table 1. *(continued)*

Class	Agent	No. of studies	Total no. of patients	No. of CR + PR	No. of toxic deaths
	cyclophosphamide	1	13	1	0
	mafosfamide	1	7	0	0
	20 agents	*44*	*1526*	*62 (4.1%)*	*4 (0.3%)*
Anthracyclines	idarubicin	5	188	7	1
	esorubicin	4	172	8	0
	menogaril	5	137	0	0
	aclarubicin	6	120	5	1
	epirubicin	3	100	6	0
	quelamycin	2	58	10	0
	zorubicin	2	42	2	0
	marcellomycin	2	40	0	0
	daunorubicin	1	40	0	0
	AD-32	1	23	2	0
	carubicin	1	19	0	0
	dactinomycin	1	18	0	0
	pirarubicin	1	15	1	0
	13 agents	*34*	*972*	*41 (4.2%)*	*2 (0.2%)*
Alkaloids	maytansine	5	237	10	4
	homoharringtonine	5	181	2	1
	etoposide	3	128	5	0
	vindesine	2	69	20	0
	vinzolidine	2	66	4	1
	thalicarpine	1	42	0	0
	indicine	1	37	0	0
	elliptinium	1	23	1	0
	8 agents	*20*	*783*	*44 (5.6%)*	*6 (0.8%)*
Platinums	carboplatin	7	227	33	0
	cisplatin	4	130	26	0
	iproplatin	2	65	8	0
	DACCP	1	45	2	0
	4 agents	*14*	*467*	*69 (14.8%)*	*0*
Natural agents	spirogermanium	4	130	4	0
	bruceantin	3	114	0	0
	taxol	4	97	7	0
	3 agents	*11*	*341*	*11 (3.2%)*	*0*
Anthracenes	mitoxantrone	6	144	7	1
	bisantrene	4	114	10	0
	ametantrone	3	55	0	0
	3 agents	*13*	*313*	*17 (5.4%)*	*1 (0.3%)*
Acridines	amsacrine	4	119	9	0
	one agent	*4*	*119*	*9 (7.6%)*	*0*

Table 1. (*continued*)

Class	Agent	No. of studies	Total no. of patients	No. of CR+PR	No. of toxic deaths
Others	anguidine	4	118	0	0
	acivicin	4	117	1	0
	DON	3	79	0	0
	methylformamide	3	71	2	0
	SoAZ	3	71	0	1
	LM985	2	57	0	0
	nafazatrom	1	48	0	0
	Ionidamine	2	46	2	0
	DAU	1	44	0	3
	caracemide	1	42	0	0
	acadazole	1	39	0	0
	neocarzinostatin	1	38	0	0
	trans-N3P3Az2	1	30	3	0
	KW203	1	22	1	2
	14 agents	*28*	*822*	*9 (1.1%)*	*6 (0.7%)*
Total	87 agents	211	6639	302 (4.5%)	31 (0.5%)

CR=complete response, PR=partial response.

Table 2. Response rate per tumor types

Tumor types	Total no. of patients	No. of CR+PR (%)
Gastrointestinal cancer	1330	31 (2.3)
Colorectal	951	14 (1.5)
Gastric	113	6 (5.3)
Others	266	11
Lung cancer	1150	39 (3.4)
Nonsmall cell	710	31 (4.4)
Small cell	67	3 (4.5)
Lung unspecified	373	5
Breast cancer	469	21 (4.5)
Genitourinary cancer	455	27 (5.9)
Renal cell	302	12 (4.0)
Testicular	51	8 (15.7)
Prostatic	45	3 (6.7)
Others	57	4
Malignant melanoma	451	23 (5.1)

(*continued overleaf*)

Table 2. *(continued)*

Tumor types	Total no. of patients	No. of CR+PR (%)
Gynecological cancer	376	47 (12.5)
Ovarian	264	38 (14.4)
Cervical	91	6 (6.6)
Others	21	3
Soft tissue sarcoma	350	13 (3.7)
Head and neck cancer	322	17 (5.3)
Hematologic malignancies	273	47 (17.2)
Non-Hodgkin's lymphoma	142	21 (14.8)
Acute leukemia	63	10 (15.9)
Hodgkin's disease	31	10 (32.3)
Others	37	6
Unknown primary	229	14 (6.1)
Brain tumors	79	9 (11.4)
Liver cancer	39	2 (5.1)
Endocrine tumors	38	5 (13.2)
Multiple primary tumors	12	0
Miscellaneous tumors	472	2

CR = complete response, PR = partial response.

ABOUT THE AUTHORS

Dr Eduard Holdener, after studying medicine at the University of Zurich, Switzerland, went on to postgraduate training in internal medicine. He wrote his thesis on ^{57}Co absorption and secretion in various anemias and he was awarded an MD in 1975 by the University of Basel.

After a Fellowship in clinical and experimental oncology in the USA he returned to Switzerland and worked for many years as senior staff member at the Kantonsspital Luzern and St Gallen, Switzerland, mainly in the in-patient service of onco-hematology. In 1986 he joined the Department of Clinical Research of F. Hoffmann-La Roche Ltd in Basel.

Since January 1991 he has been International Therapeutic Area Head in Oncology in the same department of Roche, and responsible for the worldwide clinical development of all new anticancer drugs.

Genevieve Decoster, after graduating in photography from the Institut National de Radio-Electricité et de Cinématographie of Brussels in 1968, Mrs Decoster worked as a researcher in aerial photography in the field of Roman and industrial archaeology.

In 1979 Mrs Decoster joined the Free University Cancer Center (Institut Jules Bordet) in Brussels as an Administrative Officer and a Clinical Research Assistant for the Department of Internal Medicine Investigational New Drugs Session and for the EORTC Early Clinical Trials Group.

Since 1985 Mrs Decoster has been employed by F. Hoffmann-La Roche Ltd in Basel, where she worked as a Clinical Research Associate at the Department of Clinical Oncology until 1988. In 1989 she joined the "Biotechnology—Growth Factors" Department as a Clinical Trials Specialist and is responsible for the co-ordination and training of clinical research associates and clinical research scientists.

Carol Lim, after studying natural sciences at the University of Cambridge, England, went on to study the mechanism of action of the enzyme thymidylate synthetase and was awarded a PhD in 1971. At this point she joined the Department of Medicine at the University of Manchester, England, and was involved in some of the early clinical work with 1,25- and 24,25-dihydroxycholecalciferol in patients with renal failure metabolic bone disease. In 1979 she moved to the University of Bern, Switzerland, where she studied the factors regulating the kidney hydroxylases of vitamin D.

Her move into the field of oncology occurred in 1983 when she joined the Ludwig Institute for Cancer Research in Bern, where she was involved in in vitro studies with anti-estrogens and retinoids in hormone-dependent breast cancer, and also in the measurement of hormone receptors in tissue from patients participating in the Ludwig Breast Cancer Trials.

Since 1987 Dr Lim has been employed by Hoffmann-La Roche Ltd in Basel, where she is a member of the Department of Clinical Documentation and is responsible for the preparation of clinical regulatory documentation in the area of oncology.

12 "The Uncertainty Principle": Selection of Patients for Cancer Clinical Trials

SALLY STENNING

BACKGROUND AND MOTIVATION

Randomized clinical trials remain the fundamental testing ground for new cancer treatments, and the majority of these treatments will pass through this stage before they can be introduced into clinical practice. The extent to which the results of a trial will be accepted by the clinical community is determined largely by the protocol eligibility criteria, as these determine the characteristics of the patients included in the trial. It is for this reason that the principles underlying patient selection have recently come into question.

The "uncertainty principle" defines the principle under which any patient eligible for a clinical trial should be considered for randomization. It may be defined as follows: in the setting of a randomized clinical trial, if the responsible clinician is *reasonably certain* that one of the treatments under investigation is inappropriate, for whatever reason, for a patient otherwise eligible for the trial, that patient should not be randomized, but treated in the way the responsible clinician feels most appropriate. Only if there is *substantial uncertainty* over the best treatment should the patient be randomized.

Figure 1 gives an example illustrating an important fact inherent in the principle, that the "grey area" of uncertainty will vary from one clinician to another.

The use of the uncertainty principle in clinical trials has been promoted most notably by the Oxford group (Richard Peto, Rory Collins and colleagues). Initially, this was in the field of cardiovascular disease, in particular the ISIS trials of treatment for myocardial infarction. The ISIS trials needed tens of thousands of patients to answer reliably the questions they posed, and it was recognized that, to succeed, all aspects, including the eligibility criteria, had to be simplified. In the second ISIS trial [1] this was achieved partly through having as the fundamental criterion for entry that the responsible physician was uncertain whether, for a particular patient, treatment with streptokinase or with aspirin was indicated.

The edict "only randomize if uncertain" is not a new idea—it has simply been given a name, "the uncertainty principle", which has been used

Introducing New Treatments for Cancer: Practical, Ethical and Legal Problems. Edited by C. J. Williams
© 1992 John Wiley & Sons Ltd

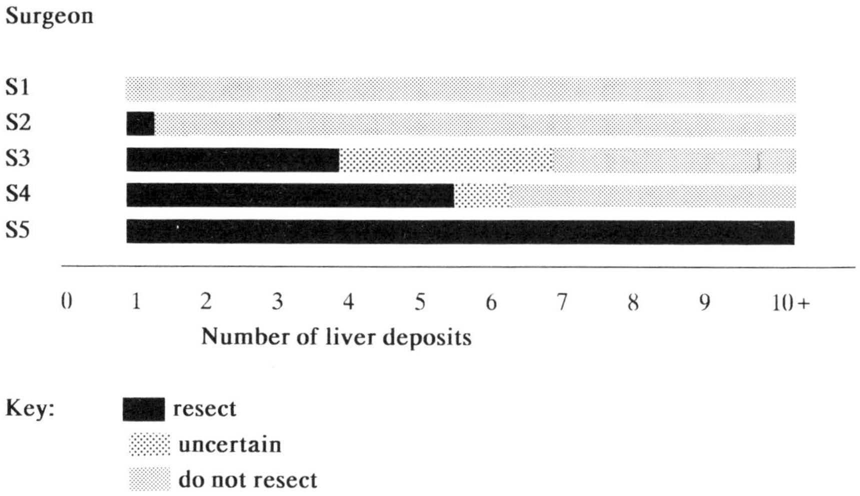
Surgeon
S1
S2
S3
S4
S5
0
1
2
3
4
5
6
7
8
9
10+
Number of liver deposits
Key:
resect
uncertain
do not resect

Figure 1. The figure illustrates the possible areas of uncertainty relating to resection of liver metastases from colorectal cancer. S1 to S5 represent surgeons with different opinions as to resectability of liver metastases. Thus, S1 never resects liver metastases while S2 only considers solitary metastases resectable—neither has a "grey area" of uncertainty. S3 and S4 represent those surgeons who would attempt resection if only a "small" number of deposits were present, but for whom the "resectable range" and the "uncertain range" are different—and are likely to differ from patient to patient for the same surgeon depending on a variety of other considerations including his own previous experience—for example, the general condition of the patient or the number of lobes of the liver involved. Finally, S5 represents a surgeon who would always attempt to resect any number of liver metastases. Thus if one was attempting to define a "resectable range" which incorporated every surgeons' opinion, perhaps for a trial comparing survival in patients with "resectable" disease which is either resected or observed, this would allow entry of patients with any number of liver deposits since this represents the "uncertain range" of the surgical population

as a peg on which to hang many ideas relating to the design and conduct of clinical trials, in particular those aspects which encourage trials to address the areas of uncertainty present in clinical practice. However, these ideas have been extended to oncology only recently, concurrently with the push towards the launch of some large trials in common cancers. The ISIS trials examined simple treatments. The circumstances where eligibility for a clinical cancer trial could be based *solely* on the uncertainty principle are rare. However, the ideas associated with the uncertainty principle as they relate to selection of patients for cancer trials are widely applicable. In fact, this simple and perhaps obvious principle has surprisingly wide repercussions for the design, conduct and interpretation of clinical trials. These repercussions are both ethical and practical. The ethical issues, which relate largely to informed consent, are discussed in more detail elsewhere, and so this chapter will concentrate on the "practical" aspects relating to selection of patients for randomized cancer clinical trials, reviewing the general aims of eligibility criteria in cancer trials, the problems of conduct and interpretation of trials if they do not reflect clinical uncertainty, how and when they may be simplified, and the consequences of this action.

UNCERTAINTY IN CLINICAL TRIALS AND CLINICAL PRACTICE

In designing a clinical trial, two areas of uncertainty in clinical practice are particularly pertinent—first, uncertainty over the potential impact of the treatment, both in the likely treatment effect the trial may demonstrate and in the size of difference which would be considered clinically worthwhile. This area of uncertainty must be addressed in the sample size calculations, taking into account what size of benefit it is *reasonable* to expect (moderate at best) and what the public health impact may be—even small survival improvements in common cancers can have a large public health impact.

The second area of uncertainty relates to the type of patient who might be considered for the treatments under examination. This area is normally addressed through the eligibility criteria listed in the trial protocol. Figure 2 gives a typical example, listing the inclusion and exclusion criteria for the Cancer Research Campaign (CRC) hepatic artery pump trial—a randomized trial comparing survival and quality of life in patients with colorectal hepatic metastases treated by continuous intrahepatic artery 5-fluoro-2-deoxyuridine (FUDR) with that of patients receiving conventional symptomatic treatment. The eligibility and ineligibility criteria listed illustrate the two principal objectives of patient selection criteria:

(1) to define patients fit to receive any of the treatments under study;
(2) to define a similar group of patients thought likely to respond to treatment in a similar way.

The first condition is often reflected in requirements for particular levels of haematological function and for the absence of certain previous or concomitant diseases. Regarding the second condition, Begg and Engstrom [2] argue that the requirement for patients to be as similar as possible results largely from an outdated and, in the field of oncology, inappropriate aim: that of approximating as far as possible the "ideal experiment", the basic requirement for which is the homogeneous experimental unit. This is simply impossible in clinical experimentation. Even the most restrictive eligibility criteria will not produce a group of patients so alike that the only explanation for one patient living longer than another is that they received treatment A rather than treatment B.

Eligibility criteria

1. Informed consent
2. Histological confirmation of:
   (a) primary colorectal carcinoma
   (b) liver metastasis (by fine needle aspiration)
3. No evidence of residual disease outside the liver on colonoscopy or barium enema, chest X-ray, CT scan of abdomen and pelvis
4. Measurable liver disease on liver CT scan, ultrasound or isotope scan
5. Karnofsky performance status >60
6. Haematological requirements: WBC >4000 mm^3,
                                                     platelet count $>100\,000$ mm^3
7. Normal bilirubin

Ineligibility criteria

1. Age >70 years
2. Severe psychiatric, emotional or neurological disturbances
3. Previous liver irradiation
4. Previous chemotherapy
5. $>60\%$ liver involvement assessed by CT scan, ultrasound, or isotope scan
6. Disease limited to one lobe of the liver which is deemed surgically resectable
7. Previous history of other malignant cancer, except squamous cell skin cancer
8. Gross ascites
9. Prothrombin time 70% or evidence of other bleeding disorders that would preclude insertion of intra-arterial catheter

Figure 2. Cancer Research Campaign Hepatic Artery Pump Trial

WHAT PROBLEMS ARE ASSOCIATED WITH RESTRICTIVE ELIGIBILITY CRITERIA?

One basic problem is that the results of clinical trials may be difficult to interpret and to act upon if patient selection criteria do not reflect normal clinical practice and decision-making procedures on treatment policy.

The principal aims of a clinical trial are often said to be:

(1) ask a good question;
(2) answer it reliably.

Perhaps to this should be added:

(3) influence clinical practice.

There are many reasons why the results of a clinical trial may not influence clinical practice. However, two points relate directly to the selection of patients for trials:

1. If eligibility criteria are too restrictive, the trial population may represent only a small proportion of the patients to whom the results are implicitly intended to be extrapolated

Where this is the case, clinicians may ignore them as being irrelevant to their typical patient, or accept them and extrapolate them to other situations, possibly without good evidence.

For example, many trials of therapy for colorectal cancer will include upper age limits. In trying to conduct a "clean" trial, and to this end setting the limit such that it will preclude entry to patients with too great a chance of dying from an intercurrent condition, it would be easy to eliminate a large proportion of patients with colorectal cancer. An upper limit of 70 years would exclude over a third of patients with the disease, and would give no information on treatment tolerance in the older patient, for example.

A similar problem can arise with the haematological function requirements included in protocols investigating potentially toxic chemotherapy. These are intended to prevent delivery of standard doses of therapy to patients likely to be intolerant to these. Guidelines are of course essential, particularly if the protocol is likely to be applied to patients in centres where there is little or no experience with the regimen concerned. But again, care should be taken not to exclude in this way a large proportion of patients who would be considered for chemotherapy *outside* of the trial—for example, an ongoing Medical Research Council trial of neo-adjuvant chemotherapy in locally advanced bladder cancer, in which patients are randomized to chemotherapy (with cisplatin, methotrexate and vinblastine) or no chemotherapy following definitive local therapy. The protocol requires that the patient's glomerular filtration rate should be at least 60 ml/min in order that he or she may tolerate the chemotherapy being given, in particular the cisplatin which is to be given at a dose of $100 \, mg/m^2$. Some time after the launch of the trial, it was found that many patients were being excluded because of renal function requirements not being fulfilled. However, many of these patients were actually receiving chemotherapy outside of the trial, albeit at lower doses than those specified in the protocol, for example cisplatin doses of $70 \, mg/m^2$. An alternative trial design might include the option of allowing patients with reduced renal function to be randomized, but receiving lower drug doses, rather than excluding them altogether.

2. If eligibility criteria demand investigations not available in many hospitals

One simple fact is that a long list of inclusion and exclusion criteria are off-putting; they take time to read and to assess with respect to each individual patient. But even the shortest list of inclusion criteria can preclude a clinician's participation in a trial if it demands an investigation not available to him. If it is not available to the majority of clinicians, it is therefore not presently being used in the routine management of the majority of patients, and should perhaps not therefore be a mandatory investigation. Even if, in addition to the therapeutic question, the trial is planned to investigate a diagnostic tool or potential prognostic factor, these can often be assessed in a subgroup of patients taken from centres with the necessary facilities.

It is known that, currently, patients in clinical trials represent a very small proportion of the whole population of patients with cancer. This was quantified in a US Veterans Administration Cooperative Group Trial of warfarin anticoagulant therapy incorporating several tumour sites [3], in which efforts were made to identify all potentially eligible patients in the contributing centres. Only 16% of patients screened actually entered the study, the majority of exclusions being related to technical ineligibility for the protocol. In just 15% of cases was failure to enter the study related to physician or patient preference for an alternative (including no) treatment. A review of cancer trials in the UK [4] suggested that, at best, 5–10% of patients enter trials. The figures are highest for those treated in specialized centres (e.g. leukaemia, osteosarcoma), and lowest for the commonest cancers—it was estimated that only 1% of lung cancer patients and 2% of colorectal cancer patients entered randomized trials.

It is often argued that if trial patients represent such a small proportion of the total, the results of such trials cannot help clinicians decide on the appropriate treatment for an individual patient. Thus there may be a case for relaxing eligibility criteria, at least to the extent that they reflect clinical practice to a greater degree than at present.

HOW FAR CAN ELIGIBILITY CRITERIA BE REDUCED?

Each eligibility criterion may be classified as a characteristic of the host or of the tumour. Within each of these categories it is possible to identify characteristics which, it may be argued, are over-restrictive.

Taking first the host characteristics, any variable that is measured on a continuous scale (such as age or white blood count) into which cut-offs are introduced can be problematic. For example, upper age limits are commonly included—but different trials of precisely the same disease often choose different limits, reflecting the fact that there is no clear dividing line such that patients below a certain age will be fit enough to receive treatment and those above will not. Every clinician's range of uncertainty will differ; within the protocol eligibility criteria, some clinicians will restrict still further the age range of patients they would include in a trial while others would consider entering a much wider range than the protocol allows. It can be argued that upper age limits should be dropped altogether, with the assumption that the aims of this restriction should be covered by the requirement that all patients should be fit to receive any of the treatments they may be allocated. Other continuous variables, such as blood counts and renal function, are much more difficult to dismiss. In chemotherapy trials they are important, but very careful consideration should be given to what the limits should be, and how a patient who is a borderline exclusion would be treated outside of the trial.

Figure 2 may be used to illustrate an argument for relaxation of a particular criteria relating to tumour characteristics. In the CRC hepatic artery pump trial, evidence of exclusion of residual disease outside the liver is required through colonoscopy or barium enema, together with chest X-ray and computed tomography (CT) scans of the abdomen and pelvis. Contrast this with the eligibility criteria for another randomized trial of chemotherapy for hepatic metastases from colorectal cancer. Figure 3 lists the eligibility criteria for a (proposed) United Kingdom Co-ordinating Committee on Cancer Research (UKCCCR) trial of chemotherapy for patients with apparently complete resection of liver metastases, and no evidence of disease outside the pelvis. The UKCCCR trial asks for "reasonable exclusion of extrahepatic metastases and local recurrence". Such an approach means that each centre would use their standard methods of excluding extrahepatic disease, and none would be excluded because of their inability to carry out abdominal CT scans, for example. Although the trials in Figures 2 and 3 are aimed at slightly different populations, both have survival as their principal end-point. It should not therefore be necessary for the CRC trial to exclude patients without "measurable liver disease on CT scan, ultrasound or isotope scan" since this is only essential if tumour response is a principal end-point. The design of the UKCCCR trial has taken into account difficulties of recruitment of trials like the first in many ways, not least in the minimization of eligibility criteria and pre-randomization requirements.

Trials in which the eligibility criteria permit entry of any patient who would potentially be considered for the treatments under investigation would be the ideal. Taking this to an extreme, the simplest trial would be one in which the uncertainty principle was the only eligibility criteria. That is, that any patient with the disease in question would be eligible for the trial if there is no definite indication or contraindication to either treatment being compared. It should be emphasized that the circumstances where such an approach is possible are fairly rare in the field of cancer chemotherapy. Any protocol which involves cytotoxic chemotherapy should include at the very least guidelines on the type of patient who may not be suitable for treatment.

Eligibility criteria

1. Informed consent
2. Apparently complete resection of liver metastasis following curative surgery for primary colorectal cancer
3. Patient fit for treatment if allocated
4. Extrahepatic metastases and local recurrence reasonably excluded

Figure 3. Proposed UKCCCR trial of resection versus resection plus adjuvant immunochemotherapy

However, the circumstances do exist. They coincide with the circumstances under which large trials of simple treatments for common cancers (which have potentially large public health impact even if the survival advantage demonstrable is small) are possible. The UKCCCR AXIS trial of adjuvant therapy for colorectal cancer is one such example. In this ongoing trial patients with colonic or rectal cancer are randomized to intrahepatic chemotherapy (5-fluorouracil) or no chemotherapy, with an additional randomization to perioperative radiotherapy or no radiotherapy for rectal cancer patients. This is one of the first cancer trials to base eligibility almost exclusively on "the uncertainty principle". This was possible because the chemotherapy—which is given directly into the portal vein for seven days postoperatively—is relatively non-toxic. There was also no clear evidence for alternative treatment strategies for different subgroups—Dukes stage for example—although the opinions of the participating clinicians as to the need for adjuvant therapy after surgery for Dukes stage A, B, C and D tumours vary quite considerably. The section on eligibility from the protocol reads as follows:

> *Trial eligibility is determined by participants, not by the protocol.* Views of British surgeons on the likely value of adjuvant therapy are widely divergent. Some surgeons are convinced of the value of radiotherapy in advanced rectal cancer, but others are uncertain. Some surgeons are convinced that chemotherapy would be an inappropriate treatment for a Dukes A tumour—others are not so sure. Because of these very heterogeneous opinions, the suitability of a particular patient for entry into AXIS is not dictated by a rigid protocol but will be at the discretion of the responsible clinician. Patients are eligible for the trial if, and only if, the responsible clinician is *uncertain* about whether or not to treat a particular patient with chemotherapy and/or with radiotherapy. Depending on the views of the local clinician, a very wide range of patients may be eligible, perhaps including many whose tumour is limited to the bowel wall, many whose tumour is locally advanced and even some where there are already overt metastases in the liver. While this might at first seem to weaken the trial by not defining precisely which patients are eligible, it is, curiously, the converse that is true. This is because—given sufficient numbers—a wide range of patients will not only answer the question of *whether* treatment is of benefit but also, if it is of benefit, may help identify *which* type of patient is likely to benefit most.

The eligibility criteria are given in Figure 4. Such entry criteria will result in a wide range of patients being entered, making it easier to generalize the results to a wide population. But, hopefully, the increase in entry is twofold: by limiting the entry criteria, the number of mandatory pre-randomization investigations are limited, and thus the number of surgeons "technically" unable to participate is reduced. The trial is *not* designed to address specific questions such as the value of preoperative radiotherapy in Dukes stage C rectal tumours. The principal aim is to randomize sufficiently large numbers of patients to enable reliable estimation of the overall survival impact of

5-fluorouracil in colorectal cancer, and of perioperative radiotherapy in rectal cancer, and as such will provide an estimate of the benefit the "average patient" will receive.

In putting forward the argument that eligibility criteria for clinical trials should more readily reflect the uncertainty in clinical practice, particularly uncertainty over the differential effects of treatment in different subgroups of patients, it is necessary to accept the hypothesis that unexpected interactions between treatment and subgroups of patients are unlikely [5]. To explain this in more detail, given a number of estimates of treatment effect, perhaps in different subgroups of patients entered into a trial, they would be said to differ *qualitatively* if in some subgroups treatment was beneficial, and others it was harmful. If the results all suggested a treatment effect in the same direction but of different sizes they would be said to differ not qualitatively but *quantitatively*. An argument in favour of the unrestrictive trial is that the *direction* of treatment difference is likely to be the same across all subgroups of patients, even though the size of the difference is likely to vary. That is, *quantitative* differences in treatment effects in subpopulations are likely: *unexpected qualitative* differences are very unlikely. Thus if due allowance is made for potentially smaller effects in some groups in the sample size calculations, this should not affect the ability of the trial to detect an overall improvement in survival which is clinically important.

It is possible to pinpoint cases where a hypothesis of different treatment effects in recognizable patient groups has later been questioned. For example, prior to the Early Breast Cancer Trialists Co-operative Group (EBCTCG) overview of treatment for early breast cancer, it was quite widely considered that patients with early breast cancer who were oestrogen receptor (ER) negative would not benefit from tamoxifen. The eligibility criteria of many tamoxifen trials included in the overview excluded ER-negative patients. However, sufficient patient numbers were available from those trials in which ER status was not a selection criteria to demonstrate that the benefit to tamoxifen in ER-negative patients was both statistically significantly greater than zero, and also not significantly different from the size of effect demonstrated in the ER-positive patients. Had the assumption that

Eligibility criteria

1. Suspected carcinoma of colon or rectum
2. Patient fit* for XRT or 5-FU if allocated
3. The surgeon is uncertain whether adjuvant treatment is indicated

*Contraindications to XRT or 5-FU are specified not by the protocol but by the responsible physician, and might include: intra-abdominal sepsis, insulin-dependent diabetes, high blood urea, pregnancy, marked hepatic impairment (contact clinical coordinator or see product data sheet if unsure).

Figure 4. UKCCCR AXIS trial of adjuvant therapy for colorectal cancer

ER-negative women would not benefit led to no such women being entered into tamoxifen trials, this would never have been disproved.

Buyse [6] demonstrates that, where there is no a priori reason to believe that the magnitude of treatment effect is different in different subgroups, the best strategy from a statistical standpoint is to include all available patients in the trial. The efficiency of a "broad" trial compared to a restrictive trial can be quantified in terms of the relative duration of the trial—that is, the time taken to detect the existing treatment effect with a smaller number of relatively homogeneous patients compared with the time if a larger number of more heterogeneous patients are included. The efficiency then depends on the treatment effect in the additional subgroup which may be included in the trial, and the proportion of the total patients it represents. If the true treatment effect in this subgroup is similar to the rest of the trial patients, the benefit to its inclusion can be quite considerable, and the benefit increases as the proportion of the total patients represented by the subgroup increases. It follows that the only circumstances where the restricted trial would be more efficient are where the true treatment benefit in the subgroup is much less than in the main group, and where the subgroup would represent a very small proportion of the total patients. Even here, the potential *decrease* in the efficiency of the broad trial is at most twofold, yet under the best circumstances the *increase* can be up to fourfold.

There are of course particular circumstances where it is important to recognize different groups of patients within a particular tumour type. For example, it would not be appropriate to include all patients with metastatic testicular teratoma in a common protocol, since strong prognostic factors have been identified to select patients with a very good prognosis (long-term survival approaching 95%) from those with a much poorer prognosis (60% long-term survival). Very different treatment strategies are appropriate for these two groups. In the former, trials addressing ways to maintain treatment efficacy while attempting to reduce the toxicity of the best standard treatment are in progress, whilst in the latter group the principal aim of current trials is to improve survival rates through more aggressive, intensive chemotherapy in comparison with the best available combinations.

BENEFITS AND COSTS OF RELAXING ELIGIBILITY CRITERIA

Any lessening of the restrictions on patient entry to a trial will of course increase the range of patients included. This has both advantages and disadvantages. If trials are sufficiently large, the heterogeneity of population and response resulting may in fact be useful, giving some indication of the impact of treatment on different subgroups of the population. This may be more useful than extrapolating results to areas of the patient population which were not included in the trial at all.

In the MRC bladder cancer trial discussed earlier, a counter-argument to the inclusion of patients with impaired renal function with a lower dose of cisplatin is that there may be dose–response relationship with cisplatin. If this is true, the inclusion of patients receiving lower doses may mean that the overall trial size must be increased to compensate for the possible dilution of treatment effect in the whole randomized group. On the other hand, it can be argued that the results of the trial as originally designed will be extrapolated to "ineligible" patients anyway, and it would be better to expand the trial and thus have some hard data on which to base the treatment of such patients.

A similar problem potentially arises with the proposed UKCCCR liver metastases trial in comparison with the CRC. The latter's more stringent requirement for exclusion of extrahepatic metastases is likely to result in a "cleaner" group of patients being entered into this trial than the UKCCCR trial. This in turn may mean that the CRC trial would be able to detect a smaller treatment difference than the UKCCCR trial *if the total number of patients randomized into the two trials is the same*. This is a crucial point. "Simple" trials have to be larger to cope with the increase in random error inherent in a heterogeneous population of patients. The hope is that by reducing the hurdles to participation patient entry will be so greatly increased as to more than compensate for any dilution of treatment effect. Large trials based on minimal entry criteria are designed to provide very reliable evidence of the overall benefit the "average" patient can expect. While this does not provide a "prescription" for any specific patient, the estimate of the overall treatment effect in the whole trial population is likely to be much more reliable than any estimate of treatment effect in a smaller, but more homogeneous subgroup, and as such should be a much better figure on which to base treatment policy for an individual patient.

CONCLUSIONS

In conclusion, the uncertainty principle is one which embodies a range of concepts related to the design and conduct of clinical trials. It is a basic, if often unwritten, criterion for randomization of any patient into any trial. In some circumstances it may be the only criterion necessary. However, the associated ideas can be extended to the majority of trials—of any size or design—such that eligibility criteria can often sensibly be made less restrictive and better able to address uncertainty in clinical practice. It is only by these means that clinical trials will succeed and have the potential to influence clinical practice, rather than simply being an end in themselves.

REFERENCES

1. ISIS-2 Collaborative Group (1988) Randomised trial of intravenous streptokinase, oral aspirin, both, or neither among 17,187 cases of suspected acute myocardial infarction: ISIS-2. Lancet, 13th August: 349–360
2. Begg CB, Engstrom PF (1987) Eligibility and extrapolation in cancer clinical trials. J Clin Oncol 5: 962–968
3. Martin JF, Henderson WG, Zacharaski LR et al (1984) Accrual of patients into a multihospital cancer clinical trial and its implications on planning future studies. Am J Clin Oncol 7: 173–182
4. Tate HC, Rawlinson JB, Freedman LS (1979) Randomised comparative studies in the treatment of cancer in the United Kingdom: room for improvement? Lancet, 22nd September: 623–625
5. Peto R (1987) Why do we need systematic overviews of randomized trials? Statist Med 6: 233–240
6. Buyse ME (1990) The case for loose inclusion criteria in clinical trials. Acta Chir Belg 90: 129–131

ABOUT THE AUTHOR

Sally Stenning has worked as a statistician for the Medical Research Council (MRC) for 5 years, joining the Cancer Trials Office in Cambridge in 1986.

Her main area of work has been the design, coordination and analysis of over 30 of the clinical trials run by the MRC's Cancer Therapy Committee. She has an interest in several tumour types, being a member of the MRC's Working Parties on Brain Tumours, Testicular Tumours, Rectal Cancer and Advanced Colorectal Cancer, and the Steering Group of AXIS Colorectal Cancer trial, run under the auspices of the United Kingdom Coordinating Committee on Cancer Research. In addition, she acts as a consultant statistician to the clinicians and scientists of the MRC Clinical Oncology and Radiotherapeutics Unit, and is a member of the recently formed panel of statistical referees for *The Lancet*.

13 Large-Scale Studies

ROBERT SOUHAMI

There is a growing awareness among oncologists of the increasing difficulties in the assessment of the value of new cancer treatments. As will be seen, the problems arise fundamentally from cancer biology and the relative insensitivity to treatment of many common tumours. The solutions demand reappraisal of our organizational, methodological and ethical approach to clinical trials [1].

Once a new drug or treatment has been found to produce responses in a tumour type, it is often tested alone or in combination with other agents (Chapter 10). This process does not usually involve a randomized comparison of the new drug, or drug combination, with other well-established treatments (although there is a great deal to be said for such controlled comparisons at an early stage). Rather there is a process of exploration of the new drug using a variety of drug schedules in different categories of patients. Finally a general consensus emerges of the effectiveness of the new agent and the appropriate dose range and schedule of administration. At this stage randomized comparisons may be made in which the tumour response to a drug combination containing the new agent is then compared with another combination or even the best single agent. These studies have two purposes. The first is that of finding the most effective treatment for advanced disease. The second, in some cancers, is to identify treatments which might be effective in increasing the cure rate when used as an adjuvant to surgery or radiotherapy.

In the period from 1970 to 1980 cytotoxic drugs were used with increasing intensity in a variety of tumours. Spectacular increases in response rate and, subsequently, in cure rate were found in highly chemosensitive tumours such as Hodgkin's disease, non-Hodgkin's lymphoma, testicular teratoma and some childhood tumours. These improvements were so large that they were observed with confidence without the need for controlled comparison against no treatment or single-agent therapy. Somewhat later, encouraged by these successes, oncologists began to use combination chemotherapy as treatment for the much more common solid tumours of adults. An increase in response rate was usually observed compared with single-agent treatment although these responses were, in general, less complete and less durable than for the less common but more sensitive cancers. Very little is known of the cellular basis which results in some tumours being sensitive to treatment and others not. A remarkable, fairly consistent, yet unexplained

Introducing New Treatments for Cancer: Practical, Ethical and Legal Problems. Edited by C. J. Williams
© 1992 John Wiley & Sons Ltd

fact of chemotherapy is that chemosensitivity is a property of tumours—both of tumour types and of the same tumour in different individuals—rather than of drugs. When a new drug is introduced, even when it is a new class of chemical structure, it will usually prove to have activity against tumours (such as lymphomas, testicular cancers) which show sensitivity to established drugs and have less activity against common, more resistant tumours (such as pancreatic and non-small cell lung cancer).

Two consequences follow. The first is that new drugs or drug combinations are now unlikely to produce dramatic improvements in response rate or survival in sensitive tumour types (since existing drugs are already relatively effective). The second is that both new and existing drugs will produce very small differences in response and survival in the relatively resistant tumours.

To some extent oncologists have been over-optimistic in the past about the likely differences in survival when drug combinations are compared in advanced disease and when systemic treatments are used as adjuvants to local therapy. As we shall see this has led to serious defects in methodology which have greatly impeded the efficiency of assessment of treatment. Conversely, the failure to observe substantial differences in survival has sometimes led to an inappropriate pessimism. The difficulties and frustrations of this aspect of clinical research in cancer treatment can be illustrated by consideration of four tumours: the chemotherapy of operable breast cancer, chemotherapy in inoperable non-small-cell lung cancer, the treatment of advanced Hodgkin's disease and the treatment of Ewing's sarcoma.

ADJUVANT CHEMOTHERAPY IN OPERABLE BREAST CANCER

It has long been apparent that advanced, metastatic breast cancer occasionally responded to cytotoxic drugs. Temporary regressions were found with cyclophosphamide and other alkylating agents, antimetabolites such as methotrexate and anthracyclines such as doxorubicin, soon after these drugs were introduced into clinical practice. Drug combinations were developed in which responses could be achieved in 50–70% of patients with advanced disease. One such combination is cyclophosphamide (usually given orally), methotrexate and 5-fluorouracil (a regimen known as CMF). This treatment has some toxicity but is reasonably well tolerated. Very few tumours respond completely, and most responses are maintained for less than a year.

The next and logical step was to pose the question, would the use of CMF (or equivalent regimen) in patients who had had a mastectomy, but who were at high risk of developing clinically apparent metastases, delay or prevent recurrence and improve survival? Women at such high risk could be identified relatively easily when mastectomy was performed. They were those who had involvement of axillary nodes. Only about 60% of these patients would be expected to be alive at five years after operation (because clinically inapparent metastases were present at the time of surgery).

Accordingly trials were started in which such women were randomly allocated into two groups—either to receive or not receive CMF postoperatively. At the time when these trials were started in the early 1970s several problems in design went unnoticed or the implications were not clearly understood:

(1) Most of the trials were started with no idea of what size of difference in survival could be expected. The responses achieved in metastatic disease could clearly not give any indication of survival benefit when used as an adjuvant since the relationship between the response rate with clinically apparent metastases and the effect on subclinical metastases was not known. Indeed one possible outcome was that no benefit at all might result from the use of adjuvant chemotherapy, otherwise the comparison with no treatment would not have been ethical. This uncertainty exists whenever chemotherapy is introduced as an adjuvant to local treatment.

(2) The trials did not attempt to define what size of difference would be regarded as of importance clinically. This question is only now receiving attention. If we ask what difference in survival, if known with certainty, would influence our practice the answer will depend on the current treatment results without adjuvant treatment, and on the toxicity and the practicability of the treatment. A 5–8% improvement in survival (from 60% to 65–68%) at five years would be regarded as well worthwhile with a non-toxic, oral treatment such as tamoxifen, but might be regarded as less compelling if obtained by a toxic chemotherapy regimen. The difficulty is that we cannot be sure what survival differences will influence general attitudes and thus be important. Furthermore these attitudes will not be the same in different cultures, and within the various branches of the medical profession. They will be different for patients and doctors (patients usually being less conservative) and will change with time and with experience of the treatment in question. Suffice it to say that, with the realization that survival improvements of 5–8% are what is attainable with chemotherapy, there has been a general agreement that such improvements are of value in pre-menopausal women with stage II breast cancer (see below).

(3) There was little appreciation of the size of trials necessary to be sure that small differences, if present, would be detected [2]. Since trials were started with no prior definition of what was likely to be observed, or what differences would be worthwhile, it is hardly surprising that the majority of studies were carried out in ignorance of the necessary size required. Furthermore there was (and is) a general level of ignorance about the statistical imperatives.

The fact is that differences of 5% (from 60% to 65%) can only be reliably detected by trials that contain thousands of patients. The reason for this is

176

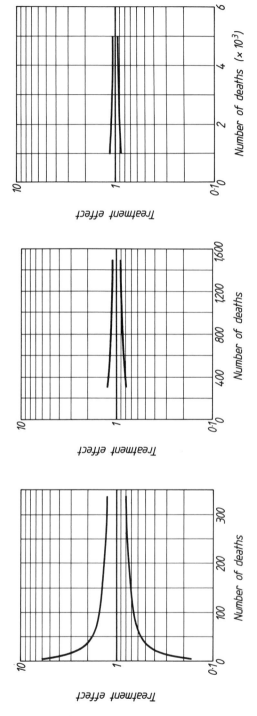

Figure 1. The relationship between number of deaths and the 95% confidence intervals of an odds ratio. For explanation see text

shown in Figure 1. This figure shows how the width of the 95% confidence interval for an odds ratio decreases with the increasing number of deaths observed in the study. The x-axis represents an odds ratio of unity which corresponds to the two treatments being compared, having equal efficacy. Points above the line indicate an advantage to treatment A (say), and points above the confidence contour indicate a statistically significant result in favour of A. The corresponding points below the x-axis favour treatment B. The width of the confidence interval is wide for very small numbers of deaths (below 200) but becomes smaller as numbers increase. It is only when the numbers of deaths reach 5000 or more that we can be reasonably sure that a survival advantage of 5–10% will be reflected in an odds ratio outside the "funnel". The adjuvant trials were from 10 to 30 times too small to detect this. The results of the large numbers of studies were confusing and appeared to show at random small benefits, significant benefits or no benefit at all. An overview analysis (Chapter 26) was able to show a survival advantage of this magnitude.

What future questions could now be posed for the adjuvant chemotherapy of breast cancer? If a 7% improvement in five-year survival is obtained with CMF in pre-menopausal women in stage II breast cancer, would there not be a chance of a bigger benefit with more active (and more toxic) chemotherapy? Alternatively, could we achieve the same benefit with less treatment?

In the overview analysis referred to above, there was no suggestion that the addition of drugs to the CMF regimen improved results, but there were too few patients in randomized studies of this kind to be sure. Although, in metastatic breast cancer, response rates higher than those achieved with CMF can be obtained with other drug regimens (such as those containing doxorubicin), it is not known how large a difference in response, above that obtained with CMF, would be needed before there was a realistic expectation that results would be improved in an adjuvant trial. Patients who respond to the new regimen will include those who would have responded to CMF. The others, who respond to the new regimen but who did not respond to CMF, are likely to have less chemosensitive tumours and the responses to be shorter lived. This is reflected in the fact that when regimens produce higher response rates in advanced disease they seldom result in significant prolongation in survival. For this reason randomized comparisons between chemotherapy regimens *in advanced disease* should be designed to look for large differences in response rate and significant improvements in survival, if the intention is to identify regimens which might improve the results currently obtained with CMF in *adjuvant* chemotherapy. Such improvements are likely to be very small in degree (possibly a change from 7% to 10%) and will therefore be detected only in very large studies. On the other hand, results similar to those currently obtained with CMF might be achieved with less chemotherapy thereby reducing the acute, and possibly long-term, toxicity of chemotherapy treatment. Trials of this kind, where equivalence is the end-point, will have to define the clinical difference which can be ignored and be of an appropriate size. It might be agreed, for example, that a difference less than 2% could be accepted (a decrease in improvement in survival from 7% to 5%). It is clear that such trials will need to be very large indeed, and the design of these trials will need to be very flexible in order to encourage wide participation. For example, if the question is the length of adjuvant chemotherapy required in stage II breast cancer a trial might allow several different chemotherapy combinations (to satisfy the differing points of view of participants), so long as the randomization was between "short" and "long". Insistence on a single regimen is unnecessary in studies of this kind.

The example of breast cancer illustrates general principles in trials of adjuvant treatment. First, that in common cancers survival benefits are likely to be small. Second, that while small improvement in survival due to chemotherapy (compared with no treatment) can be detected if trials are designed and executed appropriately (see below), studies where new adjuvant regimens are compared to existing regimens will be seeking to detect even smaller differences and will need to be larger still.

CHEMOTHERAPY FOR INOPERABLE NON-SMALL-CELL LUNG CANCER

Approximately 50% of patients with non-small-cell lung carcinoma (NSCLC) have no detectable metastases at presentation and about 15–20% of all patients can be considered for surgical resection. There remains 30–35% of patients with apparently localized but inoperable intrathoracic disease in whom radiotherapy is usually the standard treatment. In recent years combination chemotherapy regimens have been devised which are capable of producing responses in 50–70% of such patients. The prognosis with radiotherapy alone is only 10% survival at three years. It is reasonable to suggest that the addition of chemotherapy to radiation might improve survival.

Several trials of 100–250 patients have addressed the question of the value of chemotherapy in addition to radiation. Most have failed to show an advantage for less effective chemotherapy, and one, with only 150 patients, has suggested improved median survival. The chemotherapy and radiotherapy are both quite toxic, and the patients are often (but not always) elderly with chronic lung disease due to smoking. There are, however, 30 000 cases of NSCLC yearly in the UK so that there are potentially 8000–10 000 patients in the above category. A doubling of survival (from 7% to 14%) would save 600–800 lives annually (and many more in the world as a whole) although the three-year figure will not represent cure rate since relapse may occur later.

Would such an improvement be worthwhile? Once again we have only an imprecise idea of what would influence practice generally, but the certain knowledge of benefit would be likely to have an impact on the management of younger patients. The negative results in previous studies and the one positive study can be explained either by a genuine lack of effect of some drug regimens or, more plausibly, by the considerable likelihood of being unable to detect differences with the size of trial which has been so far employed.

THE CHEMOTHERAPY OF ADVANCED HODGKIN'S DISEASE

Although an uncommon cancer, the spectacular success of combination cytotoxic chemotherapy in advanced Hodgkin's disease has led to a large number of treatment trials of differing combinations of drugs in an attempt to increase the cure rate. At present the long-term results of the MOPP chemotherapy regimen indicate that about 45% of patients may be relapse free at ten or more years and may be cured. No comparable follow-up data exist for more recent regimens. MOPP will produce complete regression in 65% of cases and a partial response in another 25%. The overall response rate with other more intensive regimens approaches 100% but, as with breast cancer, this will include cases whose tumours are less sensitive and where the responses will be less durable.

To detect, with certainty, an improvement of survival from 45% to 55% with new regimens will require several thousand patients in a randomized trial of MOPP against the new treatment. Claims for such improvements have been made on the basis of small trials where the point estimate of the survival and the associated *p*-value suggests improvement but where the 95% confidence intervals are overlapping.

Only about 1000 such cases are eligible for entry into studies in the UK each year. The problem is then one which cannot be solved within national boundaries. Failure to grapple with the necessary organizational arrangements has meant that the optimum chemotherapy treatment of advanced Hodgkin's disease has remained unresolved for over a decade.

CHEMOTHERAPY OF EWING'S SARCOMA

The problem of treatment trials in advanced Hodgkin's disease is demonstrated even more dramatically in Ewing's sarcoma. Only 80–100 cases occur each year in the UK. Of these 45–60% are large tumours where the prognosis is known to be poor (30–40% cure rate) in spite of intensive chemotherapy to which the tumour is almost always initially sensitive. The smaller tumours are cured in over 70% of cases. Systemic metastasis and local recurrence are the major reasons for treatment failure.

Treatment trials, in which randomized comparisons between therapies are made, are rare and have only been carried out by the Intergroup Ewing's Sarcoma Study (IESS) in the USA. Elsewhere in the USA and in Europe, smaller national groups and even single centres have published the results of small-scale, non-randomized studies in which retrospective subgroup and regression analyses have been used in an attempt to determine which treatment policies are likely to be most effective in which group of patients. The limitations of these procedures are well known, with the ever-present likelihood of demonstrating spurious associations which are due to chance effects.

Such a rare tumour means that the 10–15% improvements in survival which may be possible at the present time (without the need to develop new drugs) will be demonstrated only by trials with international collaboration.

These foregoing examples lead inevitably to consideration of how we might make further progress in the years ahead. There are practical steps which those responsible for cancer treatment trials in the UK are now taking as a result of a more realistic assessment of likely benefits. The key to these developments lies in collaboration in clinical trials regionally, nationally and internationally. The focus of attention must be on agreement on the nature of the important unanswered questions, the design of collaborative studies in a manner which encourages participation, and on ways to increase recruitment of patients into these trials. Collaborations of this kind are possible but also require agreement on ethical issues and on matters such as interim analyses, authorship and funding.

REGIONAL COLLABORATIVE GROUPS

As in other countries there are geographical areas in the UK which, although relatively small, contain large populations (in excess of 2–3 million). The hospitals which serve populations of this size may choose to collaborate in cancer trials. The advantages of these regional collaborative groups is that they have a sense of identity, that participants can meet regularly and be involved at all stages of planning the studies, and that the results and publications are seen to bring credit to the participants. For phase II studies (Chapter 10) and non-randomized studies of combination treatment, such collaborative groups are an undisputed asset since studies can be carried out quickly. The problem for this level of collaboration lies in recognizing the point at which the attempt to limit participation to a group of this size becomes counter-productive. In some cancers with a very high death rate (such as small-cell lung cancer) randomized trials of treatment can be carried out with 500–700 patients [1], with a good chance of detecting 10% differences in survival at, say, two years.

Differences smaller than this, in this disease, would probably not be considered to be clinically interesting. For reasons discussed earlier, this would be an inadequate trial size in localized breast cancer or in resectable colorectal cancer and probably in Hodgkin's disease. By attempting studies of this size in these latter diseases small groups begin to undermine the purpose of their activity. The trial proceeds slowly and enthusiasm starts to decline; the presence of the trial inhibits discussion of whether such a trial should be national rather than regional; often the study will be terminated without reaching the desired size and a negative result is obtained which might hide a smaller than anticipated difference which might nonetheless be clinically useful. When the world literature contains five to ten such studies the issue will be seen to be unresolved (although an overview analysis (Chapter 26) may give an indication of an effect).

Regional groups form an essential basis for the preliminary testing of treatments, and for smaller-scale studies where larger differences can be quickly discovered. They also are essential participants in the next level of organization, namely larger-scale, national studies. The responsibility of the organizers of regional groups is to ask themselves which of their studies is better served by a local or a national organization.

NATIONAL COLLABORATIVE GROUPS

Organizations such as the UK Medical Research Council (MRC), the European Organization for Research and Treatment of Cancer (EORTC) or the Cancer and Leukemia Group B and the National Surgical Adjuvant Breast Project in the USA have been formed in an attempt to increase the efficiency with which trials can be carried out. Until recently none of these groups has conducted studies in common cancers of a size which truly demonstrates a national function. There have, however, been excellent trials in rarer tumours, where there is a much readier recognition nationally that no single centre or regional group can expect to carry out significant studies.

In the UK, national organizations such as the MRC have carried out valuable studies in relatively rare diseases such as leukaemia, myeloma, osteosarcoma, glioma and testicular cancer. The MRC has also conducted trials of preoperative radiotherapy in colorectal cancer but these studies would now be regarded as too small to show realistic survival differences. Useful intermediate-size studies have also been carried out in lung cancer, addressing questions of the length and intensity of chemotherapy in small-cell lung carcinoma and of the palliative effect of radiotherapy in NSCLC.

The EORTC has a similarly wide portfolio of studies completed and in progress. In general these studies have been of intermediate size and, as in the case of the UK MRC, they have tended not to show conclusive differences between the regimens being compared. The projected trials have often been optimistic with respect to the likely differences and have thus been too small, although many studies where no difference has been found have excluded differences in outcome which the trial participants would have regarded as clinically important.

National trials agencies are an essential resource. Few single centres have the statistical resources, the experience in trial design and execution or the financial backing which is necessary for the effective conduct of clinical trials. By virtue of the fact that they are "national" these larger organizations occupy a neutral territory in which participants from around the country can meet and press for new studies which are not then perceived as one person's property. They are indisputably essential for running trials in rare tumours or uncommon subgroups of commoner tumours. In common tumours these national groupings will increasingly need to focus on larger-scale studies often conducted internationally. Why have larger studies not been carried out? In part this has been due to a failure to appreciate the necessity and value of detecting small survival differences. In part it has been due to a tension between national and regional trial organizations. National organizations may be perceived by regional groups as bureaucratic, or as likely to undermine or detract from the autonomy of the participants, or as prone to carry out trials asking questions which are regarded as less exciting or fashionable. Of course this misses the point, which is that there should be little overlap between the studies undertaken by national and regional groups. In an ideal world the representatives of the regional trials groups should form part of the national trials structure.

INTERNATIONAL COLLABORATION

There is much to be said for collaboration between national groups in different countries. When agreement can be reached on the nature of the question which needs to be asked in either a very rare tumour (such as Ewing's sarcoma) or a very common tumour when a very small difference in outcome is sought, trials can be conducted much more effectively if the accrual of cases proceeds, say, ten times more quickly than is possible in a national or regional study.

The great difficulties are, first, to reach agreement on the study design and, second, to simplify administration to the bare minimum. There are many economic and cultural differences in medical practice which make collaboration difficult particularly with respect to agreement on the protocol. There are ways to avoid this problem and to understand how greater collaboration can be achieved we need to consider some of our current practices in carrying out trials which stand in the way of progress.

SIMPLICITY AND EFFICIENCY IN TRIAL DESIGN

Chemotherapists and radiotherapists are, rightly, concerned about the toxicity of the treatment they use. They are also well aware that in treating patients with a particular cancer the value of a treatment is only partly expressed in terms of its impact on overall survival of a group. They know that survival is only one end-point among many. For example, a treatment which improves the chance of freedom from local recurrence in laryngeal cancer may not improve survival (because recurrence can be treated by laryngectomy) but the preservation of speech is of inestimable benefit for the patient. Another consideration is that cancers of a particular type may be very varied in prognosis—some breast cancers, for example, grow more slowly than others. In a group of 1000 pre-menopausal women treated with adjuvant chemotherapy for stage II breast cancer, only a small minority will benefit and oncologists will, rightly, wish to know if the group who benefits can be identified so as to spare the other patients unnecessary treatment. Finally, in judging the results and "cost–benefit" of a therapy the toxicity and expense of the treatment will be considered. If resources are scarce, a complex treatment of limited benefit might have to compete with other treatments for other tumours.

These sensible concerns have, to some degree, distorted our view of clinical trials in several ways. First, they have sometimes led to rigid inclusion criteria, sometimes based on complex and expensive staging methods. This has been done to limit, or focus, the trial on a particular subgroup either considered to be at high risk, or to exclude patients who would clearly be less likely to benefit (a patient with metastases will not be helped by surgical treatment of the primary tumour). Trials have often collected elaborate details of dosage of drugs and technical details of radiotherapy as well as sequential laboratory data. While this is essential when a new drug or drug regimen is first being assessed (Chapter 10) it is not necessary when the toxicity of an established treatment, now being assessed in a randomized trial, is already known. The complexity of investigation and the tedium of form-filling has discouraged participation. Most of the information collected is unusable as far as the main point of interest of the trial is concerned which, in a large study, is survival. It is sometimes argued that, by collecting all these data, interesting subsidiary analyses can be performed which will generate hypotheses for future studies. However, while this may sometimes be true (for example, the effect of menopausal status as a determinant of the effectiveness of chemotherapy in breast cancer has been clearly shown), such analyses may be misleading. For example, relating results of the study to the dose of drugs administered or intensity of treatment is fraught with bias since many of the clinical reasons for dose modification are themselves related to prognosis (for example, dose reduction in sick or elderly patients). Similarly subgroup analyses are often misleading unless trials are very large indeed. Repeated analyses of the data will inevitably produce some spurious associations and it may not be possible to tell intuitively which are correct. The problem with collection of detailed information in a large-scale trial is that by making the conduct of a study over-elaborate the trial runs into the far greater, and ultimately self-defeating, danger of poor accrual and loss of power to detect differences. It is clear that trials must be designed in such a way as to allow wide entry criteria and ask for as little follow-up information as is compatible with the stated end-points of the study. When national groups cannot agree points of detail in designing a study, they will often do well to question whether the points of difference are not entirely compatible with a flexible trial design.

What kinds of question might be addressed in such large-scale trials? In my view the most important questions of this type are those where a major question of treatment policy is being studied. Recent examples are the use of CMF or tamoxifen as an adjuvant to mastectomy in stage II breast cancer where the control group is no adjuvant treatment. In such "yes or no" questions the effect of treatment (or lack of it) is likely to be relatively robust and the therapeutic effect of differences in detail (such as dose and timing of chemotherapy cycles) is likely to be small in comparison with the major question. In Table 1, I give examples of some studies of this type where a small benefit might save a lot of lives in some common cancers.

Overview analyses of past small, unsuccessful, trials will be helpful in stimulating large trials and in gaining support for the need for certain questions to be answered unequivocally. The entry criteria must then be kept as broad as possible and essential preliminary staging investigations kept to a minimum. These trials should allow a range of treatment techniques and not define radiotherapy or chemotherapy regimens too narrowly, thereby losing support from centres who insist on following particular methods.

ETHICAL CONSIDERATIONS

Although major questions of treatment policy are the most suitable areas for large-scale collaborative trials, they may cause ethical difficulties. The

Table 1. Questions which might be (or are) the subject of large-scale randomized trials

1. Does perioperative radiotherapy improve survival in resectable colorectal cancer?
2. Does adjuvant 5-fluorouracil improve the prognosis of operable colorectal cancer?
3. Does chemotherapy improve survival in advanced bladder cancer treated with surgery or radiotherapy?
4. Does chemotherapy improve survival in localized, but inoperable, NSCLC?
5. Does chemotherapy improve survival in advanced head and neck cancer treated with radiotherapy?
6. Does tamoxifen improve survival in breast cancer in pre-menopausal women?

approaches to treatment in the two arms of the study differ considerably. Obtaining informed consent may then provoke anxiety for the doctor and, more importantly, the patient. If, for example, the question being posed is whether chemotherapy will contribute to survival in limited-stage, inoperable, NSCLC, an explanation of the possible benefits and toxicities of chemotherapy may create anxiety and confusion if the patient is then randomized to the no-chemotherapy arm. Attempts have been made to avoid this problem by designating one treatment as "standard" and only discussing the treatment with the patient *after* randomization if he or she has been allocated to the "non-standard" treatment. However, the statistical and ethical disadvantages of post-randomization consent are such as to make this procedure generally unacceptable. Difficulties with informed consent in clinical trials are a major obstacle to recruitment. We need a much better understanding, among the public, the medical profession and journalists, of the powerful arguments to show that controlled trials are not just ethically justifiable but essential [3, 4]. Collaborative studies highlight this problem since the ethical issues have to be understood by many participants in several countries. For the participating doctors there should be no difficulty. The patient is only entered into the trial if the doctor considers that he does not know, in the case of that particular patient, or that group of patients, whether treatment A or B is the correct approach (see Chapter 12 for discussion of the "uncertainty principle").

CONCLUSION

Advances in cancer treatment will come slowly with small increments of benefit. No treatment currently available or likely to be developed in the foreseeable future will add more than a few percentage points to long-term survival. For common cancers these few points mean tens of thousands of lives saved. We have an absolute responsibility to demonstrate these differences incontrovertibly and thus change medical practice. Collaboration in the design and execution of clinical trials is an essential prerequisite for this to take place. A full understanding of the issues by professionals, politicians and the public is long overdue.

ACKNOWLEDGMENTS

I am greatly indebted to Marc Buyse for the use of Figure 1 and to David Machin for advice on the manuscript.

REFERENCES

1. Freedman LS (1989) The size of clinical trials in cancer research: what are the current needs? (Report to MRC Cancer Therapy Committee.) Br J Cancer 59: 396–400
2. Yusuf S, Collins R, Peto R (1984) Why do we need some large, simple, randomized trials? Stat Med 3: 409–420
3. Freedman B (1987) Equipoise and the ethics of clinical research. N Engl J Med 317: 141–145
4. Spodick DH (1982) The randomized controlled clinical trial: scientific and ethical bases. Am J Med 73: 420–425

ABOUT THE AUTHOR

R. L. Souhami received his undergraduate training at University College Hospital (UCH), qualifying in October 1962. After pre-registration house posts he developed an interest in the new field of clinical immunology and immuno-suppression at the MRC Rheumatism Research Unit at Taplow, and then in the Department of Connective Tissue Diseases at Johns Hopkins Hospital in Baltimore. On return to the UK he completed three years internal medicine at UCH, where he developed a particular interest in therapy of leukaemia.

A two-year period in the Department of Experimental Pathology at St Mary's Hospital Medical School followed, leading to his MD degree in Kupffer cell function and formation of mononuclear phagocytes. Returning to UCH as a senior registrar he continued his interest in leukaemia and worked in the laboratories of Professor N. A. Mitchison on aspects of tumour immunology. He was appointed Consultant Physician with a special interest in medical oncology at Poole General Hospital in 1973, but returned as Consultant Physician and Senior Lecturer to UCH in 1975. Here he set up the Medical Oncology Unit and, with Professor Peter Beverley, the ICRF Human Tumour Immunology Unit. The clinical interests were in small-cell lung cancer and bone cancer and, in the laboratory, in tumour cell antigens.

The unit expanded, and in 1987 he was appointed as the first holder of the Kathleen Ferrier Chair in Clinical Oncology at the combined University College and Middlesex School of Medicine.

The unit has continued its clinical research interest in small-cell lung cancer, osteosarcoma and glioma. Clinical research has focused on large-scale trials in lung cancer, high-dose chemotherapy with autologous bone marrow transplantation, and the development of national trials in bone sarcoma. Laboratory research programmes include molecular pharmacology of drug/DNA interaction, small-cell lung cancer antigens, and pharmacokinetic and metabolic profiles of drugs in phase II studies.

Since 1987 Professor Souhami has been Chairman of the Cancer Therapy Committee of the MRC, in which capacity he has been involved in the development of national trials in cancer.

14 Randomization before Consent: Practical and Ethical Considerations

MAHESH K. B. PARMAR

When confronted with a patient suffering from cancer, the treating clinician may have a number of treatment options available. Often, for a particular patient, he will find it difficult to choose between the competing treatments. In such cases he will rely on his clinical experience and the available evidence for and against these competing therapies. Randomized clinical trials are a major source of such evidence, and are now widely accepted as the best means of comparing the efficacy of different forms of therapy for the treatment of a human disease.

A randomized clinical trial is defined as a study in which patients are allocated a particular therapy by a chance mechanism. An important feature of this random assignment of treatments is that neither the patient nor the clinician knows the treatment allocation before the patient is entered into the study (Figure 1).

Most countries require that patients entering into such studies of comparative treatments do so after having given their informed consent. Typically, this requires the clinician to inform the patient that the treatment will be assigned by a chance mechanism, that there are at least two competing treatments on offer (one of which is the standard), and of the possible benefits and toxicities of the different forms of therapy. Many clinicians feel that such a discussion can compromise the "patient–doctor" relationship, particularly as the doctor will have to admit he does not know which treatment is best. This difficult problem often prevents clinicians and patients participating in randomized clinical trials.

It is widely accepted that recruiting the necessary number of patients to a trial is a considerable problem. It usually takes a number of years to accrue the required number of patients, and achievement of the target is often more difficult than anticipated. The patients declared suitable before the start of the trial suddenly seem to disappear when the trial actually starts. At worst, this can lead to early closure of the trial through poor accrual; more usually, the process of accrual takes longer than projected, perhaps even by two or three years. In this case, by the time trial results are published, the question being addressed may no longer be of interest and the collaborators may,

Introducing New Treatments for Cancer: Practical, Ethical and Legal Problems. Edited by C. J. Williams
© 1992 John Wiley & Sons Ltd

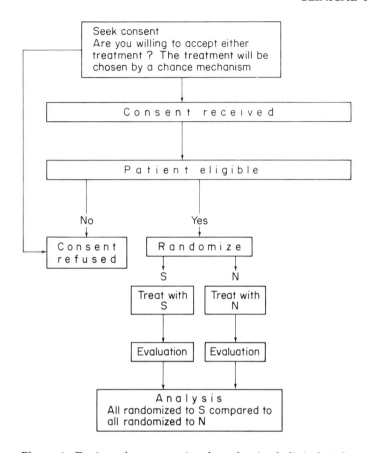

Figure 1. Design of a conventional randomized clinical trial

quite reasonably, lose interest in the trial and possibly not participate in future trials. Thus removal of any impediment to participation by either clinician or patient could prove enormously beneficial in many respects.

It was chiefly for this reason that Zelen [1] introduced the idea of "randomisation before consent". The principal feature of this approach is that before the patient's consent is obtained for entry into the study, both patient and physician *know* to which treatment the patient has been allocated (Figure 2). This design has become variously known as Zelen's design, the randomized consent design and the pre-randomization design. I shall refer to it as the randomized consent design.

In this chapter I shall describe in detail the structure and analysis of conventional randomized trials and of the two forms of the randomized consent design. I will then proceed to consider the practical and ethical considerations involved in using randomized consent designs and discuss some examples of trials in which these designs have been used.

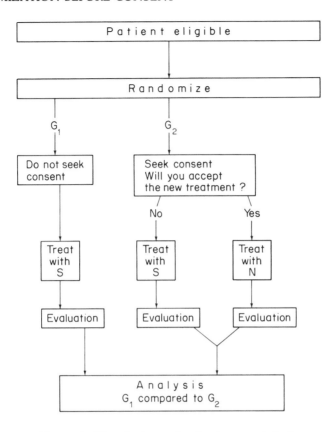

Figure 2. The single randomized consent design

A CONVENTIONAL RANDOMIZED CLINICAL TRIAL

The conventional randomized clinical trial arrangement is shown in Figure 1. Once a patient is deemed suitable for the study, informed consent must be sought. It is usual to explain to the patient the purpose of the study, the features of the treatments being compared and the basic randomization procedure. Those who do not consent will subsequently not be included in the trial and the choice of their treatment is then left to the clinician. Consenting patients will be randomized between two treatments, assumed here to be a standard therapy (S) and a new treatment (N).

THE SINGLE RANDOMIZED CONSENT DESIGN

Zelen [1] proposed an alternative to the conventional randomized design which is depicted in Figure 2. Randomization to groups G1 and G2 first takes place without the patient's knowledge or consent. Those in G1 are not told about the study and are given the best standard treatment (S). Patients in G2, having been allocated the new treatment (N), are told that they are in a trial, and their consent is then sought. Those who refuse are given the standard (S). Patients in G1 therefore receive only the standard therapy (S), whereas those in G2 may receive either the new treatment (N) or the standard treatment (S).

THE DOUBLE RANDOMIZED CONSENT DESIGN

The double randomized consent design (Figure 3) is similar to the single randomized consent design, except that patients in group G1 are now also asked for their consent. Patients in both groups will therefore receive either the standard treatment (S), or the new treatment (N), depending on their acceptance of the allocated treatment.

ANALYSIS

For a conventional randomized trial, it is normal practice to report, at the end of the study, on all patients randomized. Failure to comply with, or

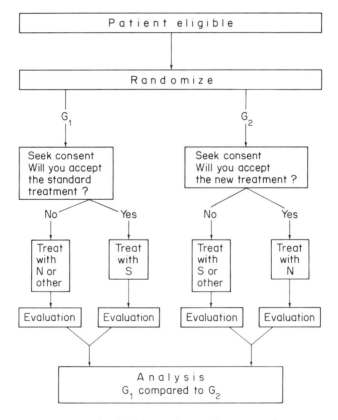

Figure 3. The double randomized consent design

even not to receive, the treatment schedule is not grounds for excluding a patient from the statistical analysis. In the analysis all patients are counted against the treatment to which they were randomized. Such an "intention-to-treat analysis" avoids biases due to treatment-related withdrawals [2]. Although consenting patients may not be fully representative of all eligible patients, the treatment groups are fully comparable, and there is *no bias* in the treatment comparison caused by those who *refuse* to participate.

The analysis of randomized consent designs causes particular problems. The reason for this is that some of the patients will refuse the treatment allocated, leading to a "dilution" in the estimated treatment effect. The two treatments will appear more similar than they actually are. This can be seen from the following example: suppose we know that the true survival rates associated with the standard and new treatments are 50% and 70% respectively. Further, suppose that 20% of patients assigned to each treatment actually refuse the treatment allocated and receive the other one. We would then expect to see a survival rate of 54% ($0.8 \times 50\% + 0.2 \times 70\%$) in patients randomized to receive the standard treatment, and 66% ($0.8 \times 70\% + 0.2 \times 50\%$) in patients randomized to receive the new treatment. Thus, the apparent difference in the treatments is 12% ($66\% - 54\%$) and not 20% ($70\% - 50\%$).

To counter this problem, it may be argued that an analysis should be performed on the treatments *actually received*, or that patients refusing treatment should be excluded from the analysis. Either approach, however, can lead to a very biased analysis. For example, suppose that in a trial there are 25% good prognosis and 75% poor prognosis patients. Further, suppose that there is *no difference* between the new and standard treatments, with both treatments giving 80% survival for good prognosis patients, and 40% survival for poor prognosis patients. Suppose also that all the good prognosis patients allocated the standard treatment refuse it and receive the new treatment instead. If we then *exclude* the patients who refuse the allocated treatment, the expected survival rates are 50% for the new treatment ($0.25 \times 80\% + 0.75 \times 40\%$) and 40% for the standard treatment ($1.0 \times 40\%$). An apparent treatment difference of 10% is therefore observed when there is in reality no difference. Similar biases can occur if an analysis is performed on the treatment actually received. As we can never know whether such biases actually exist, the only analysis that can safely be performed is the "intention-to-treat" analysis, i.e. a comparison of group G1 with group G2 (see Figures 2 and 3).

Employing this approach we must, however, consider the probable refusal rate when we design the trial, and to allow for dilution of the "treatment effect" we must plan to enter more patients into a randomized consent trial than a conventional randomized trial. In the first example presented above, a randomized consent trial would need to be designed so that the apparent difference of 12%, rather than the actual difference of 20%, can be reliably

Table 1. Total number of patients required using the double randomized consent design to have the same power as a conventional trial for various rates of refusal of the allocated treatment

Number of patients using conventional design	Percentage of patients refusing treatment allocated				
	5%	10%	15%	20%	30%
250	310	390	510	695	1560
500	630	790	1030	1390	3125
1000	1240	1570	2050	2780	6250

detected, that is with the same statistical power. Table 1 shows the total number of patients required for a two-group trial using the double-consent design assuming various refusal rates. It can be seen from Table 1 that a trial requiring 1000 patients with a conventional randomized design would require as many as 1390 patients (to have the same statistical power) using a randomized consent design with a refusal rate of 15%.

It should be noted that throughout the above (and in Table 1), we have implicitly assumed that there are no refusers after randomization in a conventional randomized trial. Our experience shows that this is generally a good approximation in most situations, as refusal rates are usually less than 5% in such trials.

If the proportion of "refusers" is small in the randomized consent trial, then clearly there is little practical difference between it and a conventional trial. However, the examples presented below suggest that a refusal rate of 15% is not uncommon in some randomized consent trials, which considerably increases the number of patients required.

Zelen [1] argues that the increase in accrual that can be obtained by using the randomized consent design outweighs any loss in efficiency due to refusal of the allocated treatment. I will consider this later with reference to examples.

Although it is possible to preserve statistical power of the trial by increasing the sample size when a significant proportion of patients refuse the treatment allocated, a further problem may arise. In such situations we have seen that the estimate of the difference between treatments is reduced. The estimate may be further reduced by, for example, poor-prognosis patients requesting the new treatment when allocated the standard and good-prognosis patients requesting the standard treatment having been allocated the new. It is not difficult to see that in such circumstances the treatments in the trial would appear even more similar than they actually are. It may be argued that this situation is unlikely to occur as a clinician is unlikely to influence a patient on their choice of treatment. The very fact that the patient is entered into the clinical trial should mean the clinician has no treatment preference for that patient. But it is possible to imagine situations in which the clinician, either consciously or subconsciously, might endorse or discourage the use of the treatment allocated. This can only happen in a randomized consent trial where the treatment is known before consent is obtained.

ETHICAL CONSIDERATIONS

The major criticisms of the randomized consent designs are:

(1) The act of randomization before consent enrols a patient into a study before they have given consent. It is clear that although a patient has a right to accept or refuse the treatment allocated, they cannot withdraw from the study altogether (to allow the intention-to-treat analysis, G1 v. G2). This may be considered to be a relatively unimportant point, but it does raise the question of voluntary participation in research.

(2) As we have seen the success of such designs is dependent upon a high proportion of patients accepting the allocated treatment. Thus, knowledge of the assigned treatment allows and perhaps encourages the clinician to present the trial, either consciously or subconsciously, in such a way that predisposes the patient to accept the assigned treatment. For example, if the patient is allocated the standard treatment, the clinician may stress the experimental nature of the new treatment and the possibility that it may be worse than the standard. Conversely, if the patient is allocated the new treatment then the clinician may stress the lack of benefit obtained using the standard and the hopes of the new treatment. That the treatment has been allocated by a random mechanism may only be mentioned in passing or not mentioned at all. In fact, it has been argued that the accrual of more patients, generally required for the randomized consent design, is practical "proof" of this concern, as patients refuse to be randomized because they have a preference for one of the treatments, and so if more patients are willing to accept a randomized treatment this must be the result of incomplete information.

The first concern is particularly relevant for the single-consent design as patients allocated the standard treatment may not be informed that they are in a trial. It has been argued, however, that there is widespread use of routine patient data for research purposes (especially for non-randomized clinical trials in which concurrent controls are used). Such data is obviously used without the patient's consent. Nevertheless, this lack of consent has made the single consent design unacceptable to several research funding bodies including the British Medical Research Council. Current federal guidelines in the United States also preclude this design (Zelen, 1991). The second concern is mainly relevant to the double-consent design.

Although these arguments may appear initially compelling, others have argued that the question of "informed consent" should be considered in the wider context of standard clinical practice. The main thrust of the argument is that a clinician enters a patient into a randomized clinical trial only when he has no treatment preference for that patient. Randomized clinical trials, although strictly research, should therefore be a straightforward extension of clinical practice, and the level of informed consent required for a trial should be similar to that required for standard practice. In clinical practice, different patients will be given varying amounts of information concerning the therapy they are receiving and any other treatment options available to them. It may be argued that imposing strict, detailed informed consent procedures on both patients and clinicians is "unethical" because such a requirement may prove severely distressing to the patient. It may also damage recruitment to a trial which may lead to an important therapeutic question remaining unanswered. It should be stressed that this argument does not state that informed consent is not necessary; only that for each individual patient, the degree and timing (before or after randomization) of consent should be governed by local considerations and the "doctor–patient" relationship (as for routine practice). This approach can be regarded not so much an argument in favour of randomized consent designs as an argument to reconsider the nature and need for informed consent. Chapter 4 introduces and discusses these ideas in more detail.

EXAMPLES OF RANDOMIZED CONSENT TRIALS

Zelen, in an update of the randomized consent design [3], reviews 12 trials conducted in the USA in which the design has been used. I shall outline four of those examples here and also present one example from a study being conducted in the UK.

AN ECOG TRIAL

The collaborative group ECOG (Eastern Cooperative Oncology Group) initiated a conventional randomized study of adjuvant chemotherapy in women with node-negative breast cancer. During the first year, accrual for this group averaged 3.9 patients per month. To increase accrual, a randomized double-consent design was adopted and the accrual rate for the next 16 months averaged 7.6 patients per month. This increase in accrual by a factor of almost two would seem to suggest that the change in design achieved its purpose. But during this period only two-thirds of the patients accepted the allocated treatment; with this level of acceptance the accrual rate would have to be increased by a factor of 9 to prove as efficient as the conventional design. Indeed, the relative inefficiency of the randomized consent design persuaded the group to revert to the conventional design with an accrual rate of 4.1 patients per month over the next 16 months. Overall, during the period the design was used, it became clear that the randomized consent design failed to achieve the increase in accrual required to overcome its lack of efficiency.

AN NSABP TRIAL I

An NSABP (National Surgical Adjuvant Breast and Bowel Project) trial comparing radical mastectomy with lumpectomy (with or without radiotherapy) achieved a sixfold increase in accrual when using a randomized double-consent design rather than a conventional design. In this study, 89% of patients accepted the allocated treatment with the randomized consent design. With this level of acceptance, an increase of a factor of 1.6 was all that was required to achieve parity in terms of efficiency. This was more than exceeded by the sixfold increase mentioned above.

AN NSABP TRIAL II

Two NSABP trials of adjuvant therapy for colon and rectal cancer were amended to permit randomization before consent one year after the start of the studies. Accrual rates increased from 16 to 20 patients per month (a factor of 1.25) in the colon study and from 3.5 to 7 patients per month (a factor of 2) in the rectal study. (This increase in accrual in the rectal study was due in part to an increase in the accrual rate of conventionally randomized patients.) In both studies, 88% of patients entered using the randomized consent design accepted the allocated treatment. This rate of acceptance requires an increase in the rate of accrual by a factor of 1.7 to achieve the same efficiency. Thus, if these accrual rates continue then the change in design in the rectal study may prove worthwhile, whereas the change in design of the colon study will not.

THE ECMO TRIALS

Two studies, in newborn infants with persistent pulmonary hypertension (PPH) comparing extracorporeal membrane oxygen (ECMO) with conventional therapy, have used the randomized single-consent design. Infants, shortly after birth, were diagnosed with PPH. In a conventional randomized trial, before treatment allocation the parents of an infant near death would need to be approached to give consent for an invasive surgical procedure (ECMO) which in the event might not be allocated. The randomized single-consent design requires only the parents of those infants assigned ECMO to be approached for consent as ECMO is not the standard treatment. All 40 of the parents in the two trials accepted the treatment allocated.

A CRC TRIAL

The UK Cancer Research Campaign Clinical Trials Centre (CRCCTC) is currently responsible for co-ordinating a randomized trial evaluating serial carcinoembryonic antigen assay (CEA) as an indicator for second-look surgery in recurrent colorectal cancer. The randomization is between surgery and no immediate treatment. In this trial informed consent is sought for all patients entering the study to allow regular blood sampling for CEA estimation, and at this stage no consent for possible randomization at a later stage is obtained. These blood samples are then sent to the CRCCTC for analysis (having not been analysed at the treating centre). If at some point a significant rise in the CEA is observed, then patients are randomized by the CRCCTC to surgery or no immediate treatment (observation alone). Both the clinician and the patient are only informed when the allocated treatment is surgery; in which case informed consent to proceed is obtained from the patient. The trial organizers do not think it necessary to inform the patient or the surgeon of the rising CEA when no immediate treatment is allocated. They give the following reasons. First, the study will cease to be "blind" and this may lead to a bias in clinical follow-up in the no-immediate-treatment group. Second, the information may cause unnecessary alarm to the patient especially if there are no other indications for undertaking second-look surgery. Third, consent to continue with conventional follow-up is implicit in the "doctor–patient" relationship and is in any case implicit in the consent received originally from all patients. This study aims to register 2000 patients and randomize 500 of them between surgery and observation alone. At the time of writing 1500 patients have been registered and 150 randomized. The CRCCTC have indicated that the number of patients refusing surgery is relatively small and certainly less than 5%.

CONCLUSIONS

Since Zelen first proposed them in 1979, randomized consent designs have been the centre of a great deal of controversy with all groups involved in clinical trials—patients, clinicians, ethicists, philosophers and statisticians alike. Zelen's proposed design is a method of addressing the difficulty of obtaining informed consent. The process of obtaining such consent in a conventional trial can be both difficult and distressing for the patient and the clinician. The advantage of randomized consent designs is the simplification in obtaining consent from patients. However, for many this advantage is seen as a major disadvantage, as it encourages clinicians—for the practical reasons of maximizing patient acceptance of the allocated treatment and for ease of explanation—to minimize the explanation of the nature of the trial and alternative treatments available.

The single randomized consent design has been used relatively rarely in the USA and then always in fairly small trials. It has probably been used a little more widely in the UK, although this is difficult to gauge as information on its use are not readily available.

The double randomized consent design has been more widely used, certainly in the USA and probably also in the UK, although again comparative data are not easily available to establish this latter point. All of these studies have by no means proved successful. The chief problem in the unsuccessful studies has been that any increase in the accrual rate using this design was more than negated by the refusal rate of the allocated treatment. In documented studies refusal of the allocated treatment has sometimes been observed to be as much as 36%. Such a high rate of refusal of the allocated treatment leads to a massive 13-fold increase in the number of patients required in the study. Even a relatively low refusal rate of 15% means that we would need an increase in patient numbers by a factor of 2. Clearly, one has to consider whether such increases in patient numbers are possible even with the implementation of this design. The cost of the study needs also to be considered since many more patients need to be entered and subsequently treated. It should be noted, however, that all of the examples of the "failure" of the randomized consent design presented here (and the others presented by Zelen) are taken from the USA, where informed consent procedures (whether given before or after randomization) are particularly onerous, generally requiring the patient to read a multipage information document and then to sign a detailed form (see Chapter 4). Such procedures, rather than the design used, may be responsible for a large proportion of refusals. Detailed examples of the randomized consent design with the number of patients randomized by this method are not as easily available in the UK. It may be that a number of trials have employed this design implicitly in individual centres or in multicentre protocols. Certainly, the British Medical Research Council guidelines, adopted by many major trials organizations, allow individual centres in multicentre trials to use the double-consent design when they and the local ethical committee think it appropriate. Thus it may be that many individual centres may use this design in some trials. If this is indeed the case then the refusal rate is not a cause for concern, being not much different from that obtained in conventional randomized trial. We should note that detailed written informed consent is becoming a more common requirement in the UK and it may not be long before procedures similar to those in the USA are generally adopted. In this case we may see a corresponding increase in the refusal rate not just in randomized consent trials but also from patients approached to enter conventionally randomized trials.

As we have seen, an important point, which is largely ignored in the medical literature, is that a significant proportion of refusers not only influences the number of patients required but also the estimate of the treatment effect. This is not the case for a conventional randomized trial. For randomized consent trials a reduced or diluted estimate of the treatment effect may be obtained. For instance, in the example described early in the chapter with a refusal rate of 20%, the estimate of treatment effect was almost halved from the true 20% to 12%. The former may prove sufficient to encourage general use of the new treatment whereas the latter may prove insufficient to persuade most clinicians to change the treatment policy. A good estimate of the difference between the two treatments is particularly relevant in the field of cancer, because the new treatment will generally be both more toxic and more expensive than the standard.

Considering the examples presented here (and in references [3] and [4]), randomized consent designs appear to be most useful when there is marked difference between the treatments being compared. Thus the trials of invasive surgery (ECMO) versus no invasive surgery in newly born infants, of mastectomy versus breast-conserving surgery in women with breast cancer, and of second-look surgery versus observation alone in patients with recurrent colorectal cancer have been very successful in employing these designs. The breast cancer study in fact saw a sixfold increase in the rate of accrual of patients with a refusal rate of 12%. The similarity between these studies is the emotive nature of the choice between treatments—to submit an infant with hypertension to surgery, whether or not a woman with breast cancer is able to retain her breast and whether or not surgery should be undertaken when a tumour recurrence is only suspected. In these situations excessively detailed consent and discussion of the options available may be both distressing and difficult for a patient; in which case randomization before consent may be a more appropriate option for some patients. This is especially true if one treatment option is regarded as the standard therapy, as is the case in the examples discussed.

It is now more than ten years since Zelen first proposed the idea of randomization before consent. Since then this design has apparently only been *explicitly* used in relatively few to my knowledge. This lack of use stems partly from the ethical concerns, to the extent that it has been regarded as unacceptable by some ethical committees responsible for reviewing research protocols. However, ethical issues are never clear cut and to impose highly detailed consent may, *in some situations*, be distressing for the patient and difficult for the clinician. It may be more appropriate in these situations, if it eases these problems, to allow randomization before consent. We should not, however, overlook the practical drawback of these designs when there are a significant proportion of patients refusing the allocated treatment (greater than 10%). This is reflected in an increase in the number of patients required and a reduced estimate of the treatment effect—a very important consideration when one needs to balance any improvement in survival with the toxicity and cost of a new treatment.

REFERENCES

1. Zelen M (1979) A new design for randomized clinical trials. N Engl J Med 300: 1242–1245
2. Gail MH (1985) Eligibility exclusions, losses to follow-up, removal of randomized patient, and uncounted events in cancer clinical trials. Cancer Treat Rep 69: 1107–1112
3. Zelen M (1990) Randomized consent designs for clinical trials: an update. Stat Med 9: 645–656
4. Ellenberg SS (1984) Randomization designs in comparative clinical trials. N Engl J Med 310: 1404–1408

ABOUT THE AUTHOR

Mahesh K. B. Parmar is a statistician who has been involved in various stages of designing, coordinating and analysing over 25 cancer clinical trials for the British Medical Research Council (MRC) since 1987. He has also set up and heads the overview section in the Trials Office, which now has a portfolio of six overview studies at various stages of completion. Before joining the MRC Cancer Trials Office he completed a thesis for doctor of philosophy in medical statistics at the University of Oxford. He has research interests in the interim analysis of clinical trial data, in the appropriate analysis of overviews and in the design, conduct and analysis of observer agreement studies.

15 Interim Analysis and Ethical Issues in the Conduct of Trials

DAVID MACHIN

It is important that when investigators are considering the design of a phase III comparative trial in cancer they have one or more key questions in mind, the answers to which will be of interest to a wider clinical community and, most crucially, have ultimate benefit to patients. It is clear too that the answers to the questions posed are not already known. At the design stage of the trial the decision is taken as to the treatments to be compared and the appropriate patient types that are to be recruited identified.

In most circumstances treatment allocation would be at random for a phase III clinical trial. In that case, provided that the treating clinician is uncertain in his own mind about which of the treatments is the better, he will accept the need for randomization for the patient before him. Thus one of the basic requirements at the planning stage of the trial is the presence of this "uncertainty" in the minds of clinicians actively involved in the management and treatment of patients with the particular tumour (see Chapter 12). In contrast, once a trial is completed, the requirement is now that most of the uncertainty about the relative merits of the treatments is removed. Once the uncertainty is removed, or at least substantially reduced, this then allows the clinician to treat his patients with some confidence with one particular treatment if, for example, it has been shown to bring survival advantage over the other treatment(s) in the trial just completed.

The method of deciding on the appropriate number of patients to be recruited to a randomized phase III clinical trial depends both on the size of the anticipated benefit of one treatment over the other and the rate at which critical events, for example deaths if survival is the end-point, occur. In addition there are statistical considerations such as the size of the associated significance test to be used when the results are available, usually denoted by α at the planning stage, and the statistical power. Once these are determined the size of the trial can be calculated by standard formulae or from tables. It is as well to remember that one is planning the size of a trial in the face of considerable uncertainty about the relative merits of the treatments proposed. Thus patient number calculations are only indications of the appropriate study size.

The next step is to decide if such a study size is a viable proposition, although some consideration will have been given to this at an earlier stage

Introducing New Treatments for Cancer: Practical, Ethical and Legal Problems. Edited by C. J. Williams
© 1992 John Wiley & Sons Ltd

as part of the original formulation of the question. There are clearly difficulties here. If the number of patients required is not achievable then several options present themselves. One of these is to re-examine the basic trial design to identify any changes that could facilitate patient entry, possibly by modification of the treatment modalities or changing patient eligibility criteria. A second is to seek a wider collaborative effort, perhaps by extending the trial from a single institution to a multicentre study. It is not acceptable to open the trial to patient entry if there is little chance that the recruitment targets will be achieved, since this exposes patients to "experimentation" without an achievable goal.

Once the target patient number is deemed achievable (even though one can never be certain of that) the objective must be to recruit the necessary patients as quickly as possible into the trial. One need for this is the natural desire to answer the question posed as quickly as possible. There are obvious reasons for this, amongst them the consideration that if a trial is prolonged then there is always the distinct possibility of a new, more exciting, question coming along which is relevant to the patient type currently under study. This is of particular concern when it seems there is a hope of a clear advantage over the treatments being compared in the current trial.

We define a clinical trial to be of prolonged recruitment if a substantial number of critical events occur during the recruitment period. For example, suppose in a particular tumour type, perhaps non-small-cell lung cancer, the majority of patients die within two years of randomization. Then in a clinical trial involving such patients, prolonged recruitment would correspond to any period in excess of two years from entry of the first patient. For other tumour types a recruitment period may have to exceed five years or more before it is deemed prolonged.

A second reason for rapid recruitment of patients, and the one that will become the focus of this chapter, is that if patient recruitment is prolonged then there is a distinct possibility that many events (deaths) will occur during the recruitment period. This implies that there may be substantial evidence already available in these events, perhaps already in the computer files of the responsible trial office, pertinent to the relative merits of the two treatments. Despite this evidence recruitment continues since the treating clinicians themselves retain the same levels of uncertainty they had when treating their first patient under the trial protocol. Should this evidence substantially favour one treatment then, were it to become general knowledge, some if not all of the "uncertainty" demanded of the investigators in order for them to randomize patients could be removed. There would therefore be an ethical dilemma for the individual clinician and the trial organizers, who must then decide if the trial is to continue. Thus prolonged recruitment can create ethical difficulties and may force the trial organizers into an "interim" analysis of the data albeit while recruitment is continuing.

There are several reasons why interim analyses are important. These include stopping a trial early when sufficient information is available on efficacy, either to prevent potential trial patients from receiving a less effective therapy or to ensure, by earlier than expected dissemination of the results, that patients at large receive the better therapy. Of particular concern is if, for example, the new treatment which should be an improvement on the old or standard treatment turns out to be worse. If the situation corresponds to one in which no difference in efficacy is observed then, in some sense, there is no ethical imperative to stop the trial early since, whichever of the treatments is given to the future patients, it has a similar effect to the other. In such cases the patient, outside of the trial, may truly have a choice and preference for one treatment may be made on the basis of other considerations. Perhaps the clinician will consider the cost of treatment whereas the patient may consider the associated side-effects. Although we shall describe some formal rules for interim analyses, it must be emphasized that untoward events should be given due consideration. For example, although there may be no formal (statistical) reasons for stopping a trial the observation that just one patient has experienced a particular side-effect may warrant cessation of patient recruitment.

It may also occur that an interim analysis is used to modify recruitment targets in circumstances where information on possible relative treatment efficacy was rather scanty at the planning stage of the trial. Such a situation may arise if the information on the efficacy of the alternatives has been based on non-randomized studies.

Whatever the reasons for an interim analysis it is usually appropriate to pass the "interim" analysis for a "decision" to a data-monitoring committee set up for the specific purpose of reviewing the trial data as they accumulate. In general such a committee would not only examine the trial data themselves but also relevant external evidence provided by the up-to-date scientific literature and other sources. The final decision of such a committee, as to whether or not to continue to recruit patients to the trial, should not rely only on a formal test of statistical significance.

It must be emphasized that the evidence collected before recruitment to the trial is complete is, by definition, less than that which would be available at the end of a trial when all the patients are entered and the corresponding critical events observed. The trial size was determined in an attempt to reduce the uncertainty about the relative benefits of the two treatments to a level sufficient to convince the majority of clinicians concerned with treating new patients of the appropriate (best) therapy. Even if the early evidence reflects exactly the benefit that the completed trial demonstrates (and one can never know that without completing the trial!) the level of uncertainty associated with that effect will still be unacceptably high. For example, the benefit at interim analysis may be estimated as 10% in favour of the new therapy, but the associated confidence interval at that stage may not exclude either a zero or even a negative benefit. The associated completed trial may also indicate exactly the same 10% benefit but will have an associated confidence interval sufficiently narrow around this 10% to persuade most investigators that a zero or negative benefit can be disregarded.

Again by definition, evidence collected part way through the trial should only be acted upon if it is of a form that is contrary to the expectations of the trial organizers at the planning stage; for example, if a new treatment perhaps known to be more toxic than the standard therapy would be expected, on biological grounds perhaps, to improve the survival experience of the patients as compared to the standard but turned out to be associated with a much greater death rate. An example of this has occurred in a randomized phase III trial comparing neutron and proton beams in the radiotherapy treatment of locally advanced cancer in the pelvis [1]. In this case the interim data were indeed contrary to expectations and this information activated a formal review of the trial data by an expert committee convened for that purpose.

A second situation is one in which even the optimistic view of a treatment's efficacy at the planning stage has been exceeded, thereby giving rise to a situation contrary to expectations. Thus Dillman et al. [2] in a randomized trial of an induction chemotherapy in patients with non-small-cell lung cancer closed recruitment after 180 of a planned 250 patients as the apparent benefit in survival at two years was twofold compared to the 50% increase anticipated at the design stage. A formal protocol-monitoring committee participated in the interim assessments of this trial. However, no confidence interval for this benefit is quoted and therefore it is difficult to say how much uncertainty remains as to the claimed benefit.

At the same time as patients are being recruited to a clinical trial, events on those entered some time ago are observed and so become available for analysis. Suppose at a particular point in time there are 100 patients randomized in a clinical trial with 50 in each of two treatment groups. If survival is the main trial endpoint then the number of deaths (events), albeit perhaps few in number, can be used in a formal statistical significance test using the logrank test to give a p-value. The associated hazard ratio (HR), with the corresponding 95% confidence interval, provides an estimate of relative treatment efficacy.

Suppose further that this comparison is repeated after a further 100 patients have entered the study. At this stage there may be many more deaths available for analysis. These comprise those deaths that were available at the first "interim" analysis, some subsequent deaths from those who were still alive at that analysis from the first 100 patients recruited, and finally the deaths amongst the second 100 patients recruited. At this stage there are now 100 patients in each treatment group, the logrank test can be repeated to provide a new p-value, and the HR and associated confidence interval once more estimated. This provides a second-"interim" analysis of the trial data. This type of procedure is known as an analysis on accumulating data.

This second statistical significance test, however, will not be statistically independent of the first since it also includes information on the survival time for the first group of deaths on which the first interim analysis was made. This formal lack of independence invalidates the statistical properties of the second test and the resulting p-value cannot be interpreted in the usual way. For example, if the first test gave a p-value of 0.01 this could be interpreted as indicative of evidence against the null hypothesis of equal treatment efficacy, although there remains a one in a hundred chance that we have falsely rejected this hypothesis. However, if the second test were also to give $p=0.01$ then this can no longer be interpreted in terms of a conventional significance test as we did for the first test. In fact the true second p-value will be larger than 0.01—by how much depends in a complex way on the proportion of "new" deaths available for the second analysis and the extra survival time observed on the first 100 patients recruited.

There is an additional difficulty if a decision on whether or not patient recruitment to the trial should terminate was to be based on the result of the first interim analysis. Had this first test been "very significant" then the trial may have closed and the second 100 patients not recruited at all! However, although new patients are no longer being recruited, information on those of the 100 patients, who were still alive at that analysis point, could be collected until such time as all deaths had occurred. Unfortunately the p-value from the final test of significance based on the survival times of all 100 patients could not be interpreted in the standard way either since the decision to stop the trial was conditional on the results of the interim significance test. There are corresponding difficulties with the interpretation of the final estimate of the HR and its associated confidence interval.

Despite the difficulties inherent in the statistical consequences of interim analysis they may well be an essential element in the ethical surveillance process for the majority of phase III clinical trials. The procedures for interim analysis should be written into the study protocol. These paragraphs will address not only the frequency of such analyses but the consequential steps to be taken if such an analysis is deemed "statistically significant".

There are several ways in which one can devise formal procedures for interim analysis which overcome the problems described and maintain the overall test size as specified at the planning stage of the trial. We shall describe in detail three of these.

The first method begins by fixing the overall test size required for the final treatment comparison in advance of starting patient recruitment to the trial. This will usually be part of the routine of estimating the trial size as described earlier. We assume this test size, often referred to as the nominal test size, to correspond to a value $\alpha=0.05$. Following this, and once the trial has opened and patients recruited to the trial, one performs as many "interim" analyses as one likes. These interim analyses could be planned for every six months, after every 100 patients recruited or after every 100 deaths observed, or quite haphazardly implemented. However, at each of these analyses a decision to stop recruitment to the trial would only be made if an "interim" p-value was less than an "interim" test size set to 0.001. If no such decision is made the trial is completed, and the final test comparison made with the significance level of $\alpha = 0.05$ as planned. This simple procedure, of using a very extreme "interim" test size for analysis, preserves the overall significance level for the final logrank, or other test, at the end of the trial and the corresponding p-value then obtained can be interpreted in the standard way. The usual estimates of the HR and confidence interval remain unaffected. If the trial is stopped early then this rule guarantees a p-value less than the significance level.

What are the disadvantages of such a procedure? The obvious one is that this device almost certainly implies the trial will not close early except in the most extreme of circumstances! We illustrate this by means of an example.

Suppose we have designed a randomized trial to assess the difference in response rates given by two treatments. We have planned the study size as 1000 with 500 patients per treatment, which is sufficient to detect a difference in response rates of the two treatments of 7% with test size $\alpha = 0.05$ and power 0.9. For a 34% response on the standard therapy an improvement over that of 7% implies an odds ratio (OR) $= (41/59)/(34/66) = 1.35$ in favour of the new treatment. Suppose we perform an interim analysis using a χ^2 test after 50 patients have been recruited to each treatment in this study. Then we would need to have a difference in response rates in excess of 20% at this stage for the statistical test to produce $p < 0.05$ and our comparison to be statistically significant at test size $\alpha = 0.05$. This situation corresponds to an OR $= (54/56)/(34/66) = 1.87$. However, for the same comparison to give a test result with $p = 0.001$ at the same stage of the trial, the difference in response rates observed would have to be in excess of 33%. Such a difference would be equivalent to an estimated OR $= 4.13$ in favour of the new therapy—an advantage very unlikely to occur in phase III trials especially of cancer therapy.

It might be argued therefore that such a method is intrinsically unethical as it is tantamount to adopting no stopping rule at all since such differences are never going to be realized. However, our example describes only the first such "interim" analysis where the number of patients is small in relation to the planned study size. At this stage it is sensible to argue that only the most extreme of differences should prevent the trial continuing. If the next interim analysis is after a total of 200 patients, then an OR $= 2.68$ will be required for the second interim analysis to be significant at $p = 0.001$. This is much smaller than the required OR $= 4.13$ for the first analysis.

In the second method of interim analysis the number of "interim" analyses to be carried out while patient recruitment continues is fixed in advance at the planning stage of the trial. The best way of doing this, from a statistical point of view, is to base the interval between successive analyses on the occurrence of a fixed number of new events (deaths). Thus in a trial anticipating a total of 1000 deaths, interim analysis could be performed on nine occasions at intervals of 100 deaths, with a final analysis following the last death using the planned significance level of $\alpha = 0.05$ unaltered. The number of interim analyses planned determines the constant test size to be used on each occasion. This will always be less than α. Table 1 shows how this nominal test size varies with the number of interim analyses planned.

Thus, as in our example, if nine interim analyses are planned as well as the tenth and final analysis using test size $\alpha = 0.05$ for statistical significance, Table 1 suggests these "interim" analyses would only be regarded as statistically significant if $p \leqslant 0.011$. Such a result at any of the planned interim analyses would institute a formal review of the progress of the trial with the possibility of closure. The final analysis, corresponding to the tenth look at the data, would be assessed as statistically significant if $p \leqslant 0.05$ in the usual way. If just one interim analysis was planned this would be regarded as statistically significant only if $p \leqslant 0.029$.

It can be seen from Table 1 that the first method of interim analysis described is also part of this second procedure and corresponds to a very large (infinite) number of planned interim analyses.

Suppose for the response rate trial discussed before in which we were looking for a 7% treatment benefit nine interim analyses were planned. These analyses would be conducted after each 100 patients had been recruited. Then, if we use the $p = 0.011$ suggested by Table 1 above, a statistically

Table 1. The nominal significance level required for repeated interim analyses to preserve an overall test size corresponding to $\alpha = 0.05$ (after Pocock [3])

Number of interim analyses planned	Required p-value at each interim analysis for $\alpha = 0.05$
1	0.029
2	0.022
3	0.018
4	0.016
5	0.014
6	0.013
7	0.012
8	0.011
9	0.011
14	0.009
19	0.008
∞	0.001

significant result at the first interim analysis would occur if a difference in response rates of 26% between the two treatments was observed. This corresponds to an OR$=2.91$, which is a more credible value than the OR$=4.13$ required for the first method to be significant at the first interim analysis, albeit still much more than anticipated by the design value of OR$=1.35$.

One difficulty with the second procedure is that it does assume that there are approximately equal numbers of events available between successive analyses. In practice clinical trial co-operative groups usually prefer interim analyses to coincide more with the calendar of meetings than on more scientific criteria. For trials concerned with survival as the end-point it does not take account of the data that will subsequently become available on those patients still alive after the trial has been closed following a statistically significant interim analysis. This is also true of the simple $p=0.001$ procedure but this is unlikely to be influenced more than marginally by these outstanding data.

So far we have described methods of interim analysis that use stopping rules that do not directly utilize clinical opinion. They are merely statistical rules in which the final decision consequent on a p-value below a certain critical value is transferred to a data-monitoring committee for their consideration.

Clearly clinical opinion is incorporated into the original study design of all phase III trials. This involvement can be extended to the formalization of this opinion into appropriate stopping rules to be used at interim analysis. The method requires, at the design stage of the study, that clinical opinion is obtained and summarized on what difference in the two treatments, for example, new and standard therapies, under study is required for the new treatment to replace the standard. In forming this opinion the individual clinician will consider many factors. If the main outcome of interest is survival then any improvement in survival, even a very modest advantage, brings benefit. However, this presumes there are no other considerations involved. For example, if the standard treatment is no treatment, then the marginal advantage of an "active" therapy could well be questioned. The active therapy may involve the patient returning for therapy on a regular basis with associated "costs" in patient concern as well as monetary costs of the treatment itself. Perhaps more realistically if the new treatment is more toxic than the old then the new treatment would have to bring sufficient gain in survival to outweigh in some sense the short or longer-term reduction in the quality of life consequential on receiving the treatment. Only if this gain could be clearly demonstrated would it be appropriate for the new treatment to come into everyday clinical practice.

In developing appropriate stopping rules the clinicians are therefore asked to give their opinion of the level of improvement which exactly compensates for the other, real or perceived, shortcomings of the new treatment. Without going into details, essentially the investigators planning the new study are asked to provide a range of equivalence of the therapies under test. They first do this on an individual basis and then meet collectively to produce a consensus range of equivalence for the trial. This is then used to construct an appropriate stopping rule.

In a similar way to the previous interim analysis methods described it is also necessary to decide on the number of interim analyses that are intended. This then provides an appropriate interim analysis significance level, again analogous to the corresponding value in Table 1, but now which also depends on the "range of equivalence" provided by the investigators. The implementation of the method requires the calculation of a confidence interval (CI) at each interim analysis.

For a particular trial the standard (95%) CI is replaced by a wider CI dependent on the number of interim analyses proposed and the range of equivalence specified. For example, if the number of interim analyses is set at 9 and the range of equivalence is set to a width of one unit of treatment difference, then the nominal test size would be adjusted to $\alpha = 0.0119$ (compare with 0.011 in Table 1) and a 98.81% or approximately 99% CI used, rather than the 95% CI which is reserved for the final comparison at the end of the trial. A unit of treatment difference is the actual difference anticipated divided by its standard deviation. How this procedure works in practice is shown in Figure 1.

Thus the protocol design team identify that if the benefit to the new treatment is less than δ_1 they would stick to the standard therapy but were it larger than δ_2 they would utilize the new therapy in subsequent patients. If the advantage to the new therapy was between δ_1 and δ_2 they would deem the therapies of equivalent value for treatment of patients. The value $\delta = 0$ corresponds to the treatments being of equal efficacy. Suppose at a particular interim analysis the (wider) CI "starts" in the range of equivalence and "ends" indicating an advantage to the new treatment. In this event the trial is closed to patient entry and the new treatment recommended. This

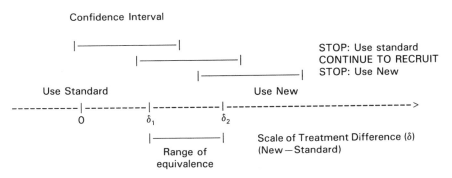

Figure 1. Graphical representation of stopping rules based on the range of equivalence provided by the protocol writing team (after Freedman, Lowe and Macaskill [4])

is illustrated by the CI labelled : STOP : Use New, in Figure 1. If on the other hand the CI "starts" in the region for which the standard will be retained and "ends" in the range of equivalence, then the trial would also close to patient entry. This is indicated by the CI : STOP : Use Standard in Figure 1. This time the standard therapy would be recommended. Finally if neither "end" of the CI lies in the range of equivalence the trial continues. Detailed tables for the "interim" significance levels required for a specific test size, number of interim analyses and range of equivalence are given by Freedman et al. [4].

It should be noted that the notions of "start" and "end" of a CI are somewhat misleading since a CI is not guaranteed to contain the true difference between the treatments. Thus treatment differences below the "start" and above the "end" of any CI cannot be ruled out albeit they are thought to be unlikely.

The first method for interim analysis described is very simple and can be implemented with the minimum of planning. It does not require equal spacings, either of time, patients recruited or events, between "interim" analyses, and it ensures that trials are not closed too early with associated high levels of uncertainty on treatment efficacy remaining. It can be applied whatever the outcome measure, survival time, response rates or some laboratory value and does not change with the statistical test used. It has the added advantage that it can be easily explained. It may, however, miss in the early stages of a trial the opportunity of stopping the trial if a new therapy is doing worse than the standard. The other methods described are more complex, particularly that which requires a range of equivalence to be specified. Their implementation requires in advance of patient recruitment the often unrealistic specification of the precise number of interim analyses planned. The appropriate significance levels used are also dependent to some extent on the type of data, survival time, response rates or continuous outcome variables being used for the treatment comparison. The obvious advantage of involving the clinicians in the formulation of appropriate stopping rules requires no justification, however.

This latter method of developing stopping rules can be used directly to assist decision making consequential on the results of randomized phase III clinical trials in cancer as it attempts to bring the decision-making process nearer to the "real life" clinical situation. In contrast the earlier methods have been "single end-point" related and have merely passed over a statistically significant effect at an interim analysis to another group, the data-monitoring committee, for a final judgment.

Now it is clear that the statistical evidence is important in any decision-making process but as such is only part of the "evidence" that the monitoring committee must evaluate. The members of such a monitoring committee should be wholly or at least mainly distinct from the trial organizers, so that they can act with appropriate authority and independence as the occasion arises. The committee will reflect opinion and uncertainty which may be different from involved clinicians. There are few formal rules for how the ultimate decision to close a trial or to continue patient recruitment to a trial should be taken. The magnitude and direction of the observed effect will be one important influence on this process. Other criteria will vary from trial to trial. Decisions will no doubt be influenced by the particular experiences of the individual members of the committee. The published literature will be relevant to this process as will "gossip" as to the benefits or shortcomings of the relevant treatments. Whatever the process used in arriving at a decision, a trial should *not* be stopped if it leaves the level of uncertainty about the relative efficacy of the alternative treatments at an unacceptably high level. In some circumstances a trial may be stopped, not because of efficacy but because the associated toxicity is so high as to be life threatening for many patients. However, as we have already mentioned, this fact would provide grounds for ceasing the use of the particular therapy in question without any reference to its efficacy. Such problems should be "unexpected" by definition else the phase III trial should not have started. If indeed the level of toxicity was truly "unexpected" then this might suggest a modification to the protocol treatment schedule or dose rather than the cessation of recruitment, thus providing a quite different but legitimate alternative to closure in appropriate circumstances. The monitoring committee must therefore balance the ethics between continuation of a trial, perhaps denying half the patients treatment, against discontinuation of a trial which leaves the levels of uncertainty unacceptably high. Is the evidence, although there is some, yet sufficient to close to patient recruitment?

A randomized phase III trial should never be closed in the early stages of recruitment merely because it is failing to reach the anticipated "minimal" benefit envisaged at the design stage of the study. This is because early closing of a study in these circumstances will leave the associated CI unacceptably wide thereby indicating the possibility of a plausible, and maybe worthwhile, advantage to one therapy even when there is no true difference in treatment efficacy. In such circumstances the level of uncertainty remains unacceptably high.

Whatever method of interim analysis is implemented it is of paramount importance that the data and hence the interim analyses themselves are as up to date and complete as possible [5]. If "interim" analyses are planned rather than performed on an "ad hoc" basis then not only can the responsible trials office prepare for the successive analyses in advance, it can warn the clinicians from the participating centres so that the data available within a particular clinic can be passed to the trials office without delay. Inevitably some delay is unavoidable; for example, data may have to be posted or a data item verified, but these delays can be reduced to a minimum by careful planning, good data management procedures and, above all, active involvement of the investigators. It is important too that the data once within the trials office is immediately verified and checked for consistencies with earlier data, and transferred as quickly as possible to the computer file accessed by the interim analysis. Any analysis based on incomplete data is by definition not up to date and at worst may be misleading. If there are several key end-points of concern in a trial together with perhaps detailed but more secondary data, it may be that the trials office gives more emphasis and urgency to being up to date with these items and allowing "fast track" methods for their processing. The ethical requirement that the clinician does his best for the individual patient during treatment extends beyond the clinical activity, to responsibility for the quality, accuracy and despatch of that data without delay. At that stage, responsibility for the ethics is transferred to the analysis team and then to the interim analysis review committee.

In summary there is a clear ethical need to monitor the progress of randomized phase III trials by means of successive "interim" analyses. The simplest procedure is to do as many interim analyses as is thought appropriate, without rigidly defining the rules on frequency, number of patients or events, and to use a significance test of size $\alpha = 0.001$ on each occasion. The final report on the trial would then give a valid estimate of the relative treatment effect and associated 95% CI, at whatever stage the trial is stopped, whether early or after planned recruitment has been achieved.

This procedure recognizes the realities with, in particular, multicentre trials in that many trials are not up to date at the time of planned interim analyses. Experience suggests that if one such analysis is "significant" this prompts an urgent request for outstanding data, which then initiates a further and extra "interim" analysis. If the planned number of interim analyses is fixed, either by time or numbers of events, then this additional analysis does not have the properties of the scheduled interim analysis (Table 1 and Figure 1) unless the extreme nominal level, here set at 0.001, is adhered to. This recommendation therefore reflects the practicalities of co-ordinating a randomized phase III trial in cancer, hopefully involving many patients, from many centres, treated by numerous investigators.

REFERENCES

1. Errington RD, Ashby D, Gore SM et al (1991) High energy neutron treatment for pelvic cancers: study stopped because of increased mortality. Br Med J 302: 1045–1051
2. Dillman RO, Seagren SL, Propert KJ et al (1990) A randomised trial of induction chemotherapy plus high-dose radiation versus radiation alone in stage III non-small-cell lung cancer. N Engl J M 323: 940–945
3. Pocock SJ (1977) Group sequential methods in the design and analysis of clinical trials. Biometrika 64: 191–199
4. Freedman LS, Lowe D, Macaskill P (1984) Stopping rules for clinical trials incorporating clinical opinion. Biometrics 40: 575–586
5. COMPACT Steering Committee (1991) Improving the quality of data in clinical trials in cancer. Br J Cancer 63: 412–415

ABOUT THE AUTHOR

David Machin is Chief Statistician in charge of the MRC Cancer Trials Office in Cambridge. His office co-ordinates over 40 randomized trials on behalf of the MRC Cancer Therapy Committee. He was formerly Head of Medical Statistics and Computing at the University of Southampton and before that a Senior Statistician for the EORTC Data Center in Brussels, Belgium. He is a statistical consultant to the Human Reproduction Programme of WHO and Senior Visiting Fellow at the University of Surrey Institute of Public Health. He is the author with M. J. Campbell of two books—one on sample sizes for clinical trials and one on medical statistics. He is an editor of *Statistics in Medicine* and a member of the editorial board of *Clinical Oncology*. He is an examiner for the Faculty of Radiologists.

16 Experiments on the Dying

GRAHAM THORPE

HUMAN GUINEA PIGS

In 1967 the debate concerning the medical ethics of research on patients was fuelled dramatically by the publication in Britain of a book, *Human Guinea Pigs*, by M. H. Pappworth [1]. He drew attention to the fact that the human being was the only animal that doctors could experiment upon without a licence, and demonstrated a wide gap between the doctor's care of the patient and his pursuit of knowledge. A chapter was devoted to each of the following vulnerable groups: infants and children, pregnant women, mental defectives and mentally sick, prison inmates, the dying and the old, and patients awaiting or undergoing operations.

Looking back 25 years, much of the research cited involved puncture and catheterization of blood and other vessels, an indication of the frontier of medical progress at that time. Numerous examples of exploitation and abuse were given. With respect to the dying and the old, Pappworth lists the new techniques of splenic puncture to measure blood pressure in the splenic vein in patients with liver disease and percutaneous splenoportography, percutaneous transhepatic cannulation of a hepatic or portal vein, arterial and cardiac catheterization, and cannulation of the thoracic duct.

Other research involved the production of temporary anuria by the injection of large volumes of water intravenously to induce haemolysis, the measurement of oxygen consumption in paralysed men exposed to cold, and rib puncture with the injection of contrast medium to outline the azygos veins.

In some of the patients, many of whom had advanced cancer, there were complications ranging from minor to serious, and several died as a direct result of the experiments. In a number of instances a new investigational procedure was first practised on cadavers and then on an ill patient with a poor prognosis. If he should die in the course of perfecting the technique or improving the operator's technical skill, then that would be unfortunate, but a lesser loss than a fitter patient or normal subject.

All this research was non-therapeutic and of no benefit to the persons concerned and Pappworth argued that patients seriously ill with advanced disease should not be treated as expendable, but they were entitled to the best possible palliative care. As for experiments and research they should be regarded as prohibited subjects. To this end acknowledged and observed

Introducing New Treatments for Cancer: Practical, Ethical and Legal Problems. Edited by C. J. Williams
© 1992 John Wiley & Sons Ltd

safeguards should be introduced otherwise abuses would inevitably continue.

A SECRET TRIAL

Fourteen years later in 1981 an anterior resection of a carcinoma of the rectum was performed on an 84-year-old widow who had previously enjoyed good health. She died 15 days later from acute bone marrow depression induced by 5-fluorouracil (5-FU). At the inquest it emerged that the patient had been an unwitting participant in a randomized controlled trial (see Chapter 5 for further discussion).

Following earlier work which suggested that the infusion of 5-FU into the portal vein would reduce the incidence of liver metastasis, a new multicentre study had been set up. After an operation to remove a primary carcinoma of rectum had been performed, patients with no evidence of metastatic disease were allocated randomly into three groups. In one there was no further treatment. In the second group, as heparin had been given with the 5-FU in the previous study, to determine whether this drug alone had any effect a heparin infusion was given via the portal vein twice daily for seven days. In the third group 500 mg of 5-FU was infused with heparin as in the second group.

Careful consideration had been given by ethical committees as to whether patients and their relatives should be informed of the existence and details of the trial, and it had been decided that they should not be informed and therefore their consent was not sought.

Writing about this case in *The Lancet* the barrister Diana Brahams stated:

> I find the concept of secret random control trials wholly unacceptable, and the reasons offered to justify them both unconvincing and unsatisfactory. It is usual to tell patients and obtain their consent apparently, but where the end measure is death and cancer is involved the doctor thinks he knows best.

At the inquest evidence showed that the trial protocol which required blood counts every other day after operation had not been followed and therefore the bone marrow depression which had occurred was not detected at an early stage. The coroner brought in a verdict of misadventure and stated that the whole idea of concealed controlled trials should be brought to the public notice so that proper discussion could take place.

ETHICAL PRINCIPLES

The ethics of administering a potentially lethal treatment to patients who may have been cured of their disease is outside the compass of this chapter, but the above case demonstrates clearly that in 1981 a group of research workers considered it acceptable practice to embark on a secret trial of a novel therapy. Patients and families were not informed of the existence and nature of the trial and their consent was not sought. Committees established to maintain ethical standards, to protect subjects of research from harm and to preserve their rights gave approval to this trial.

History teaches us that from time immemorial the human race has been divided and redivided into groups with labels. One result of such division is that a member of one group perceives a member of another group as "other than" and "different from" himself. This is a situation in which exploitation arises easily. Thus, having attached the label of "cancer" or "dying" to a patient, he can be treated differently from other patients and may be included in a secret trial without being asked to give his consent.

Most people, and doctors are no exception, find it easy to pass on good news but have difficulty in communicating bad news. At the time the above trial was being set up, Ian Kennedy was giving the Reith Lectures, and discussing honest communication with the dying said:

> People do not want to die, neither do they want to know they are dying, nor could they tolerate being told they are dying, nor do they know they are dying. Some or even all of these assumptions may be well-founded on occasions but they are unsupported by any evidence. They reflect the anxieties of the healthy.

And later:

> The doctors realised that some patients may indeed have wished to know the truth but, since without asking they could not know which patients, they managed the problem by not telling anyone. This may have proved the ideal coping mechanism for the doctors. But it meant that only the patient who insisted on the truth and was confident enough to be persistent, got his way.

Cancer patients and dying patients are a forceful reminder of our own mortality and it is not surprising that there are communication problems when we meet them.

Has the situation changed ten years on from the Reith Lectures? Indeed it has. It is now recognized more widely that part of the doctor–patient contract is the provision of information about the illness, and that the well-informed patient is much more likely to co-operate in the management and treatment of his disease.

Some patients prefer a paternalistic approach by their doctor, trusting him to act in their best interest. In such circumstances the doctor, having discussed this matter with the patient and defined their relationship, should then respect his attitude and act accordingly (see Chapter 4). However, most patients today expect to be kept informed about their illness and its progress, and wish to share in the decision making, thus working in partnership with their doctor throughout. The development of the hospice movement over the past twenty years and also the advent of medical oncology departments have fostered open and honest communication in the context of cancer and other lethal diseases.

The two important ethical principles with respect to medical research are patient autonomy and informed consent. The report of the Royal College of Physicians, *Research involving patients* (see Chapter 3), sets out clear guidelines. Special attention is drawn to certain groups of patients, namely children, mentally handicapped people, mentally ill patients, prisoners, severely ill or unconscious patients, pregnant patients and elderly patients. These are remarkably similar to Pappworth's vulnerable groups although dying patients are not specifically considered as a separate group.

This document also states: "There are some circumstances in which it is justifiable to initiate research without the consent of the patient." Reference is made to observational research totally without risk, innocuous research involving comprehension and the examination of anonymous specimens. In the companion report of the Royal College of Physicians, *Guidelines on the practice of ethics committees in medical research involving human subjects* [2], there exists a similar loophole. Referring to research without consent this document states: "There are some research activities which an Ethics Committee may agree can be carried out without consent of the subject." One category is:

> Where it is the investigator's medical opinion that disclosure of the information that would be adequate for consent would be so harmful that it would be unjustifiable, this can only be a decision about individual patients and only in therapeutic research and only if the option is approved by the Ethics Committee.

This was the exact situation with respect to the secret trial described above in that it was considered harmful to tell patients that they had cancer or to inform them of the serious nature of their disease: ironically, the widow who died in fact knew that she had cancer. Thus, even in the present more enlightened climate and with up-to-date guidelines on research and ethics committees, although less likely, it remains possible for patients, including terminally ill patients, to be included in trials without their knowledge.

Raanan Gillon, writing on autonomy and consent in *Moral dilemmas in modern medicine* [3], states:

> Whenever one imposes decisions upon people without consulting them, let alone against their will, whether or not these decisions are designed to be beneficial, one is treating them as things or animals or as children, but not rational agents, not as ends in themselves.

Proper consent is the cornerstone of ethical medical research. Although those responsible for the Royal College of Physicians reports *Research involving patients* and *Guidelines on the practice of ethics committees in medical research involving human subjects* were not prepared to make informed consent an absolute condition of all research, for the full protection of the patient with advanced and lethal disease such consent should be mandatory.

Where children are concerned, whether or not they are dying, *Research involving patients* gives clear guidance. Research which could equally well be done on adults should never be done on children. Except in rare circumstances, non-therapeutic research in children should not carry greater than minimal risk. There must be no financial or other inducement. Where a child is capable of giving legally valid consent for a research procedure, the advice is that the approval of a parent or guardian should still be obtained for a child under the age of 16 years. Where the child is not competent to give consent, although the law is unclear, the prevailing view is that as it is the duty of the parent to act in the best interests of the child the investigator can properly rely on the consent of a parent or guardian with respect to research. If, when parental approval has been obtained, a child were to object to the procedure himself, then the investigator should reconsider whether it would be appropriate to proceed.

What is the situation then with respect to adults, or even children, where there is mental impairment and the individual is not able to give consent? A number of terminally ill patients have primary or metastatic cerebral tumours or metabolic states that cloud consciousness and it might well be on occasion that there are good reasons for wishing to undertake research in them. Where a mentally handicapped person is not competent to give consent, *Research involving patients* states that there is no provision in law providing for another individual to give consent on his behalf. Referring to a recent decision of the House of Lords which established that a doctor may proceed with treatment in such circumstances without the patient's consent, provided that he acts in the best interests of the patient in accordance with a practice accepted by a responsible body of medical opinion, it is suggested that the principles enunciated might apply where the research involves treatment chosen for the patient by the exercise of the investigator's clinical judgment. The relatives should also be consulted.

Pappworth concluded that patients with a poor prognosis or dying should be protected from taking part in any research whatsoever. But are dying patients different from other patients? For the purposes of research, no. All patients should be treated in the same way and research protocols discussed with them and their consent and participation invited.

PRACTICAL PROBLEMS

One of the criticisms of those involved in the remarkable development of palliative care over the past twenty years has been the paucity of research.

Treatments have tended to proceed by fashion rather than by critical judgment. For example, prochlorperazine, which had pride of place as the general anti-emetic agent of choice, has now been replaced in many centres by haloperidol. Both are effective, but which is better remains uncertain. In patients with advanced disease of various kinds vomiting may be due to one or more of a long list of causes, but a well-conducted trial comparing several anti-emetic drugs has never been done to provide evidence on which rational choice can be based. By contrast, in medical oncology trials of anti-emetic agents for the treatment of vomiting induced by chemotherapy appear almost weekly!

Again, for the patient unable to take oral drugs their administration by the subcutaneous route via a syringe driver has to a large extent replaced the rectal route, but there are no studies comparing these two methods of administration.

What then are the problems which have hampered research in palliative care? One obvious difficulty is the brief and uncertain prognosis. However, well-designed short-term studies can provide useful information.

Many patients are ill and weak and face progressive deterioration. They find it difficult to concentrate for any length of time and research involving the completion of questionnaires or visual analogue scales on a regular basis may prove too demanding as their disease advances.

The perception of the pioneers of the hospice movement was that terminally ill patients were not being provided with good care. As a result of their commitment and that of those following them, undoubtedly there has been a tremendous improvement in the standard of palliative care. However, it is easy to regard these patients as a special group and once labelled to treat them differently. Probably the major problem with respect to research in palliative care has been the desire of the carers to protect their patients. In an extreme form the patient is tucked up in bed and loved to death, never being allowed the option to develop fully as an individual at this time of potential growth. No one would want a modern hospice to become like Bedlam long ago where patients with mental illness were put on display, as in a zoo, for all and sundry to gawp at and comment upon. But a sensible balance has to be struck.

Hospices have been encouraged to develop as teaching centres but sometimes a barrier of protection created by staff has made medical students and other learners unwelcome, the view being taken that it is unfair for dying patients to be exploited for teaching purposes. In actual fact most hospice patients enjoy meeting students and others, and are only too happy to discuss their illnesses and feelings with them. Medical students at Southampton Medical School undertake in their fourth year a simple research project under supervision as part of their education, and a number have chosen to do this work at Countess Mountbatten House, a palliative care unit for cancer patients within the National Health Service. Lacking the inhibitions which appear to come with qualification they have entered into this research with enthusiasm, often exploring difficult areas such as communication and the awareness of patients and relatives of the serious nature of the illness. Not only has some useful work been accomplished but almost without exception patients have been keen to participate in these projects.

The devotion of the staff to the care of patients with advanced disease together with a powerful protective instinct can easily result in their becoming, not as was considered earlier, a vulnerable group, but instead an invulnerable group within a zariba unable to be approached by any research worker. Obviously such carers will not be undertaking any research themselves!

Within the hospice movement some useful research has been undertaken. As far as drugs are concerned the major interest has been in the opioids, with Twycross and Hanks taking the lead. Much more remains to be done and there is ample opportunity. Over 130 000 patients in Britain die from cancer every year and the proportion included in research projects is minuscule. Those working in the field of palliative care should consult together and agree on a number of simple questions which need to be answered. Then appropriate research protocols can be devised and programmes implemented, if necessary on a multicentre basis.

A HEROIC DEATH?

Basing decisions on assumptions is as hazardous as walking on thin ice. If terminally ill patients were allowed to speak for themselves a different story might be heard. They do not present as a clone but as a wide range of individuals. Some will certainly wish to be left alone and will decline participation in any research; however, a majority would be only too pleased to share in a project, which even if it did not help them might benefit other patients. As with telling the truth the only way to determine the patient's wishes is to ask him. With regard to research, only by entering into some discussion, explaining the project and inviting participation can the individual patient's views be obtained.

In an age of transplant surgery many people are prepared to sign donor cards giving permission for organs to be used in the event of their death. Some patients with great altruism press hard a request that after death their bodies be used for medical science and research. Such offers are nearly always an embarrassment to the doctor concerned. Rarely can a grateful recipient for such a unique gift be found amongst research workers and even medical schools, now that students have given up dissection, no longer seek cadavers.

Some societies, usually those with warlike propensity, encourage the placement of a high value on a heroic death. This was the case with the

Japanese kamikaze pilots in the Second World War, and more recent examples have been the Moslem fanatics on suicidal missions driving vehicles filled with explosives at selected targets in Lebanon, and children in the name of Islam bravely marching forward across minefields in the Iran–Iraq war. Their powerful motivation required to achieve self-sacrifice is based not on any humanitarian principle but is a religious fervour created by a vision of post-mortem glory and reward. But in many people from less belligerent backgrounds there is the desire for their death and dying to have meaning. Part of this search for meaning may be realized in undertaking some act which will benefit their fellow human beings. An invitation to a dying person to take part in a research project, even though it may not provide any benefit for himself, can create a good opportunity for contributing something of value to society as well as achieving a degree of personal satisfaction.

CONCLUSION

The egregious atrocities of the Nazi party during the Second World War were exposed at the Nuremburg trials and included criminal medical experiments on unwilling prisoners in the name of research. The Nuremburg Code was then drawn up, which made it clear that the voluntary consent of the human subject was absolutely essential for participation in any medical research. Patient autonomy and informed consent have underpinned the ethics of all medical research, and clear guidelines were embodied in the World Medical Association declaration of Helsinki in 1964 and subsequently revised in 1975.

Much research needs to be done in the field of palliative care and there is ample opportunity. Dying patients can so easily become isolated from their family, friends and even professional staff responsible for their care. It is their right to be treated as people who are able still to make significant contributions to those around them. Most of these patients will be only too pleased to share in research if invited to do so. In this way they may bequeath to those who come after them something of value, and likewise the research worker must bequeath an unimpeachable ethical standard.

REFERENCES

1. Pappworth MH (1967) Human guinea pigs. Routledge & Kegan Paul, London
2. Royal College of Physicians (1990) Guidelines on the practice of ethics committees in medical research involving human subjects, 2nd edn. RCP, London
3. Gillon R (1985) Autonomy and consent. In: Lockwood M (ed) Moral dilemmas in modern medicine. Oxford University Press

ABOUT THE AUTHOR

After 12 years as a general physician on the Isle of Wight **Dr Graham Thorpe** was appointed Consultant in Palliative Medicine at Countess Mountbatten House in 1980. At this busy National Health Service unit, in addition to clinical work, he has been responsible for the expansion and development of an educational programme for a wide range of disciplines engaged in palliative care. He is Chairman of the Association for Palliative Medicine.

Section III

INDUSTRY AND COST OF TREATMENT DEVELOPMENT

Notes on Section III

This section is introduced by a chapter on evaluation of the general costs of cancer therapy. **Bengt Jönsson** and **Göran Karlsson** clearly outline the complexity of evaluating the costs of new treatments. A proper cost–benefit analysis takes many factors into account, not just the cost of the new therapy itself. Comments in the rest of this section regarding the high cost of new therapies must be viewed with this in mind. Unfortunately, analysis of cost/benefit is complex and must potentially fail if only estimates of comparative efficiency are available or if inappropriate comparisons are made. Other costs in the equation, such as patient time, are difficult to measure so that the final result is a best approximation. Hillman and colleagues (*New England Journal of Medicine*, 324: 1991, 1362–5) have warned about pitfalls in cost-effectiveness research particularly when this is sponsored by pharmaceutical companies.

The following chapters in this section discuss various aspects of the role of the pharmaceutical industry in the clinical development of new treatments for cancer. In order to put these into context it is important to consider how they fit in with national and academic approaches to this problem. In past years most clinical cancer research was funded nationally or by universities, often supported by cancer charities. The way this worked has obviously varied around the world depending on the health system in operation. For instance, the National Cancer Institute in the USA has in the past provided large sums of money to support clinical research in a private health care model which is predominantly based on reimbursement by insurance companies. In contrast, the National Health Service (NHS) in Britain has paid for patient care whilst academics supported by cancer charities have conducted the trials.

At present both of these systems (and others around the world) are threatened by economic restraints. In the USA the *Journal of the National Cancer Institute* regularly includes articles with titles such as "Viability of cancer clinical research: patient accrual, coverage and reimbursement", "What's going on with project grant funding at NCI?" and "Researchers deal with funding frustrations", whilst *The Lancet* in Great Britain carries papers such as "Clinical research: disturbing present, uncertain future". These bemoan the relative scarcity of funding and the small slice of the cake awarded to cancer research. In Britain the advent of the current major reorganization of the NHS is seen as a very real threat. Patient treatments will need to be costed and patients won in a new era of competitive

Introducing New Treatments for Cancer: Practical, Ethical and Legal Problems. Edited by C. J. Williams
© 1992 John Wiley & Sons Ltd

contracting. As yet, some months after implementation of the government White Paper, there is no mechanism in place to support clinical research.

In the past (ten or more years ago) there was a honeymoon period in the relationship between the pharmaceutical industry and researchers. Nearly all the drugs were new and many were covered by patents, and researchers were in a position to fund their own trials via grants—the industry seemed happy to let them get along with this. **Phil Schein** (Chapter 17) alluded to changes in this relationship when, as president, he addressed the American Society of Clinical Oncology a decade ago. His words have been prophetic—especially as he now writes representing the view of the pharmaceutical industry!

Since academic medicine appears to have a decreasing power to fund its own clinical research, the industry has stepped into the breach—at a price to the scientific impartiality of research. One of the problems of current research methods has been the ever-increasing costs of drug development. The introduction of a new agent may cost £100–150 million. This is bound to be reflected in a very high cost of the drug if it is released commercially—when it often has a relatively short patent life. The problem is worsened in cancer because the drug either works and helps or cures the patient within a few treatments when it is stopped, or rapidly fails and is stopped even earlier. Thus the potential profit from treating a single patient is small unless each treatment is very expensive—this is in marked contrast to, say, a beta-blocker used for heart problems which may be taken for years. Since the manufacturer needs to recoup the same development costs and make a profit from both drugs, we have a situation where six injections of a new anticancer drug may cost £4000 whilst years of daily heart tablets costs the same. To those assessing treatment costs cancer treatments will instantly appear a poor buy, even before their efficacy is assessed. With few exceptions drug treatment of cancer is only partially effective, so that managers and insurance companies may look at expensive new treatments with a jaundiced eye.

One of my objectives was to persuade an expert within the pharmaceutical industry to write a chapter on pricing of new drugs; unfortunately I was, perhaps for obvious reasons, unable to get anyone to put pen to paper. However, in discussion it does appear that pricing of new drugs uses some of the theories generally applied in pricing any goods or services.

Clearly this is a complex area but the basic decision of a drug company is how to make as big a profit as possible from their investment in development of the new drug. The problem is, does high pricing and smaller volume yield a better profit than low pricing/high volume? Whilst marketing of a new drug must be intrinsically different from selling a new model of a car there remain similarities in approach. Whether these are desirable remains open to question.

Image is all important in selling products and a high price often adds to image—car makers such as Jaguar are not afraid to sell their cars as expensive luxury items, whilst Volkswagen make a point in emphasizing that their cars are good buys. In selling a new drug the company concerned needs to convince doctors that this is the Rolls Royce medicine for the condition concerned. Once convinced, the price is less important—indeed, expensive drugs may be seen as more powerful, especially by patients. This is currently exemplified by a very expensive new antisickness drug (ondansetron) used to reduce nausea and vomiting caused by anticancer drugs. In newspaper articles this drug was lauded by a celebrity with cancer as a highly effective new drug not available (an inaccurate statement) to the NHS because of its price. Since then many patients have demanded this treatment—often in inappropriate circumstances. In this situation the high price probably played a part in boosting the image of the drug as the best treatment available. The decision as to the real efficacy of a new drug should depend on the results of properly randomized trials and not on the image created by marketing divisions of pharmaceutical companies.

The pharmaceutical market is not an open market—new drugs are often under patent so that initially there is a monopoly; the number and attitudes of buyers is also restricted since the drug must be prescribed by doctors. Non-regulated monopolies are free to price at what the market will bear, though this may be curbed by fear of government regulation and desire to penetrate the market faster with a low price. The relationship between price and demand is referred to as *price elasticity*. If the quantity demanded falls rapidly with increasing price this is described as elastic demand. Up until recently in the UK many pharmaceutical compounds have had an inelastic demand, price not making a major difference to demand. This has been because the cost of the drug has been distanced from the patient and physician since the NHS picks up the bill. Similarly in the USA insurance companies and doctors have in the past been less concerned about drug pricing. In this situation it is easier to price new drugs high even if the data on improved efficacy are not available. This state of affairs is, and should be, changing.

When pricing an innovative product companies can choose between two alternatives: market skimming and market penetration. Many pharmaceutical companies set high initial prices to "skim" the market. Such a company estimates the highest price it can charge given the *apparent* comparative benefits of its new drug. They set a price at which it is worthwhile some segments of the market using the drug, and when initial sales slow down they lower the price to draw in the next price-sensitive layer of customers. In this way they maximize profit from each segment of the market. In the drug world markets do vary from country to country and within the private/insurance-based, national health service and government and charity aid sectors.

The alternative is to adopt a low price, hoping to attract a large number of buyers in order to maximize profit. In financial terms price skimming is sensible if there are: (1) sufficient buyers with a high demand; (2) the cost of unit production in a small volume is not so much higher as to cancel out the advantage of charging what the market will bear; (3) the high price supports the image of a superior product. A strategy of low pricing is favoured by: (1) the market being highly price sensitive, with low price stimulating market growth; (2) production costs falling quickly with long production runs; (3) low price discouraging competition.

To date buyers of new anticancer drugs have had little impact on the pricing strategies of companies, which has resulted in a policy of market skimming. If we wish to change this we need to show that product image is based on actual results from controlled trials and not the promoted image of the marketing division. We also need to show that we are price sensitive—something that is likely to happen in these times of financial cutbacks.

There is an international awareness that the process of drug development needs to be improved (Meeting of the Royal Society of Medicine, 19 March 1990, *Journal of the Royal Society of Medicine*, 1991, 84: 52–55) and that the interface between researchers, pharmaceutical companies, regulatory authorities and the market needs strengthening (How drugs get to market, *Drug Therapeutics Bulletin*, 1990, 28: 101–104). Clearly, a major concern of regulatory authorities is the need to ensure that the new drugs are safe—a function that was highlighted by the devastating and unexpected thalidomide disaster. This aspect of new drug development is of paramount importance, though the emphasis on safety is probably even greater for, say, a new anti-arthritis drug compared with a new treatment for acute leukaemia. This difference in emphasis means that toxic drugs can be used for potentially fatal diseases that would never gain a licence for less serious indications. However, these may also be used as a way of gaining a tacit acceptance of a new drug without demonstrating whether it is beneficial to the patients. Traditionally new anticancer drugs have been submitted for licensing on the basis of demonstrating the rate of tumour shrinkage (percentage response rate). Such data have not demanded that it be shown that patients feel better or live longer for their treatment. The decision as to whether drugs be used has been left to the discretion of the individual clinician, market forces (including drug company promotion) and to a lesser extent clinical trials or "directives" (see Chapters 27 and 29) from governmental bodies or research organizations.

Whilst demonstration of a simple response rate was undoubtedly sufficient evidence for licensing anticancer drugs in the past, this practice is now questionable. There is a real dilemma: requirement to demonstrate efficacy would markedly increase the already great burden of the cost of drug development on pharmaceutical companies who we already rely on for producing sorely needed new compounds. Even if they can maintain current research programmes drug companies will in turn have to pass on the cost in yet higher prices for new products. However, the current practice of willy-nilly use of new drugs based on inadequate and uncontrolled data is hardly defensible. Whether this is the remit of licensing authorities is debatable. One aspect might be: a licence is usually provided for a specific indication (e.g. cisplatin (Paraplatin) for ovarian carcinoma and small-cell lung cancer in the UK); despite this such drugs rapidly become used in a much wider variety of conditions (though drug companies cannot promote such use). So far regulatory authorities have turned a blind eye to this; indeed daunorubicin, the standard first choice in acute myelogenous leukaemia, has *no* licence in the UK. These authorities and possibly medical defence societies need to ask whether drugs should be used routinely in unlicensed ways. To date, the concept of "clinical freedom" has allowed physicians to prescribe in such circumstances with impunity. Perhaps one way around this is to have a drug licence which operates at two levels. Initially the drug could be licensed for sale provided it is only used for the condition indicated and in studies designed to test whether it is beneficial to patients. Such trials would by their very nature have to be very simple in their concept (see Chapters 12 and 13). Such post-marketing studies would be a necessary prerequisite to the granting of a full licence which would be given on demonstration of patient benefit.

It seems likely that most regulatory authorities would feel that this approach was beyond their remit, in which case there is still a need for post-marketing studies to decide on the worth of new therapies. Since over 90% of cancer patients are treated outside of cancer trials it would be a worthwhile goal for national cancer institutions (where they exist) to organize large, simple studies of current therapies (leaving specialist centres to develop innovative new treatments) in an attempt to define "best current practice". Such trials may well cross national boundaries. In the UK the introduction of the changes in the NHS structure should demand that money is set aside for such research. If one of the aims of the new philosophy of the NHS is cost effectiveness then methods of assessing drug effectiveness will need to be provided—the only valid way to test new treatments is in randomized clinical trials. Decisions on treatment effectiveness and use cannot simply be left to market forces.

This long preamble brings us to Chapter 18 by **Bill McCulloch** and **Phil Schein**, who discuss the role of industry in clinical research. They make the point that the pharmaceutical industry has a huge stake in new drug development; they invest more than any government agency and have funded large intra- and extramural development programmes. Despite this, the authors point out that the industry sees cancer as a difficult and potentially risky market. Amongst the problems they point out, the relatively restricted market is the most worrying. Although cancer is the second leading cause of death, there are hundreds of different tumours and a drug may only by useful in a few. For instance, there is little incentive for a drug company to develop a new drug for cancer of the adrenal gland; this is very rare, so that at best sales would be very small and the cost of drug development (£100 million) would be counter-productive. Schemes (orphan drug legislation) designed to give incentives for development of such drugs are available in some countries and may offset this problem to some extent.

McCulloch and Schein emphasize the need to streamline drug development (a consensus decision of the Royal Society of Medicine meeting mentioned above). They point out the need for discussion between company and researchers in order to overcome conflicting interests. Whilst this makes common sense it may be optimistic in the current climate to assume that there will be equable agreement. Since researchers may rely wholly on the company for the supply of the drug and for reimbursement of each patient treated (per capita payment) which may pay the salary of research nurses or fellows, it is likely that the piper will "pay the tune". As mentioned in the notes on Section I, one way around this would be for such monies to be handled through a central independent organization, though this would not overcome the problem of drug supply. However, inclusion of regulatory authorities at these design stages of new drug development might be a useful way of conciliation between the two parties which produces a plan providing the best scientific result and which satisfies the regulatory authority and drug company.

This chapter refers to the need for good clinical practice and the importance of pivotal studies. There is no doubt that these are essential, though as referred to above there is often doubt about patient benefit from a new therapy, so that a new type of pivotal study is needed—the really large-scale phase III trials previously discussed. Although the authors allude to such trials carried out under the auspices of sponsoring companies there are few if any true large-scale studies of this type and their completion has nearly always been hampered by the need for good clinical practice.

This is the topic of Chapter 19 by **Frank Wells** who is the Director of Medical Affairs at the Association of the British Pharmaceutical Industry (ABPI). Over the past decade there has been increasing appreciation for the need for care in carrying out clinical research in patients, though it is surprising that he singles out cancer research—where he suggests it may not be in the patients' best interest to be told that they are taking part in a clinical trial. This has resulted in voluntary (and in some countries legal) schemes designed to ensure the very highest standard of practice and data recording. Wells discusses the British approach to good clinical practice and the likely effects of new European legislation. This welcome approach to improving early clinical research can, however, appear at times too inflexible. There seems, to the clinician, too little discussion with regulatory authorities and drug companies as to the requirements for good clinical practice in the trial to hand. Thus, a study of a new drug for peptic ulceration may require a different pattern of development from, say, a new drug for a highly lethal tumour such as lung cancer. Regulatory authorities seem to play an essentially passive role—setting general standards and assessing trial data when a submission for drug registration and licensing is made. To date they have usually not wished to soil their hands or impugn their impartiality by being involved in advising on the design of drug development. This risks inefficiency, inappropriate goals and unnecessary red tape. Whilst the demands of good clinical practice discussed by Wells are sacrosanct in early drug development, it might be appropriate at the stage of phase III development to loosen the requirements in order to maximize patient numbers. This difficult interface between drug development and routine clinical practice was discussed above. If for instance a new drug is seen to have substantial activity in non-small-cell lung cancer (say 40% response rate), an early randomized trial of hundreds of patients would ensure that the true response rate in routine clinical practice would be defined with narrow confidence intervals and that survival could be assessed compared with standard current practice. In this way the real worth of the drug alone would be quickly established. Such trials are not possible using "good clinical practice"; they are only feasible using the principles outlined in Chapters 12 and 13 and these may not be acceptable to regulatory authorities because of their "loose" nature.

Renzo Canetta and his colleagues discuss strategies for development of analogues of existing drugs in Chapter 20. This problem was mentioned by McCulloch and Schein. There has been much work done attempting to see if drugs with a slightly different structure from their parent compound will either have greater efficacy or will be less toxic. Demonstration of less toxicity is easy but testing of efficacy is more problematic. If the drug proves to have activity where the parent compound is inactive there is no problem; the real difficulty lies in showing that it is equal to or more effective than the parent compound when that drug is already standard therapy. In this situation the ethics of testing the new compound need full discussion. Cisplatin and other drugs are curative in the majority of patients with advanced teratoma. Substitution of carboplatin for cisplatin would be desirable since it has less unpleasant side-effects but if it lowers the cure rate even marginally this would be disastrous in these young patients. Since demonstration of a 5–10% reduction in long-term survival would require many hundreds of patients the difficulty becomes obvious. Ethical problems are less acute when treatment is essentially palliative in nature. For instance, as discussed by Canetta and colleagues, cisplatin is the most active drug in ovarian carcinoma but is rarely, if ever, curative. Comparison of carboplatin with cisplatin is thus not going to affect the chances of cure though it might still result in shorter survival. Trials of this sort have so far been far too small to assess this, though they have proven acceptable to regulatory authorities. A meta-analysis of 2061 patients in 11 trials has been carried out by the Advanced Ovarian Cancer Trialists Group (AOCTG), who met in Cambridge, England, in June 1990. Even with this large collection of data the AOCTG were only able to make a preliminary statement suggesting very similar survival patterns with both drugs—there was a small advantage for cisplatin after two years but too few patients had prolonged follow-up to make definitive conclusions.

The final chapter (21) in this section is by **Karen Antman**, who chairs a committee of the American Society of Clinical Oncology on this topic. She presents an American perspective on health costs and points out the perceived need in a number of countries to change their system. Within the USA there has been change and a recognition of the problem of the uninsured or under-insured and of minorities. Antman documents the refusal of some third parties (insurance companies) to cover patients treated in controlled trials or to take on the expense of procedures such as bone marrow transplantation ($150 000). She discusses some of the solutions to this: patient payment, government payment and support from the pharmaceutical industry, but finds each wanting. The Institute of Medicine in the USA concluded that clinical research in that country was under severe threat—a finding applicable to a number of other countries including the UK.

Antman also discusses the disincentives for young physicians considering entering academic medicine. She concludes by summarizing the position of the cancer patient and their physician in the USA—squeezed between large insurance companies, large pharmaceutical companies, governmental cutbacks and "competitive pricing". In this situation the patient may not get the best deal and clinical research may be severely damaged. Not only will this prevent us from developing new and more effective treatments, it will stop us from finding out which of our current therapies are truly cost effective. *Effective* new treatments are very likely to be extremely cost efficient. Our current problem is the high cost of ineffective or palliative treatments. Development of curative treatments may help and demonstration that costly treatments are ineffective *should* result in more effective use of precious resources.

17 Economic Evaluation of Cancer Treatments*

BENGT JÖNSSON and GÖRAN KARLSSON

THE ECONOMIC IMPACT OF CANCER

Cancer is an important cause of death and illness. In Sweden more than one-fifth of all deaths are due to cancer. The prevalence is 1% (84 000), the incidence approximately 0.5% (38 000), and about 8% of all patients discharged from hospitals have a cancer diagnosis [1]. The incidence for the USA is approximately the same [2].

The occurrence of cancer leads to pain, suffering and psychological harm to the patients and their families, but it is also an economic issue. Resources are used to prevent, cure and mitigate the effects of cancer. Illness also leads to loss of production due to morbidity and mortality. A distinction is often made between direct and indirect costs. Traditionally, direct costs are defined as the resources used in the treatment of the disease. Typical direct costs are costs of staff time, drugs, equipment and buildings. Indirect costs represent resources foregone due to the treatment and illness. The most important indirect cost is probably the value of the patient's time. A commonly used estimation of the time costs is the goods and services not produced due to cancer.

Costs of illness, distributed among direct costs and indirect costs, have been calculated [2–6]. Table 1 summarizes the costs of neoplasm.

Estimations for the USA, using an incidence approach in contrast to the more commonly used prevalence approach, give direct costs of 6.4 billion US dollars, indirect costs of 16.7 billion US dollars and total costs of 23.1 billion US dollars; all figures for the year 1975 [2]. Another study has calculated direct costs in 1977 of 7.2 billion US dollars and indirect costs at 18.8 billion US dollars [5]. Although the authors do not use identical methods, the results are approximately the same.

About 5% of the resources within the health care sector are used to treat, prevent or mitigate the effects of cancer. The importance of cancer on indirect costs, especially mortality costs, are even larger compared to other diseases. Notice that the indirect costs, especially the mortality costs, dominate the

*Reprinted with permission, from ESO Monographs. Drug Delivery in Cancer Treatment III, Ed. Domellöf, L., pp 63–84 (1990). Jönsson, B./Karlsson, G.: Economic evaluation of cancer treatments. © 1990 Springer-Verlag Berlin–Heidelberg.

Introducing New Treatments for Cancer: Practical, Ethical and Legal Problems. Edited by C. J. Williams
Published 1992 by John Wiley & Sons Ltd

Table 1. Costs of neoplasm; current prices

Country	Year	Direct costs	Indirect costs			Total costs
			Morbidity	Mortality	Total	
Sweden	1975					
	SEKᵃ	1 189	1332	3 117	4 249	5 438
	%²	5.3	3.0	24.3	8.3	7.4
	1983					
	SEKᵃ	3 300	1900	6 000	7 900	11 200
	%ᵇ	5.1	2.6	24.4	8.0	6.9
USA	1975					
	US$ᵃ	5 279	1105	15 974	17 079	22 079
	%ᵇ	4.5	1.9	18.2	11.7	8.5
	1985					
	US$ᵃ	18 104	7170	47 220	54 390	72 494
	%ᵇ	4.9	8.9	20.8	17.6	10.7
Finland	1975					
	FMKᵃ	102	128	518	646	748
	%²	6.9	1.4	14.0	5.1	5.3

ᵃMillions.
ᵇPercentage of all diseases for the specific type of cost. Source: references [4–6].

total costs in this type of study. Seventy-five to 85% of the total costs of cancer are made up of indirect costs and up to 93% of the total indirect costs are made up by mortality costs. Table 1 indicates that the cost shares of neoplasm have slightly decreased between 1975 and 1983.

So far, economic analyses and studies of costs of different treatments of cancer have been rare. The lack of interest in economic studies of cancer can, to a certain degree, be explained by the rapid development of alternatives in treating cancer patients. As long as the efficacy and effectiveness of different therapies have been uncertain, the need for cost estimations has been limited. However, when the number of realistic alternatives grows, knowledge about costs as well as the consequences are necessary in order to be able to make rational choices. It is not primarily the substance of the resources which determine whether an economic problem exists or not, but rather the appearance of previously unknown alternatives.

In this chapter we will discuss the economic evaluation of chemotherapy, pain relief, total parenteral nutrition and home care versus hospital care in the treatment of the terminally ill cancer patients. Drug delivery constitutes an important part of these treatments. However, it is difficult to evaluate solely drug delivery without taking into account other components in the treatment process. We will first present a framework appropriate for an economic analysis of cancer treatments. We proceed with a literature review of studies published within this field and conclude with a discussion on the economic efficiency of different types of cancer treatment.

METHODS FOR ECONOMIC EVALUATION

THE PROCESS OF CANCER TREATMENTS

Cancer treatment is a multidisciplinary therapy consisting of surgery, radiotherapy, chemotherapy and immunotherapy. The treatment sometimes has a curative intent, sometimes a palliative intent. Cancer treatment can be regarded as a process involving various interventions. These interventions support each other: adjuvant chemotherapy is used as a complement to surgery [6, 8], intensive use of chemotherapy for acute leukaemia is supported by antibiotics and leucocyte transfusion [9, 10] and home care in terminal cancer also requires professional input [11, 12].

But these interventions are also substitutes: radiation can be used instead of surgery [13] and home care replaces hospital care for terminally ill patients [14]. The treatment process of cancer is illustrated in Figure 1. It should be noticed that only some interventions are included in this figure. In order to be complete, all processes involved in the treatment of cancer, including radiation and endocrine therapy, should be represented.

Examples of therapies which define a treatment process are given in Figure 1. There is a strong interdependence between these therapies. Pain relief with parenteral use of narcotics can, to a larger degree, facilitate home care instead of hospitalization [15]. In some cases, for example, chemotherapy is the primary treatment, in other cases it supports other activities.

Chemotherapy, pain relief and total parenteral nutrition (TPN) are genuine therapies in a treatment process, while home care and hospital care refer rather to the place of treatment. Furthermore, hospital care can be carried

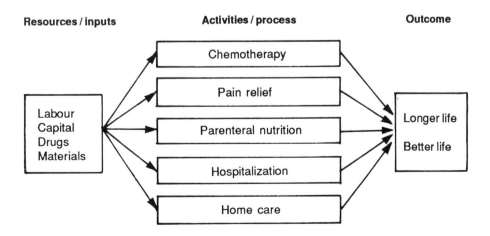

Figure 1. Illustration of the treatment process of cancer

PLACE OF TREATMENT

		Home	Hospice	Hospital		
				Out-patient	Inter-mittent	In-patient
TREATMENT ACTIVITY	Chemotherapy					
	Pain relief					
	TPN					

Figure 2. Illustration of different activities in the cancer treatment process

out in different ways: from inpatient treatment through intermittent care to outpatient treatment. Hospice care can be regarded as treatment which tries to combine the home atmosphere with round-the-clock access to professional medical management. In Figure 2 we illustrate the different characteristics of these activities. The place of treatment and the sectors in the treatment process are, however, strongly interdependent. The choice of the place for administering treatment puts special demands on the therapy, and the choice of the combination of treatment to be adopted may facilitate home care instead of hospital care.

Each activity requires resources, or some input, such as nursing time, the physician's time and other labour time, capital, drugs and materials. Traditionally in economic evaluations, costs within health care are related to different kinds of resources which, as input in a treatment process, have the ultimate goal of increasing the life-span and/or improve the quality of life for the patient. If possible, all costs should be related to the ultimate goal. The study of the treatment process is a step in that direction.

An advantage in this multidisciplinary approach to the treatment process lies in the fact that changes in prices and productivity for different aspects, or technological changes in the treatment process, can be analysed explicitly with regard to costs as well as to outcome. This reduces the risk of a too narrow approach to cost analysis of alternative treatments. The possibility of alternating different kinds of activities and inputs to facilitate unchanged or better outcome is of special interest.

DIFFERENT TYPES OF ECONOMIC EVALUATION

An economic assessment can be performed in different ways depending on the viewpoint of the study. Most economic studies contain an evaluation of the resources used—the costs. However, the way to handle the outcome

Table 2. Different types of economic assessment of medical technologies

Type of economic evaluation	Benefits evaluation
Cost-minimization	No benefit assessment Assumed to be the same for all alternatives
Cost-effectiveness	Unidimensional physical outcome measure, e.g. life-years gained
Cost–utility	Multidimensional physical outcome measure, containing quantity and quality of life
Cost–benefit	Monetary outcome measure, i.e. willingness to pay

differs. In Table 2 we show four types of commonly used economic evaluations within medical care classified from different ways to handle the outcomes—or benefits—of the treatment.

In cost-minimization studies, the outcomes of the alternatives are assumed to be identical.

In a world with scarce resources, the treatment with the lowest cost should be chosen. All resources used in the treatment process should be included in the costs. For example, time costs for the patient and his/her family and costs paid by others outside the health care sector, such as costs for travel, are relevant costs [16, 17]. In cases where the outcome differs between alternative treatments, cost-minimization studies are inappopriate. It is necessary to take the outcome into consideration.

In cost-effectiveness analysis, the outcome for alternative treatments is assumed to be of the same type, possibly to be expressed in a unidimensional physical measure. Treatments which produce the same type of outcome can be compared in this type of study. In cancers where the mortality rate is high, life expectancy is a good measure of effectiveness. A commonly used outcome measure in cost-effectiveness analysis is life-years gained. If the ultimate goal of medical care is to produce as many life-years as possible from a fixed budget, regardless of who gains or who pays, treatments with low costs per life-year gained should be given priority over treatments with high cost per life-year gained. In cost–utility analysis, not only the number of life-years but also the quality of these years are taken into account. The underlying idea is that there exists a trade-off between the duration and the quality of life. Traditionally, it is estimated by assigning different utility values to different states of health. Full health is given the utility value 1 and a health state of less than full health a value of less than 1. Assume, for instance, that a health state is given a utility value of 0.6. That means that one year in that state is equivalent to 0.6 year in a state of full health. The utility values are used to construct quality-adjusted life-years—QALYs—

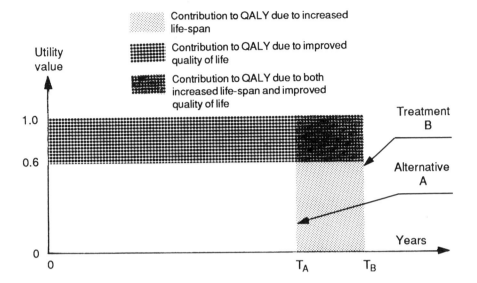

Figure 3. Illustration of the construction of quality-adjusted life-years (QALYs)

which is the outcome measure in cost–utility analysis. The idea of the construction of QALYs is shown in Figure 3.

Figure 3 illustrates two alternatives in treating a patient: with alternative A the patient has a health state with utility value 0.6 and a remaining life-span of T_A years. Treatment B takes the patient to full health with utility value 1 and gives a remaining life-span of T_B years. The difference between the two areas is the QALYs gained with treatment B compared to treatment A. How many QALYs a treatment produces is partly due to the improved quality of life and partly due to the increased life-span. However, there are still conceptual problems as well as problems of measurement connected with the use of QALYs. For further descriptions of the construction of QALYs, the measurement of quality of life and discussions of the strengths and weaknesses of utility analysis, we refer to the growing literature within this field [18–20].

In a cost–benefit analysis, all the components in the evaluation, costs as well as outcome, are evaluated in monetary terms. Actual prices of the outcome, i.e. the health improvement, do not exist and therefore it is necessary to construct "shadow prices" to convert the physical outcome to a monetary value. Lack of consensus in the construction of shadow prices and, hence, in measuring the outcome in monetary terms, together with some doubtful ethical implications, have caused cost–benefit analysis to be used rarely in economic evaluations within the health care sector.

However, methods to reveal the willingness to pay for non-market goods and services—the contingent valuation method—have been developed [21].

This method has been tested in the health care sector [22], with promising results. There are obvious practical problems with the method, but it may be worthwhile to try if a valuation in monetary terms is essential for the assessment.

Which one of the assessment methods is to be preferred depends on the issue. Cost-minimization, cost-effectiveness and cost–utility analysis handle the question how to reach a given goal as cheaply as possible. If we accept the goal, the measurements of valuation give valuable information for decision-making concerning which one of several alternatives ought to be chosen. These analyses can, however, never answer the question whether a treatment is desirable or not. The resources could be better used in another field. To answer that question, we need to measure all the components in monetary terms, i.e. by a cost–benefit analysis.

MODEL FOR ECONOMIC EVALUATION OF CANCER TREATMENTS

We will emphasize that a too narrow perspective of an economic evaluation can lead to doubtful or incorrect conclusions. It is important that costs of all activities in the treatment process are included as well as outcome measures if they differ between alternatives. Figure 4 illustrates some problems and potential mistakes in evaluating medical care. A new therapy is compared to an old one.

As has been pointed out earlier, the construction of the evaluation measure is calculated from the *difference* in outcome as well as the *difference* in costs

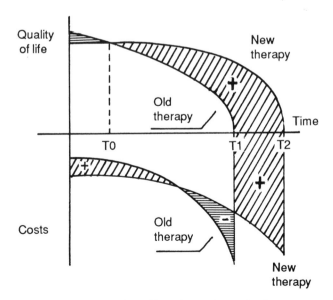

Figure 4. Example of the time profile of benefits and costs in the treatment of a disease

between the therapies during the entire treatment episode. Areas labelled "+" in Figure 4 show that the quality of life or the cost of the new therapy exceeds the old therapy. Accordingly, "−" indicates lower quality of life or lower costs for the new therapy.

The evaluation measure in a cost–utility analysis is cost per QALYs gained, e.g. $\partial QALYs/\partial COST$. In Figure 4 it is the ratio between the difference in QALYs and the difference in costs. Notice that the result depends on the time-span. If the study follows the whole treatment episode, e.g. T_1 for the old therapy and T_2 for the new therapy, the new therapy produces more QALYs, but is more expensive than the old therapy. But if the estimation period only lasts to T_0, the old therapy appears as cheaper and seems to produce more QALYs. Hence, it is important to include the whole treatment episode.

COSTS OF PROSTATIC CANCER AND ACUTE MYELOID LEUKAEMIA

In a Swedish cost study of prostatic cancer, the whole treatment episode, where the costs are distributed over different interventions, is analysed [23]. The treatment cost is estimated for patients treated at Linköping University Hospital, Sweden, for prostatic adenocarcinoma from the time of diagnosis to death for all patients who died in 1984–1985. The total number of patients was 101. Table 3 and Table 4 show the time profile of the costs and the distribution of the intervention costs. The study also shows that the treatment cost is concentrated in the last years of life; on average, the last year of life takes up 51% of the total cost and the last three years 85%.

In another study, the whole treatment episode is followed and the costs from diagnosis to death were calculated in the treatment of patients who died from acute myeloid leukaemia [8]. The patients were treated with chemotherapy and none received bone marrow transplantation. The mean survival was 259 days, ranging from two to 1227 days. The average costs are summarized in Table 5.

Table 3. Cost in relation to time after diagnosis of prostatic cancer, 1985 (Swedish kronor)

Years after diagnosis	No. of cases	Average cost per case
1	101	18 000
2	98	16 700
3	72	13 600
4	59	16 100
5	41	11 200
6+	32	66 100
Total	101	78 800

Source: reference [23].

Table 4. Distribution of cost among activities in the treatment of prostatic cancer

Activity	Average cost per case	
	(SEK)	% of TC[a]
Hospitalization* (hotel cost)	56 700	72
Laboratory investigations	2 000	2
Radiology	4 500	5
Surgery	3 100	4
Drugs	12 600	16
Oestrogen (incl. oestramustine phosphate)	8 600	11
Other chemotherapy	700	1
Analgesics	600	1
Antibiotics	200	1
Other drugs	2 500	3
Total	78 800	100

[a]TC = total cost; *includes physician and nursing costs.
Source: reference [23].

The "main treatment" of acute myeloid leukaemia—cytotoxic chemotherapy —takes up only 6% of the resources used in the treatment process. Supporting treatments, due to side-effects of chemotherapy, and especially the hotel costs are more costly than chemotherapy in itself. The importance of the hotel cost is also shown in the treatment of prostatic cancer [23] (see Table 4). These two examples illustrate the danger of limiting the calculations only to one activity, for instance the drug costs.

Table 5. Average cost of treating acute myeloid leukaemia, 1980 (Swedish kronor)

Activity	Costs	
	Kronor	% of total treatment cost
Hospital/hotel*	72 200	70
Blood products	10 600	10
Laboratory tests	3 100	3
Drugs		
Cytotoxic chemotherapy	5 700	6
Antibiotics	4 500	4
Cultures	2 100	2
Other activities	4 900	5
Total treatment cost	103 100	100

*Includes physician and nursing costs.
Source: reference [9].

ASSESSMENTS OF CANCER TREATMENTS

CHEMOTHERAPY

There are few economic studies on chemotherapy including both costs and benefits in the same study. In fact, we found only one study based on a randomized trial which provides complete cost–benefit and cost–utility analysis [24]. Chemotherapy has been compared to bone marrow transplantation in the treatment of patients with acute non-lymphocytic leukaemia in a cost–benefit study [25]. The patients are, however, not randomized. One study shows cost–benefit measures on leucocyte transfusion during intensive chemotherapy, but not on chemotherapy in itself [26]. An early example of cost-minimization analysis suffers from methodological weaknesses, which is why it is difficult to conclude anything from this study [27]. Both costs and effectiveness are discussed in a study, where some data also are presented [28]. Others [29–32] provide conceptual frameworks, or ask for economic studies of chemotherapy, but have no estimates on costs or benefits.

COSTS OF CHEMOTHERAPY

Some studies present cost or effectiveness measures separately on chemotherapy. Several cost studies underline that cancer treatment is a multidisciplinary process, of which chemotherapy is only one. The studies presented earlier [9, 23] are examples.

Treatment costs of breast cancer and testicular cancer, distributed over different activities, have been calculated [33]. The main results are shown in Table 6. The drug cost as the share of the cost of chemotherapy varies between 19% and 61%, and as the share of the total treatment cost between 7% and 38%.

However, the method used is unclear. The cost of the main treatment and the cost of different kinds of chemotherapy are calculated separately and the total treatment cost is calculated to the sum of these types of costs. Whether the total costs are prospective or retrospective estimates based on actual treatments, or hypothetical treatments constituted by different combinations of the main treatment and chemotherapy, is not clear. Neither the duration of treatment nor the year(s) of treatment are reported.

Costs are also reported in the treatment of small-cell lung cancer, where chemotherapy is employed: of the total treatment costs of 3650 US dollars, the cost of diagnosis amounts to 550 US dollars, the cost of chemotherapy to 2000 US dollars and radiotherapy to 1100 US dollars. Hence, the cost of chemotherapy is 55% of the total treatment cost [33].

The costs vary markedly between diagnoses as well as within the same diagnosis. In the treatment of acute myeloid leukaemia, the total treatment

Table 6. Activity costs in different cancer treatments; shares of total treatment costs, expressed as a percentage

Activity	Diagnosis						
	Operable		Breast cancer Advanced metastatic			Testicular cancer Advanced	
	CMFP[a]	P+Tam[a]	AC[a]	Tam[a]	Tam/AC	PVB×5	Mainten- ance V
Main treatment	522	65	32	45	29	38	34
Hospital/hotel	38	48	—	—	—	—	—
Operation	8	11	—	—	—	5	5
Investigations	6	7	—	—	—	—	—
Chemotherapy	47	35	68	55	71	62	66
Drugs	9	7	23	17	31	38	38
Investigations	17	21	22	28	20	10	10
Drug admin.	10	—	11	—	10	2	4
OPD attendance	11	7	12	9	11	13	14
Total treatment cost	100	100	100	100	100	100	100
In Australian dollars	6438	5145	11 024	7795	12 389	6656	7364

[a]Shows different regimens of chemotherapy.
CMFP: cyclophosphamide, methotrexate, fluorouracil, prednisone;
P+Tam: prednisone and tamoxifen;
AC: doxorubicin/cyclophosphamide;
PVB: cisplatin, vinblastine, bleomycin.
Source: reference [33] and estimations of our own.

costs range between SEK 49 050 and SEK 160 450 depending on age group and whether the patient goes into a state of remission or not [9].

In treatments where chemotherapy is employed, it is only a part of an overall process. Misunderstandings regarding the treatment as a process might lead to incorrect conclusions—even if the cost of chemotherapy is correctly estimated it must be related to the outcome of the treatment.

EFFECTIVENESS OF CHEMOTHERAPY

The efficacy and effectiveness of chemotherapy in solid tumours are ambiguous. In a prospective, randomized trial, no advantage in survival of adjuvant chemotherapy in gastric cancer could be seen compared to patients undergoing only surgery [11]. Based on a review of the large amount of literature regarding adjuvant chemotherapy for breast cancer, it was concluded that trial data available to 1986 justify the routine of six months' combination of cyclophosphamide, methotrexate and 5-fluorouracil (CMF) in premenopausal women with histologically involved axillary lymph nodes; for other patient groups and for other forms of adjuvant chemotherapy, the treatment was considered as experimental [6]. The uncertainty of the effectiveness of chemotherapy has been underlined by the statement concerning chemotherapy in the treatment of superficial bladder cancer that "neither its exact role nor the optimal dose or schedule of administration have been established. To date, no dramatic differences in efficacy between the agents commonly used for intravesical chemotherapy . . . have been appreciated" [34].

Comparisons between continuous infusion and bolus therapy have been carried out [35, 36]. After reviewing the literature of continuous infusion, it was concluded that the majority of agents studied have failed to demonstrate any improved effectiveness over bolus therapy [35]. On the other hand, two randomized studies have indicated that the infusion schedule is superior [36].

Most cancer chemotherapy is given with palliative rather than curative intent [37]. The existence of side-effects makes it necessary to weigh the life-prolonging effect against adverse side-effects. It has been argued that, if there is a chance of a curative or life-prolonging effect, the choice of rather aggressive chemotherapy is justified [38]. However, it is important to take into account also the patient's point of view.

The importance of the preferences of the patients and their families in health care is evident from many studies [39]. In a study concerning trade-offs between quality and quantity of life in laryngeal cancer, 20% of healthy volunteers would choose radiation instead of surgery in spite of a shorter expected remaining life-span [13]. The reason is that radiation permits a higher quality of life, as the ability of normal speech remains, while surgery does not.

Side-effects of chemotherapy occur regardless of the type of treatment be it curative, palliative or adjuvant. Quality of life and side-effects of patients treated with either a single agent (chlorambucil), or a five-drug combination postoperative adjuvant chemotherapy have been investigated [40]. Forty-two per cent of the patients receiving a single agent and 79% of the patients receiving a multi-drug treatment experienced side-effects, including nausea, vomiting, malaise and alopecia, severe enough to interfere with their life-style. Twenty-nine per cent of the patients treated with multi-drug treatment stated that the treatment was unbearable, or that they could never go through it again. In a review of adjuvant chemotherapy, more severe side-effects were found as compared to placebo [7]. However, palliative cytostatic therapy can give a good pain relief [41].

Adjuvant chemotherapy has a character of investment with uncertain payoff. Most patients with operable breast cancer relapse and die of the disease [42]. Figure 5, taken from Gelber and Goldhirsch [42], illustrates different stages after the operation. Between surgery and relapse, the patients enjoy a rather symptom-free period (TWiST). Adjuvant chemotherapy at the beginning of the treatment period can prolong the recurrence-free interval. However, whilst undergoing adjuvant chemotherapy, the patient

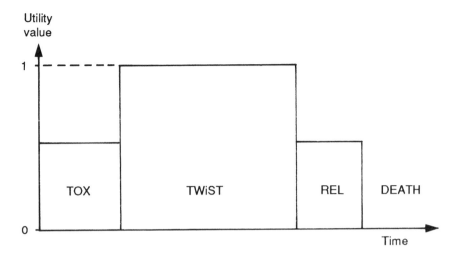

Figure 5. TOX = toxicity; TWiST = symptom-free period; REL = relapse. Quality-adjusted survival relative to TWiST

can suffer from toxic effects such as nausea, vomiting, anorexia, infections, etc. The period with toxic effects is labelled TOX and the period with relapse is labelled REL in Figure 5.

Four hundred and sixty-three patients with axillary N + breast cancer who were randomized into Ludwig Trial III to receive either chemoendocrine therapy (CMFp + T) for one year *or* endocrine therapy alone (p + T) for one year *or* no adjuvant therapy at all (Observation) were analysed in a quality-of-life approach called TWiST [42]. The average times in TOX, TWiST and REL (Figure 5) for the three strategies were estimated over a period of seven years. The authors fixed the utility value for TWiST to 1, for TOX and REL to 0.5. The highest possible outcome value, Q-TWiST, is hence seven years or 84 months, which is the length of time without symptoms or toxic effects. The average number of months in different stages, and the quality-adjusted months (Q-TWiST) during the 84 months, are shown in Table 7.

Table 7. Components of Q-TWiST in treatments of breast cancer (months)

	CMFp + T	p + T	Observation
TOX (unweighted)	9.6	2.0	0.0
TWiST	50.3	47.1	41.5
REL (unweighted)	7.1	12.9	20.9
Q-TWiST	58.7	54.6	51.9

Source: reference [42].

Table 7 shows that the most aggressive strategy (CMFp + T) gives the longest symptom-free period (TWiST) as well as the best outcome measure (Q-TWiST). The outcome measure depends on the utility values for TOX and REL and the duration of the study. This is pointed out by the authors, who also provide a sensitivity analysis for the utility values.

The existence of side-effects connected with chemotherapy shows that measurements of patients' quality of life are highly relevant in evaluation studies. The fact that different regimens provoke different types of side-effects of different severity underlines the importance of quality-of-life measures.

COST-EFFECTIVENESS OF CHEMOTHERAPY

The cost studies have shown that costs of treatments employing chemotherapy vary between different cancer diagnoses but also within diagnoses. Studies of efficacy and effectiveness show contradictory results. In an economic evaluation of chemotherapy it is important, therefore, to specify the treatment for a specific patient group, as well as the alternative, and calculate the difference in cost and effectiveness compared to the alternative.

A new measure of evaluation has been introduced, called notional patient benefit year (NPBY) cost [28]. It is defined as:

$$\frac{\text{Mean total}}{\text{cost}} \times (100/\text{response rate}) \times \begin{pmatrix} 12/\text{mean duration in months} \\ \text{of response or survival} \\ \text{prolongation} \end{pmatrix}$$

Taking the example of the author, if the cost of an abdominoperineal resection for colorectal carcinoma is £2000, the cure rate 33% and the mean life expectancy without carcinoma 12 years, then NPBY cost is:

$$£2000 \times (100/33) \times (12/12 \times 12) = £500$$

The evaluation measurement can be interpreted as cost per response year. Notice that the type of response can differ between diagnoses and treatments. If response is life prolonging, the evaluation measure is cost per life-year gained—the traditional measurement of evaluation in cost–benefit analysis. If response is, for example, pain relief, then the evaluation measurement accordingly is cost per pain relieved year gained; if response is improved physical mobility, the evaluation measurement is cost per improved physical mobility year gained. As seen, the outcome may differ in different treatments and for different diseases. The author points out that NPBY cost is a crude concept, since it takes no account of the quality of life. However, the weakness of the evaluation measure is that it is not able to discriminate between different types of effects. Survival, pain relief, improved physical mobility, or other improvements in quality of life, all are given the same weight [1] in NPBY. Treatments with high NPBY costs might be given priority to treatments with low NPBY costs if the types of effects are valued differently. For example, survival might be valued higher than pain relief. NPBY costs for different treatments might, therefore, mislead rather than facilitate rational choices. Nevertheless, we present some NPBY costs in Table 8. However, if decision-making should be based on the outcome measures, they have to capture the same type of effects for different treatments.

Chemotherapy has been compared to bone marrow transplantation in the treatment of patients with acute non-lymphocytic leukaemia [25]. All patients in the study received induction chemotherapy. Of these, 17 patients underwent transplantation and those for whom no related donors were available underwent chemotherapy only (19 patients). The cost estimations started with the induction of chemotherapy and extended over a five-year period. The two groups had equivalent use of resources over this period except for a tenfold increase of the intensive care unit for transplanted patients. The effectiveness measure was life-years gained but calculated in two ways: over the five-year period and extrapolated to the life expectancy. All survivors were assumed to be cured as they had been in continuous complete remission for at least seven years and the last death occurred three years after induction of chemotherapy. The results are presented in Table 9. Transplantation appears to be cost effective. If one is willing to pay $64 000 ($22 900 in the longer time frame) per life-year gained for chemotherapy, one also ought to be willing to pay a further $59 300 ($10 000 in the longer time frame) per life-year gained for transplantation.

Table 8. NPBY costs for different cancer treatments

Treatment	NPBY cost (£)
Potentially curative	
Surgery and radiotherapy for stage I seminoma	80
Cytotoxic chemotherapy for metastatic teratoma	110
Outpatient radiotherapy for glottic laryngeal carcinoma	120
Abdominoperineal resection for rectal carcinoma	500
Palliative	
Tamoxifen for advanced breast carcinoma	380
MRC phase II study of cisplatin and methotrexate in T4b bladder carcinoma	16 000
Chemotherapy for metastatic non-small-cell bronchogenic carcinoma with cyclophosphamide, doxorubicin and etoposide	18 000
Chemotherapy for advanced, previously treated, non-small-cell bronchogenic carcinoma with vindesine, etoposide and cisplatin	112 000

Source: reference [28].

Table 9. Cost–benefit of chemotherapy and transplantation for acute non-lymphocytic leukaemia, 1989 (US dollars); discount rate = 5%

Time length	Chemotherapy v. no treatment[a]	Transplantation v. no treatment[a]	Transplantation v. chemotherapy
Five years			
Average cost	136 000	193 000	57 000
Cost per life-year gained	64 000	62 500	59 300
Life expectancy			
Average cost	136 000	193 000	57 000
Cost per life-year gained	22 900	16 600	10 000

[a]No treatment is assumed to give zero cost and immediate death.
Source: reference [25].

Table 10. Costs and effectiveness in two treatments of small-cell lung cancer, 1984 (Canadian dollars)

Cost–benefit measures	Standard arm	Alternating arm	Difference
Costs for the hospital			
Chemotherapy			
Drugs	1 942	2 663	721
Fixed costs	772	782	10
Hospital (hotel cost)	10 666	10 004	−662
Clinic (fixed outpatient cost)	1 235	1 468	233
Radiation	780	790	10
Sum	15 395	15 707	312
Costs for other agents			
Drugs	72	73	1
Local transport	52	62	10
Out-of-town transport	178	193	15
Accommodation	167	198	31
Sum	345	391	464
Costs for the patient			
Miscellaneous non-medical	676	767	91
Sum total costs	16 416	16 866	450
Effectiveness measures			
Survival months	8.1	9.7	1.6
Quality adjusted months	3.5	4.7	1.2
Cost–benefit measures			
Cost/life-year gained			3372
Cost/quality gained			4495

Source: reference [24].

In a randomized trial, economic evaluation in terms of cost–benefit and cost–utility in the treatment of small-cell lung cancer has been carried out [24]. Six courses of intravenous cyclophosphamide, adriamycin and vincristine (CAV) alone at three-week intervals ($n = 40$)—the standard arm—is compared to CAV alternating with etoposide and cisplatin on days 1 to 3 ($n = 34$)—the alternating arm. The cost and effectiveness were calculated from the time of randomization to death. Utility measurements were performed on six health states that occur in the trial using the category scaling technique. Two proxy groups were used as respondents: 7 patients and 14 health professionals. The utility values were obtained by pooling the values from the two groups. Table 10 displays the main results.

The table shows that the alternating arm is more costly than the standard arm, but the difference is only 450 Canadian dollars, or 3%. Keeping in mind the uncertainty that always exists in cost estimations, the difference, however, might not be significant.

The alternating arm is also better both in terms of months gained and quality-adjusted months gained. The reason why the number of months gained is less when they are quality adjusted depends on the fact that the patients perceive part of the time as a health state worse than full health. Using the alternating arm instead of the standard arm costs 3400 Canadian dollars per life-year gained, and 4500 per quality-adjusted life-year.

Table 11. Evaluation measures of different selected therapies

Programme	Cost/QALY gained in US dollars, 1988[a]
Post-partum anti-D	1 400
Coronary artery bypass surgery for left main artery disease	5 000
Neonatal intensive care, 1000–1499 g	5 300
Chemotherapy, alternating arm in small-cell lung cancer	6 700[b]
Preoperative TPN in severely malnourished patients with localized stomach cancer	10 000[c]
Treatment of severe hypertension (diastolic >105 mmHg) in males age 40	11 100
Preoperative TPN in severely malnourished patients with localized oesophagus cancer	32 700[c]
Neonatal intensive care, 500–999 g	37 600
Continuous ambulatory peritoneal dialysis	55 700
Hospital haemodialysis	63 800
Preoperative TPN in well-nourished patients with metastatic oesophagus cancer	791 800[c]

[a]The table is taken from reference [18].
[b]Source: reference [24].
[c]Source: reference [43].
The 1988 US dollars are obtained by using the exchange rate and then inflating according to the US consumer price index.

Is the treatment cheap or expensive? As a comparison we indicate some results from other cost–utility analyses in Table 11. The evaluation measures must, however, be interpreted with great care, because the studies are not conducted with identical methods and, furthermore, costs are estimated in different currencies in different years.

An early cost–benefit study of chemotherapy in advanced malignant diseases has been performed [27]. Estimations of costs, calculated by hospital days, for all patients during 1973–1977 at a clinic treating cancers were performed. Chemotherapy was introduced from the end of 1974. The number of hospital days per patient decreased by 16 days, or 3200 US dollars, and the overall mortality rose from 26% to 31% from 1973 to 1977. The authors argue that the only alternation during the period was the introduction of chemotherapy in advanced cancers and, therefore, the reduction of cost must be due to chemotherapy. They also argue that the increased mortality rate was due to an increased number of malignant diseases, which should imply that the effectiveness of the treatments was unchanged. They conclude that chemotherapy induces lower costs. However, it is hard to know to what extent the chemotherapy, or the increased number of malignant diseases, affected costs and mortality rate.

PAIN RELIEF

Economic studies of pain relief are rare. In an uncontrolled study, the use of three types of continuous subcutaneous infusion (CSCI) for administration of narcotics in patients with cancer pain is evaluated [44]. The three methods of CSCI were the travenol infusor (70 patients), a non-portable pump (28 patients) and hypodermoclysis (10 patients). The total number of patients was 108. All patients were allowed to receive extra doses of narcotics. Pain control was considered adequate when the patient needed less, or equal to two extra doses of narcotics per day. Eighty per cent of all 108 patients experienced adequate pain control according to the definition of the authors. Seventy-five out of 79 patients (94%) preferred CSCI to their previous analgesic treatment after 48 hours of CSCI. The mean daily dose in 54 patients increased by 2.4% compared to their previous treatment. Systemic toxicity was found in 9% and local toxicity in 9% of the patients.

An estimation of the cost of three methods of CSCI gives daily costs for the pain relief treatment as 340 US dollars for travenol infusion, 310 US dollars for non-portable pump and 356 US dollars for hypodermoclysis for inpatient treatment and 102 US dollars for outpatient treatment. The authors conclude that CSCI facilitates outpatient treatment and, hence, reduces the cost.

The patients seem to prefer CSCI compared to their previous treatment, but the results are difficult to interpret. The outcome measurements refer to different subgroups of patients and, furthermore, it is not possible to separate the measurements for the three different methods of CSCI. Hence, the outcome is compared to the previous analgesic treatment, but the costs are implicitly compared to no analgesic treatment at all. As cost and outcome are not compared to the same alternative, it is impossible to make any cost–benefit judgements based on the study.

TOTAL PARENTERAL NUTRITION (TPN)

It seems to be uncertain to what extent parenteral nutrition for cancer patients gives favourable clinical benefits. After an evaluation of 17 trials of parenteral nutrition as an adjunct to chemotherapy or radiation treatment, it has been concluded that none of these studies has shown any favourable effect on survival [45]. Parenteral nutrition might have clinical benefits in perioperative care of patients with upper gastrointestinal cancer, but many trials of parenteral nutrition for cancer patients even show a better outcome for the control groups.

A cost-minimization study on TPN based on secondary data has been provided [46]. The charges for receiving ten days' TPN was calculated as 8000 US dollars and the benefits in terms of saved costs due to avoided wound infections and other major complications was estimated as 9720 US dollars [45]. The cost was estimated on representative charges in five hospitals and the reductions in complication rates were pooled from two trials. Hence, it is rather the expected than the actual costs and benefits that are estimated.

A cost–utility analysis of preoperative TPN in patients with upper gastrointestinal cancer has been carried out [43]. TPN reduces the risk of postoperative complications such as poor wound healing, infection, fistula formation, phlebitis and death. By using a decision-analytic approach (decision tree), four strategies were analysed: (1) no patients are administered TPN; (2) screening and only patients who are severely undernourished are

Table 12. Cost–utility measurements for preoperative TPN. Marginal cost per QALY gained, 1986 (US dollars)

Type of cancer	Cost per QALY gained for a strategy that moves from treating no one to treating:		
	Severely undernourished	Moderately undernourished	Well-nourished
Stomach			
Localized	9 300	20 700	54 400
Regionalized	57 300	127 700	335 500
Metastatic	116 700	259 900	682 900
Oesophagus			
Localized	30 400	67 800	178 100
Regionalized	86 600	193 100	507 300
Metastatic	125 700	280 300	736 400

Source: reference [43].

given TPN; (3) screening and patients who are severely or moderately undernourished are given TPN; (4) no screening, but all patients are given TPN. The probabilities in the decision tree were derived from meta-analysis, where results from different studies were pooled. The main results from the study are displayed in Table 12.

The results are interesting in that they illustrate in what way cost–utility analysis can support decision-making. If the capacity to offer TPN is limited, one ought to give priority to severely undernourished patients with localized stomach cancer, if the goal is to produce as many QALYs as possible with scarce resources. If the programme is to be expanded, the next least costly patient group—i.e., also moderately undernourished—should be offered TPN. Compared to other treatments, TPN appears to be very cost effective for some patient groups, but extremely expensive for other groups (see Table 11).

There are other economic studies, mostly cost-minimization studies, but they concern partial nutrition support [47, 48]. Since they are based on secondary data the results must be interpreted with care. They, however, show that different regimens and strategies vary in costs for different indications. It is important, therefore, to specify the strategy and the indications when TPN is economically evaluated.

HOME CARE VERSUS HOSPITAL CARE OF TERMINALLY ILL CANCER PATIENTS

As one of the major costs of treatment of cancer in hospital often is the hotel cost [9, 23, 33], one might suggest that home care would decrease the cost of treatment. In treatments of different diseases, studies suggest that outpatient instead of inpatient treatment reduces the treatment cost, due to the aforementioned hotel cost [49–51]. However, the picture is ambiguous. In an early review of the literature of outpatient versus inpatient care, it was found that only 4 out of 134 relevant papers provided enough data on both cost and efficacy, and only 2 of these showed outpatient care to be as effective as inpatient care and less costly [52].

In treating terminally ill cancer patients, alternatives to hospital care exist. In the mid-1970s, 65% of cancer patients died in hospitals, 15% in nursing homes and 20% at home [14]. A trend away from patients dying at home to nursing homes was noticed [14], a trend which can be explained by the fact that the majority of cancer patients need effective symptomatic and supportive management [53], which homes normally cannot provide [54]. Assumptions that terminally ill patients cared for in their homes experienced more dignity and comfort were also claimed [55].

Home-based hospice care tries to provide extensive supporting resources facilitating home care for terminally ill patients. The care is organized by

Table 13. Economic studies on home care, hospice care and hospital care for terminally ill patients

Study	Study period	Costs results[a]		Effectiveness results
[57]	1980–83	Home care:	66	Quality of life comparable
		Hospice care:	84	
		Hospital care:	100	
[58]		Hospice care:	99–115	No differences in survival rate
		Hospital care:	100	Comparable quality of life
[59]	1979	Hospice care:	58	No measures
		Hospital care:	100	
[60]	1978	Home care:	9	No measures
		Hospital care:	100	
[61]	1981	Home care:	60	No measures
		Hospital care:	100	
[62]	1979–81	Hospice care:	22	No measures
		Home care:	15	
		Municipal hospital:	100	
		Teaching hospital:	121	
[63]	1981–82	Hospice care:	56	No measures
		Hospital,		
		Scatterbed:	167	
		Autonomous unit:	100	
[64]	1980–81	Hospice care:	56	No measures
		Hospital care:	100	
[9]	1973–80	Partly outpatient:	81	No measures
		Hospital care:	100	
[65]	?	Home care:	35	No explicit measures
		Hospital care:	100	
[11]	1983	Home care:	100–113	Indications on longer survival time
		Hospital care:	100	
[66]	1980–81	Home care:	20	No measures
		Hospital care:	100	
[67]	?	Home care:	30	Difficult to interpret
		Hospice care:	79	
		Hospital:	100	
[68]	1975–82	Home care:	100	No measures
		Hospital care:	100	

[a]Index=100 for conventional care.
Source: estimations of our own, based on the references.

a multidisciplinary team, which visits the patients and their families at their homes [11, 53, 56]. Patients receiving hospice service are, if needed, referred to hospital care at different stages of their illness. Hence, the hospice care might require as much professional effort and resources as hospital care and it is not possible on *a priori* grounds to conclude that hospice care would save costs compared to hospital care. In Table 13 we display results of economic studies of hospice-based care compared to conventional hospital care.

The methodology differs between the studies. Only one uses a randomized control trial [58]. Two studies [11, 60] perform match-control studies, but the number of patients is small—only 19 pairs—in one of these [60]. Multiple regression analysis is used in two studies [9, 64]. One study [68] provides a quasi-experimental time series design, where mean costs and utilization between time periods were compared and tested for statistical significance using chi-square tests. The rest of the studies are retrospective uncontrolled studies estimating costs of treatment, which imply methodological problems including bias in patient selection. Studies which take these factors [11, 58, 68] into account do not show lower costs for home care, while many of the studies indicating lower costs for hospice care than for hospital care suffer from methodological weaknesses. Another randomized study, not included in Table 13, where only one-fifth of the patients were terminally ill, shows slightly lower costs for home care compared to a control group, but the difference is not significant [69]. Hence, the cost advantage for hospice care might hold only for patients not requiring intensive medical care.

Some of the studies use billed charges as proxies for costs. As costs and charges often differ [70], it is necessary to interpret the results with care.

The comparability of the studies is also limited due to a different duration of the period of care (for a discussion on what constitutes terminal illness and how long this period of care usually lasts, see reference [71]). For example, in one study [9], the length of care was on average 259 days; in another, two weeks [60]. There is evidence that the costs for medical care grow exponentially as death approaches [65, 72], especially for hospital care. Differences in the results might be due to differences in the length of time of care.

Furthermore, the concept of cost differs between studies. As home care requires participation of the patient's family in the treatment process, there are good reasons to assume that costs are paid to a larger extent by the family as compared to hospital care. One study includes income loss for family members in the costs, which amounts to 13% of the total cost for home care [60]. Costs to patients and their families associated with outpatient chemotherapy has been investigated [73], where mean costs for treatment weeks were 73 US dollars and for non-treatment weeks 46 US dollars. Approximately 45% of these costs were out-of-pocket expenses and 55% wages lost. Another study has found that family out-of-pocket expenses add about 50% to the total cost in the care of children with malignant neoplasms [74]. Most studies do not include family costs in their estimation of costs. It is not clear to what extent and to what amount family costs occur in home and hospital care for terminally ill patients.

To summarize, most studies indicate lower costs for home care than for hospital care for terminally ill cancer patients, but these studies often suffer from methodological weaknesses. Two studies, which control for bias in patient selection, show that the cost for hospice care is hardly lower than for hospital care. Another randomized study, however, only with a small proportion of terminally ill patients, supports this conclusion. Hence, from cost studies so far it is hard to make any certain conclusion whether home care saves costs or not. However, the main advantage with home hospice care might be a better outcome, i.e. a better quality of life or a longer life for the patient and the family. How to measure quality of life, especially for terminally ill cancer patients, is discussed and developed elsewhere in the literature [75, 76]. Some of the references in Table 13 present outcome data, as well as cost data. We will review outcome measures for these studies and for some further studies analysing outcome only.

One of the studies found no significant difference between patients receiving hospice care and patients receiving hospital care in measures of pain, symptoms, activity of daily living, anxiety or depression [58]. Hospice patients, however, expressed more satisfaction with interpersonal care and involvement in care.

An earlier study [77] found that home-centred care was associated with more pain than hospital-centred care. On the other hand, home-centred patients had better mobility, less confusion and better insight in the prognosis.

A longer survival time for the hospice patients has been found [11]. However, it was not possible to find out why but, according to the authors, it might be due to bias in patient selection.

Comparable participation rates have been reported in social activities for home care patients and hospital patients, but hobbies and crafts are pursued more by home patients and they also have a more realistic insight in their prognosis [67]. The home patients also appear to maintain their independence by less difficulty in walking and bathroom activities. However, pain is a greater problem for home patients than hospital patients.

In order to identify satisfaction with home care service, surviving relatives and physicians were interviewed and asked to fill out questionnaires [12]. The relatives of patients using home care reported less satisfaction with the availability of care and expressed that the patient experienced more pain than relatives of patients receiving hospital care. The study also highlights problems in communication and shows that family members need to be assured of around-the-clock availability of care.

The characteristics of 100 patients, although not only cancer patients, of which 55 died at their homes and 45 in institutions, have been analysed [78]. The patients dying at home did not experience more pain than patients dying in institutions, but there is an obvious bias in patient selection as patients dying at home had asked to receive care at home.

CONCLUSIONS

Cancer treatment is a process constituting many activities. There is a risk of a too narrow approach in economic evaluations of cancer treatments, if the assessors do not take into account all activities in the process.

The studies of chemotherapy show that the cost of the treatments vary markedly between different diagnoses, but also within the same diagnosis. Also the outcome seems to vary and it is difficult to come to any certain conclusion about the cost–benefit of chemotherapy in the treatment of cancer patients. For some patient groups, chemotherapy tends to be a cheap alternative in relation to the outcome, but for others it must be regarded as a costly treatment.

So far, full economic evaluations of chemotherapy, where both costs and outcome are included in the same study, are rare. To increase our knowledge of the implications of the use of chemotherapy on costs and outcome, controlled studies on specified patient groups are necessary. Furthermore, a full economic evaluation must include cost and outcome evaluation of a reasonable alternative treatment.

Economic evaluations on pain relief are even more rare than for chemotherapy. Studies on outcome have shown that the effectiveness is uncertain. Without knowledge about the effectiveness it is, of course, impossible to assess the cost–benefit of pain relief.

The effectiveness of TPN is uncertain. However, some economic studies have been carried out. They show that TPN for some patient groups are highly cost effective, but for others extremely costly in relation to the outcome. This underlines the importance of extending a therapy to well-selected patient groups for an optimal use of scarce resources.

Many cost studies have been performed on home care versus hospital care of terminally ill cancer patients. Most of them indicate lower costs for home care compared to hospital care. Some authors conclude that home care requires less resources than hospital care. However, the majority suffer from methodological weaknesses including bias in patient selection. Studies which control for bias in patient selection rather show that home care requires as many resources as hospital care. Outcome measurements point out some advantages with home-based care compared to institutional care. Patients treated at their homes seem to be more independent and have more active lives than patients treated in hospitals. On the other hand, problems with pain control and communication problems between the patients and their families and the home-care team have been reported. There are good reasons to assume bias in patient selection; any conclusion must, therefore, be taken with care.

However, a traditional study design which randomizes patients to home care and hospital care, respectively, can be questioned. There are good reasons to believe that different people have different preferences concerning the place of care. Today, there is a great variability among hospice programmes, with different types of organizations, different facilities and different patterns of services [79]. The variety of hospice programmes is probably, at least to a certain extent, a reaction of different preferences of the patients and their families. Probably, a better strategy is to offer the patient and his/her family the opportunity to choose between alternatives rather than to try to find the one and only "best" alternative for all patients. To find a flexible organization which satisfies different preferences for different patients and evaluates its costs and benefits appears to be a fruitful approach.

For terminally ill patients, it is obvious that the process of care and the outcome of care are strongly integrated. The use solely of standard methods for evaluating outcome with utility-based quality of life described in the literature [18, 19] might be less appropriate in cases where process and outcome are strongly integrated. Attempts to evaluate the quality of long-term care [80] and the quality of mental care [81], other examples of strong integration between process and outcome, using the structure–process–outcome model [82], have been performed. To a certain extent, the structure–process–outcome model has been employed in evaluating the care of terminally ill cancer patients [12]. A synthesis of the two approaches might be worth considering in a formal evaluation of the care of terminally ill cancer patients.

The care of terminally ill patients has only a palliative intent. Cost–benefit analysis, using the contingent evaluation method to estimate the willingness to pay, might be more appropriate for this patient group, receiving care not cure, than for many other patient groups.

REFERENCES

1. SCB (1988) Hälsan i Sverige. Hälsostatistisk årsbok 1987/88 Stockholm
2. Hartunian NS et al (1980) The incidence and economic costs of cancer, motor vehicle injuries, coronary heart disease, and stroke: a comparative analysis. Am J Public Health 1980: 1249–1260
3. Lindgren B (1981) Costs of illness in Sweden 1964–1975. Lund Economic Studies, Malmö
4. Lindgren B (1989) Costs of illness and benefits of drug treatment. The Economic Impact of Illness. Satellite Symposium to the IV World Conference on Clinical Pharmacology and Therapeutics, Mannheim
5. Hodgson TA, Rice DP (1982) Economic impact of cancer in the United States. In: Schottenfeld D, Fraumeni JF (eds) Cancer epidemiology and prevention. Saunders, Philadelphia, pp 208–228
6. Rice DP et al (1989) The economic burden of cancer, 1985: United States and California. In: Scheffler RM, Andrews NC (eds) Cancer care and cost. Health Administration Press Perspectives, Ann Arbor, Michigan
7. Henderson IC (1987) Adjuvant systemic therapy for early breast cancer. Curr Probl Cancer 11: 125–207
8. Allum WH, Hallissey MT, Kelly KA (1989) Adjuvant chemotherapy in operable gastric cancer. Lancet i: 571–574
9. Andersson F, Brodin H, Stalfelt AM (1988) Kostnader för behandling av akut myeloisk leukemi: En analys av kostnadsvariationer över tiden. Linköping University, CMT Rapport, p 8
10. Rosenheim MS et al (1980) The cost effectiveness of therapeutic and prophylactic leukocyte transfusion. N Engl J Med 302: 1058–1062

11. Gray D, MacAdam D, Boldy D (1987) A comparative cost analysis of terminal cancer care in home hospice patients and controls. J Chronic Dis 40: 801–810
12. McCuster J (1985) The use of home care in terminal cancer. Am J Prev Med 1: 42–52
13. McNeil BJ, Weichselbaum R, Pauker SG (1981) Speech and survival tradeoffs between quality and quantity of life in laryngeal cancer. N Engl J Med 305: 982–987
14. Flynn A, Stewart DE (1979) Where do cancer patients die? A review of cancer deaths in Cuyahoga County, Ohio, 1957–1974. J Community Health 5: 126–130
15. Bruera E et al (1988) Use of the subcutaneous route for the administration of narcotics in patients with cancer pain. Cancer 62: 407–411
16. Russel LB (1987) Is prevention better than cure? Brooking Institution, Washington DC
17. Jönsson B et al (1987) Cost–benefit analysis of hepatitis-B vaccination: a computerised decision model for Spain (manuscript)
18. Torrance GW (1986) Measurement of health state utilities for economic appraisal. A review. J Health Econ 5: 1–30
19. Torrance GW (1987) Utility approach to measuring health-related quality of life. J Chronic Dis 40: 593–600
20. Loomes G, McKenzie L (1989) The use of QALYs in health care decision making. Soc Sci Med 28: 299–308.
21. Cummings RG, Brookshire DS, Shulze WD (eds) (1986) Valuing environmental goods: an assessment of the contingent valuation method. Rowman & Allanheld, Totowa, pp 1–110
22. Thompson MS (1986) Willingness to pay and accept risks to cure chronic disease. Am J Publ Hlth 76: 392–396
23. Carlsson P et al (1989) The cost of prostatic cancer in a defined population. Scand J Urol Nephrol 23: 93–96
24. Goodwin PM et al (1988) Cost-effectiveness of cancer chemotherapy: an economic evaluation of a randomized trial in small-cell lung cancer. J Clin Oncol 6: 1537–1547
25. Welch HG, Larson EB (1989) Cost effectiveness of bone marrow transplantation in acute nonlymphocytic leukaemia. N Engl J Med 231: 807–812
26. Rosenhein MS et al (1980) The cost effectiveness of therapeutic and prophylactic leukocyte transfusion. N Engl J Med 302: 1058–1062
27. Mattsson W et al (1979) Cancer chemotherapy in advanced malignant disease: a cost benefit analysis. Acta Radiol Oncol 18: 509–520
28. Rees GJ (1985) Cost-effectiveness in oncology. Lancet ii: 1405–1407
29. Guess HA, Rudnick SA (1983) Use of cost-effectiveness analysis in planning cancer chemoprophylaxis trials. Controlled Clin Trials 4: 89–100
30. MacDonald EA (1987) Cost-effectiveness of cancer chemotherapy: risks/benefit ratio—socio-economic and ethical considerations. Cancer Treat Rev 14: 345–350
31. Sudovar S (1985) Economic aspects of treatment of superficial bladder cancer. Urology 26: 57–61
32. Timothy AR et al (1988) Cost versus benefit in non-surgical management of patients with cancer. Br Med J 297: 471–472
33. Tattersall MHN, Friedlander ML (1982) Cost considerations in cancer chemotherapy. Aust Health Rev 5: 21–24
34. Torti FM, Lum BL (1984) The biology and treatment of superficial bladder cancer. J Clin Oncol 2: 505–531
35. Vogelzang NJ (1984) Continuous infusion chemotherapy: a critical review. J Clin Oncol 2: 1289–1304
36. Lokich JJ (1985) Optimal schedule for 5-fluorouracil chemotherapy: intermittent bolus or continuous infusion? Am J Clin Oncol 8: 445–448

37. Coates A et al (1983) On the receiving end: patient perception on the side-effects of cancer chemotherapy. Eur J Cancer Clin Oncol 19: 203–208
38. Nagel GA, Wander HE (1986) Verantwortbare Risiken bei der Wahl der palliativen Chemotherapie. Onkologie 9: 225–230
39. Veenhoven R (1984) Conditions of happiness. Reidel, Dordrecht
40. Palmer BV et al (1980) Adjuvant chemotherapy for breast cancer: side effects and quality of life. Br Med J 281: 1594–1597
41. Hafström L et al (1981) Organisation zur Untersuchung, Behandlung und weiteren Betreuung von Patienten mit gastrointensitalem Karzinom. Zentralblatt Chir 106: 1289–1296
42. Gelber RD, Goldhirsch A (1989) Comparison of adjuvant therapies using quality-of-life considerations. Int J Technol Assess Health Care 5: 401–413
43. Goel V, Detsky AS (1989) A cost–utility analysis of preoperative total parenteral nutrition. Int J Technol Assess Health Care 5: 183–194
44. Bruera E et al (1988) Use of the subcutaneous route for the administration of narcotics in patients with cancer pain. Cancer 62: 407–411
45. Koretz RL (1986) Nutritional support: how much for how much? Gut 27: 85–95
46. Twomey PL, Patching SC (1985) Cost-effectiveness of nutritional support. J Parenteral Enteral Nutr 1985 9: 3–10
47. Jenteg S et al (1987) Clinical and economic aspects on nutritional supply. Clin Nutr 6: 185–190
48. Roberts D (1982) Parenteral and enteral nutrition: a cost–benefit audit. Minnesota Med 65: 707–710
49. Bloom BS, Kreuger N (1988) Cost and quality effects of outpatient cataract removal. Inquiry 25: 383–387
50. Jönsson B, Karlsson G, Maller R (1988) Ekonomisk utvärdering av antibiotika. Linköping University. CMT Rapport, p 3
51. Evans RG, Robinson GC (1980) Surgical day care: measurements of the economic payoff. CMA J 123: 873–880
52. Berk AA, Chalmers TC (1981) Cost and efficacy of the substitution of ambulatory for inpatient care. N Engl J Med 304: 393–397
53. Rosenbaum EH, Rosenbaum IR (1980) Principles of home care for the patient with advanced cancer. JAMA 244: 1484–1487
54. Ryder CF, Ross DM (1977) Terminal care: issues and alternatives. Publ Health Rep 92: 20–29
55. Putnam ST et al (1980) Home as a place to die. Am J Nurs 80: 1451–1453
56. Vinciguerra V et al (1980) Home oncology medical extension: a new home treatment program. CA-A Cancer J Clin 30: 183–185
57. Mor V, Kidder D (1985) Cost savings in hospice: final results of the national hospice study. Health Serv Res 20: 407–421
58. Kane RL et al (1984) A randomized controlled trial of hospice care. Lancet i: 890–895
59. Adamo A, Cronk BA, Mileo R (1979) Cost of terminal care: home hospice vs hospital. Nursing Outlook 27: 522–526
60. Bloom BS, Kissick PD (1980) Home and hospital care of terminal illness. Med Care 1980 18: 560–564
61. Brooks CH, Smyth-Staruch K (1984) Hospice home care cost savings to third-party insurers. Med Care 22: 691–703
62. Morgan NC (1984) An analysis of selected hospice programs. J Risk Insur 51: 99–114
63. Hannan EL, O'Donnel JF (1984) An evaluation of hospices in New York State hospice demonstration program. Inquiry 21: 338–348

64. Spector WD, Mor V (1984) Utilisation and charges for terminal cancer patients in Rhode Island. Inquiry 21: 328–337
65. Vinciguerra V et al (1986) Comparative cost analysis of home and hospital. Adv Cancer Control: Health Care Financing Res 216: 155–164
66. Haid M et al (1984) People and dollars: the experience of one hospice. South Med J 77: 470–472
67. Kassakian MG et al (1979) The cost and quality of dying: A comparison of home and hospital. Nurse Practitioner 4: 18–23
68. McCusker J, Stoddard AM (1987) Effects of an expanding home care program for terminally ill. Med Care 25: 373–385
69. Zimmer JG, Groth-Juncker A, McCusker J (1985) A randomized controlled study of a home health care team. Am J Publ Hlth 75: 134–141
70. Bloom B (1987) Is hospice care least expensive for the terminally ill? Hospice J 3: 67–76
71. McCusker J (1984) The terminal period of cancer: definition and descriptive epidemiology. J Chronic Dis 37: 377–385
72. Long SH et al (1984) Medical expenditures of terminal cancer patients during the last year of life. Inquiry 21: 315–327
73. Houts PS et al (1984) Nonmedical costs to patients and their families associated with outpatient chemotherapy. Cancer 53: 2388–2392
74. Bloom BS et al (1985) The epidemiology of disease expenses: the costs of caring for children with cancer. JAMA 253: 2393–2397
75. McCusker J (1984) Development of scales to measure satisfaction and preferences regarding long-term and terminal care. Med Care 22: 476–493
76. MacAdam DB, Smith M (1987) An initial assessment of suffering in terminal illness. Palliat Med 1: 37–47
77. Parkes CM (1978) Home or hospital? Terminal care as seen by surviving spouses. J R Coll Gen Pract 28: 19–30
78. Groth-Juncker A, McCusker J (1983) Where do elderly patients prefer to die? Place of death and patient characteristics of 100 elderly patients under the care of a home health care team. J Am Geriat Soc 31: 457–461
79. Torrens PR (1985) Hospice care: what have we learned? Ann Rev Public Health 6: 65–83
80. Kane RA, Kane RL (1988) Long-term care: variations on a quality assurance theme. Inquiry 25: 132–146
81. McGlynn EA et al (1988) Quality-of-care research in mental health: responding to challenge. Inquiry 25: 157–170
82. Donabedian A (1988) The quality of care: how can it be assessed? JAMA 260: 1743–1748

ABOUT THE AUTHORS

Bengt Jönsson is Professor of Health Economics at the Department of Economics, Stockholm School of Economics, Sweden. He earned his PhD in economics from the University of Lund. In 1979, Dr Jönsson was the Director of the Swedish Institute for Health Economics. Subsequently, he was Professor of Health Economics at the Department of Health and Society, Linköping University. His research in health economics includes cost–benefit analysis, international comparisons of health care systems and pharmaceutical economics. He is an associate editor of the *Journal of Health Economics* and a member of the editorial board of several other scientific journals.

Göran Karlsson BA is presently a doctoral student at the Department of Health and Society, Linköping University. He is specializing in health economics, and his dissertation, "Economic evaluation of dental implants", was presented in November 1991.

18 The Role of Industry in Cancer Research

WILLIAM McCULLOCH and PHILIP S. SCHEIN

The pharmaceutical industry has the potential to make substantial contributions to medical research both directly, by developing new, effective treatments, and indirectly by funding both basic and clinical investigation in related areas. Large multinational corporations are working with research and development budgets in excess of $200 million [1] and, collectively, their financial support for research exceeds that of any government agency including the National Institutes of Health (NIH) of the USA [2]. Some of the more profitable corporations have used their acquired funds to establish large intramural research programs which, in some cases, resemble traditional research institutes in an academic environment. The programs of the large corporations are complemented by the cottage industry of small, entrepreneurial pharmaceutical companies, many of which operate in the biotechnology field. These smaller companies make important contributions to the diversity and overall creative process, in part due to their necessary focus on the practical development of new research discoveries being made in laboratories of molecular biology, genetics and immunology. Overall, the pharmaceutical industry research effort may be of staggering magnitude if it is brought to bear on a single problem [1].

Despite the fact that oncology represents a large and unsatisfied market for the pharmaceutical industry, very few companies have made tangible and lasting commitments to cancer research. Several factors contribute to the general lack of enthusiasm. First, therapy development in oncology still represents an empirical science to some degree without the highly defined molecular targets that are present for many other diseases. Second, the market opportunity is perceived by some to be small, given the fact that cancer represents many different diseases and even a successful single product may gain only limited application. Lastly, cancer is viewed as very different from many other disease states, requiring a separate and dedicated commitment of strategic resources, not only in research and development but also in marketing, in order to make significant contributions to the field.

The basic mission of a pharmaceutical company is to discover, develop and market products that will make a contribution to medical care as well as to the financial position of the company. Although the former will generally lead to the latter, the reality is that a corporation that does not

Introducing New Treatments for Cancer: Practical, Ethical and Legal Problems. Edited by C. J. Williams
© 1992 John Wiley & Sons Ltd

generate profits will not only find its research and development efforts shrinking, but will also find the future of the company and its employees at risk. This leads to a bias in the approach industry brings to cancer research funding, with the emphasis placed on patentable novel treatments and new chemical entities based on the rationale that these are more likely to provide for long-term financial growth. In addition, neither the regulatory agencies nor the practising medical profession are interested in so-called "me too" products which do not possess a distinguishing profile. In the academic environment, substantial effort may be applied to elucidating properties of, or juggling with combinations of, older, established and maybe generic compounds with, perhaps quite properly, little regard for the magnitude of the resulting economic impact. In industry, because of the need to generate profits and justify resource allocations, the primary focus in most companies is on large market opportunities; in oncology this means lung, breast and colorectal cancer, rather than, for example, lymphoma or gliomas. One defense for these priorities is based in the recognition that the resources required to develop a product for a relatively small number of patients with a relatively rare form of cancer may be roughly equivalent to those required for a disease in which the patient number, and therefore market expectation, is much greater. It is currently estimated that a total expenditure of $100–125 million is required to bring a drug from a discovery program through development to marketing approval [3]. In addition, a large corporation (annual sales in excess of $1 billion per year) is less likely to develop drugs with limited market potential which cannot make a measurable impact on earnings. As a consequence, in the past many useful drugs have languished for failure of sponsorship or full commitment. Many countries have attempted to correct this situation with the adoption of "orphan drug" legislation, pioneered in the USA, which provides incentives to sponsors of drugs for which the number of candidate patients is small [4]. The advantages provided to industry include a greater number of years of exclusivity in the market and tax incentives to offset development costs, while the benefits to the medical profession and patients are obvious. It is of interest that most cancer drugs, because of their application to only a limited number of disease states, qualify as orphan drugs.

The potential sources of new products for pharmaceutical development in oncology are vast. While the research programs of many companies have developed an "NIH" (not invented here) syndrome in the past, resulting in an unwillingness to develop other than their "own" compounds, this can be extremely short-sighted. There is a wide range of important therapeutic research efforts worldwide, based in universities, private research centers and government-sponsored research institutions, as well as in the pharmaceutical industry. The challenges for the pharmaceutical industry are to be aware of important research developments taking place throughout the world, to make judgments about the potential importance of a new discovery in relationship to its ability to provide a safe and highly efficacious product, and, of course, to seek an exclusive licence. This offers many opportunities for academic centers and pharmaceutical companies to work together in an agreement by which both parties benefit; the academic center typically receives both short-term support for the continuation of its research program and the future benefits of royalties resulting from the full commercialization of their discoveries, while the pharmaceutical industry is provided a source of new products to both develop and market. Importantly, any new discovery made in the research laboratory cannot make its full impact in the overall management of a disease until it is made available to the broadest possible physician and patient audience through the process of commercialization. Recognizing the opportunities that exist for such collaboration, it is essential that investigators and their administrative offices ensure that patents are submitted on potentially important medical discoveries before disclosure of data. Premature disclosure cannot only jeopardize the opportunity to achieve a position of exclusivity, but also result in a loss of interest of the commercial sector, who must commit vast resources and financing to bring the discovery to the marketplace.

Regardless of the source, when candidate drugs have been identified the ensuing development program must be highly focused to ensure that the products are brought to registration and the market in the shortest possible time, and with the most efficient use of available resources. The development program must focus on two principal needs if it is to be successful. First, it must fulfill the requirements of regulatory agencies following precedents that have been set by prior drug approvals. This may not always coincide with the goals of investigators, who may wish to adopt alternative study designs or address questions of personal scientific interest which do not directly bear on the fundamental issues of safety and efficacy. It is important to recognize that the future of a potentially important new treatment can be placed in doubt by a poorly designed or executed trial which can readily provide data which unnecessarily damages the product's profile. It is for this reason that many companies are unwilling to provide a new drug to investigators without some control over the design of the study, including important details of dose, schedule and treatment duration. Compromises, if necessary, can almost always be achieved by discussion, which hopefully results in the incorporation of complementary concepts and approaches. The focus of industry in regard to study design represents an absolute necessity. Safety and efficacy are the pivotal regulatory and research questions that need to be addressed for any new therapy, and serve not only as the basis for drug-marketing approval by regulatory agencies but also physician acceptance. A development program which fails to address such fundamental research questions is one that not only delays the eventual introduction of an agent into widespread medical use, but may also subject needless numbers of patients to the risk of an experimental therapy for which there is ultimately no demonstration of compensatory benefit. Investigators also have to recognize their obligations to the development effort and the need for both them and the pharmaceutical company to comply with regulatory requirements. In societies with a litiginous environment, such as in the USA, the failure to conform to dosages, schedules and required measurements specified in a protocol may place both the pharmaceutical company and the individual investigator at risk of legal action by patients who may have in fact, or perceive that they have, been damaged by their participation in the trial. Defense of such an action would incur significant cost. The price of insuring against such an eventuality is a regular financial burden which pharmaceutical companies bear; such insurance is very difficult to obtain, and the extent of coverage never negates the potential risk. The details of the conduct of each trial, which may be perceived as a nuisance to many investigators, must be adhered to if maximum benefit is to be derived from each patient entered. Such practical details as drug accountability, obtaining informed consent and ethical committee ("IRB") approval, with written evidence of such, which must be available for review by representatives of a regulatory agency if an audit is ever conducted, are the dual responsibility of the investigator and the sponsoring company who monitor the trial. Indeed, in some countries such as the USA, participation in what is recognized as a pivotal trial for drug approval ensures that representatives of the Food and Drug Administration (FDA) will visit the institution to examine source documents, as well as other administrative details relating to the conduct of the program. Investigators must recognize in advance that participation in a study may place their program under the intense scrutiny of such auditors although this is not the case in all countries. If investigators do not adhere to the protocol or provide accurate and timely data, the overall study may be jeopardized despite appropriate contributions by other participating institutions. Invalidation of a critical trial results in attendant direct costs to the sponsor, in addition to indirect cost due to the time that is lost and which cannot be recovered. The possible necessity to repeat a very large and important clinical trial can mean that many hundreds of patients may needlessly be placed at risk of drug toxicity. The sponsoring pharmaceutical company typically attempts to relieve the investigators of some of the burden of providing data of high quality through the provision of funding for ancillary staff. This is obviously of considerable direct benefit to investigators, and must be taken into consideration along with more indirect benefits such as early access to important new therapies and opportunities to gain recognition through the resulting publications and presentations.

The second major responsibility of the development program is to elucidate, if possible, the competitive profile for the new drug. Through carefully designed clinical trials, specific distinguishing features of the new drug must be established when compared to other drugs which are already available. This often requires that specific studies be conducted in which a new treatment is directly compared to an established drug in order to demonstrate, with statistical precision, whether advantages for the new product exist either in regard to efficacy or safety. In cancer chemotherapy, small differences, which may be important to physicians and patients, especially if they relate to survival or quality of life, may require the expenditure of enormous resources for full demonstration.

While the emphasis in industry is the development of new and innovative therapies with long patent lives for cancer, it is also recognized that there are many opportunities to improve either the safety or efficacy of existing drugs, or identify additional indications for their use. Many themes have recently emerged in clinical oncology, including reduction of tumor cell resistance, biochemical modulation and dose intensification. This offers further opportunities for collaboration between the pharmaceutical industry and academic oncologists. In addition to testing established drugs in a broader spectrum of tumor types, attempts to enhance the efficacy of established therapies provides a potential new lease of life to drugs that have had only limited application in the past. For example, there is now a major effort to enhance the efficacy of 5-fluorouracil through the process of biochemical modulation using agents such as leucovorin or N-(phosphonacetyl)-L-aspartic acid (PALA) [5, 6]. In the field of radiation therapy, there is considerable interest in establishing the role of both radiation sensitizers to increase efficacy, as well as radioprotectors to reduce both acute and late toxicity. The general theme of protection of normal tissues against the toxic effects of chemotherapy, while maintaining antitumor efficacy, is currently a subject of intense interest and is being pursued with compounds such as WR-2721 (amifostine), ICRF-187 and ORG-2766. This field of chemoprotection is complemented by current development of bone marrow colony-stimulating factors (CSFs), which cause more rapid recovery of granulocyte levels, thereby reducing the risk of infection that results from protracted periods of profound leukopenia [7]. Both the protectors and the CSFs serve as major adjuncts to dose escalation, with the intent of improving the efficacy of existing cancer drugs. Importantly, their development represents a joint academia–industry undertaking, as do parallel efforts in supportive care including the development of new antibiotics, anti-emetics and new forms of nutritional supplementation.

From the above it is clear that, while the pharmaceutical industry is in a position to make a major contribution to the funding of cancer research, this cannot be done in isolation and that, in order to procure medical advances, the industry must work closely with investigators in academic centers. The relationships are delicate, and require a good deal of understanding of the goals of each party in the collaborative effort to ensure that the needs and prerogatives of each are prospectively addressed. In the past, there has been an uneasy relationship between academic medicine and the pharmaceutical industry, with perhaps a misguided impression that one side was attempting to maintain integrity, freedom of thought and the pursuit of non-economic ends while the other side was forever seeking to undermine these moral and ethical objectives in pursuit of ever greater profits. These polarized positions, if they ever did exist, have been softened in the more recent past so that all have realized that a co-operative approach will be more successful and that moral and ethical requirements in order to advance medicine are not incompatible with the financial needs of the pharmaceutical industry. It is not uncommon now for senior scientists and researchers to act as consultants to the pharmaceutical industry, which gives them a better perspective. In addition, there are many researchers with distinguished careers in both the basic sciences and clinical medicine who now work full time within the industry and who, by dint of their previous experience, can appreciate better the different objectives of industry and academia. All of this must lead to better co-operative efforts and the achievement of mutually satisfying goals. This softening of polarized positions has been reflected in receptivity of researchers and physicians to collaborate with the pharmaceutical industry when, in the past, they disparaged their colleagues in industry on the grounds that they had "sold out". It is now recognized that there are many worthy investigators working within the industry and concrete evidence of this was provided when, in 1988, the Nobel Committee awarded the Nobel Prize in Physiology and Medicine to Gertrude Elion, George Hitchings and Sir James Black, all of whom had made their major contributions to science while working within a pharmaceutical industry environment. It is of interest to note that one of the contributions cited for the prize was the discovery of the anticancer agent 6-mercaptopurine [8].

To some researchers, it is the wide scope of opportunity within the industry which is attractive. For pharmaceutical physicians, the ability to take a compound from pre-clinical promise through a clinical development program and define its contribution to medical care is much more rewarding than operating within the limitations of a single institution's academic program. The relative security of industry funding, at least in successful companies, can be more reassuring than the constant battle for the ever-shrinking, peer-reviewed, grant-derived support which beleaguers researchers in other environments. However, it should be recognized that in industry, as in academia, programs and individuals are ultimately judged by their productivity.

We are currently in a period of reduced governmental funding for research and, increasingly, investigators are looking to the pharmaceutical industry as a source of support for their research programs. This brings both opportunities and concerns. It is essential that appropriate safeguards be set in place to ensure that the ethical integrity of investigators is not compromised, and that the balance of applied versus basic non-directed research, so necessary for future discoveries, is not upset. Needless to say, investigators should never participate in a study which they feel is either badly designed or unethical. Although there may be the temptation of funding, participation in substandard development or a promotional program with no scientific basis may cause irreparable damage to both their reputation and career. In this regard, the institutions in which research is being conducted, and their institutional review (ethical) committees, bear responsibility for ensuring that research being conducted in the institution is not only of high scientific merit but will not place patients at unwarranted risks. The process of informed consent, while difficult to effect, is the best means of ensuring that a potential participant in a clinical trial fully understands the benefits versus risks they may encounter by their participation.

Publication of results, even negative results, of all research is essential to the overall research mission. This should be the prerogative of the investigator and agreed upon in advance of conducting the research program. The sponsoring company often requests that it be allowed to review all manuscripts and abstracts for some finite period prior to the actual submission for publication and presentation. This ensures that information that is truly proprietary is not accidentally disclosed, thus compromising either the patent or any competitive position of the product. This also enables the company to assist the investigator by providing additional analyses and interpretations. Both the investigator and the company must be treated with fairness, with the end result being the complete and objective disclosure of the data.

Multi-institutional trials, particularly those carried out in several countries, require the use of a single statistical and data management center, which not only coordinates the study but also monitors the results, reports serious adverse reactions to both investigators and regulatory agencies, and provides analysis of the final data. For most large phase III clinical trials this function is served by the sponsoring company, which is ultimately responsible for the conduct of the study, as well as adherence to national regulations and monitoring activities for quality control. In such an arrangement, investigators must be assured that the company will treat the data with complete objectivity both in its analyses and reports. Society has placed important checks and balances on this process, and a company which does not fully report or misrepresents data places itself in both legal and economic peril. Relationships with national regulatory agencies, who have responsibility for granting marketing approval, and also the medical and lay public are at risk and no sensible company would wish to have these relationships disrupted. Publication of the final results is almost always a co-operative effort involving both the principal investigators of the study and representatives of the company, with the former having the dominant role in the final interpretation and publication.

While there are many challenges to establishing and maintaining a strong and co-operative relationship between the pharmaceutical industry and academic centers, the potential rewards for the public are vast. Importantly, the system works, and it is salutary to consider the number of therapeutic advances in cancer management that have taken place in the last two decades, and the overall contribution of the pharmaceutical industry in this regard.

REFERENCES

1. Pharmaceutical Manufacturers Association Statistical Fact Book (August 1988) Ch 2, pp 2–4, Pharmaceutical Manufacturers Association, Washington, DC
2. Budget of the United States Government (fiscal year 1991) Office of Budget and Management, US Government Printing Office, Washington, DC
3. Wiggins SN (June 1987) Costs of developing a new drug. Office of Policy Analysis, Pharmaceutical Manufacturers Association, Washington, DC
4. The Orphan Drug Act, P.L. 97–414 (4 January 1983)
5. Petrelli N, Douglass HO Jr, Herrera L et al (1989) The modulation of fluorouracil with leucovorin in metastatic colorectal carcinoma: a prospective randomized phase III trial. J Clin Oncol 7: 1419–1426
6. Ardalan B, Singh G, Silberman H (1988) A randomized phase I and II study of short-term infusion of high-dose fluorouracil with or without N-(phosphonacetyl)-L-aspartic acid in patients with advanced pancreatic and colorectal cancers. J Clin Oncol 6: 1053–1058
7. Laver J, Moore MAS (1989) Clinical use of recombinant human hematopoietic growth factors, J Nat Cancer Inst 81: 1370–1382
8. Marx JL (1988) The Nobel prize for physiology or medicine. Science 242: 516–517

ABOUT THE AUTHORS

Dr William McCulloch is the Vice President for Clinical Research and Development of US Bioscience of West Conshohocken, Pennsylvania, and has wide experience of oncology drug development within the pharmaceutical industry. He obtained his medical degree from Glasgow University in Scotland and, after gaining a diploma from the Royal College of Obstetricians and Gynecologists, studied and became a member of the Royal College of Physicians of the United Kingdom. In his clinical practice his main interests were malignant hematology, especially in children, and pediatric oncology. He joined the Bristol-Myers Company in the United Kingdom in 1984 and has held several positions within the pharmaceutical industry, including Medical Director at Celltech Limited, a British biotechnology firm, and Director of Clinical Research in Oncology for Astra AB in Sweden. He obtained the Diploma in Pharmaceutical Medicine in 1986.

Dr Philip Schein US Bioscience's CEO and President, is widely regarded as a leading international authority in the treatment of cancer. Formerly he was Vice President of Worldwide Clinical Research and Development, Smith Kline & French Laboratories, where he had responsibility for all SK&F clinical research and development activities. His previous appointments were at Georgetown University School of Medicine in Washington, DC, where he was Scientific Director of the Vincent T. Lombardi Cancer Research Center. He also served as Senior Investigator and Head of the Clinical Pharmacology Section of the Medicine Branch, National Cancer Institute, Bethesda, Maryland. Dr Schein has authored over 300 articles and texts relating to basic and clinical cancer research and drug development. He is a recipient of numerous scientific and medical awards and honors and a member of many scientific societies. He served as President of the American Society of Clinical Oncology and he has chaired the Food and Drug Administration's Oncology Drugs Advisory Committee, where he received the Commissioner's Special Citation and the Harvey W. Wiley Medal. Furthermore, he has served as a member of the board of directors on the American Board of Internal Medicine, where he chaired the Medical Oncology Committee, and has been a member of many international cancer research programs. Dr Schein received his AB degree from Rutgers University and his MD degree from Upstate Medical Center in Syracuse, New York. He is a Fellow of the Royal College of Physicians of London and the Royal College of Physicians and Surgeons at Glasgow. His current academic appointments include Adjunct Professor of Medicine and Pharmacology at the University of Pennsylvania School of Medicine, Clinical Professor of Medicine and Pharmacology at the Georgetown University School of Medicine, and Adjunct Professor of Medicine at Brown University School of Medicine.

19 Good Clinical Research Practice

FRANK WELLS

Good clinical research standards must be maintained for all studies in whatever clinical field they are conducted. That means that, even in the context of cancer research, such standards must apply, if possible following guidelines agreed by all those involved in conducting the research. The pharmaceutical industry in the UK has adopted voluntary guidelines on good clinical research practice (GCRP), and it is on these guidelines that this chapter is based, with comments on their relevance in the context of cancer research and research into novel therapies. It is also timely to bear in mind the regulations coming into force from the European Commission which will apply mandatorily to clinical research.

In late 1984 the Association of the British Pharmaceutical Industry (ABPI) set up a working party to study the subject of good clinical research practice with a view to preparing a report and position paper as guidance for member companies of the ABPI. The report was circulated in 1986 as an ABPI statement, revised in the spring in 1988, and then issued as definitive ABPI policy [1]. Since then they have been operated by pharmaceutical companies voluntarily, but reasonably effectively, and it has proved invaluable to have these guidelines established as a UK voluntary policy during discussions and negotiations which have taken place regarding mandatory European policy guidelines that have recently been published. It is important to make this point at this stage, because the voluntary nature of the UK guidelines has enabled companies to adopt rational policies when conducting research into cancer therapy which may not be permitted under European legislation.

As well as forthcoming European policy, a similar mandatory policy already operates in the USA. However, the UK voluntary guidelines are proving to be suitable and acceptable, being compatible with Food and Drug Administration (FDA) requirements, insofar as they operate for pivotal studies conducted in the UK. Certainly they have proved to be suitable and acceptable to the medical profession and the licensing authority, as well as to the pharmaceutical industry, in the UK.

The guidance applies to all four phases of pharmaceutical industry research, but does not refer to post-marketing surveillance. That is the subject of separate guidance published in the *British Medical Journal* in February 1988 [2]. Additionally, more specific guidance on phase I studies appears in two further ABPI policy documents on the conduct of human non-patient volunteer studies [3], and on minimum standards for facilities at which such

Introducing New Treatments for Cancer: Practical, Ethical and Legal Problems. Edited by C. J. Williams
© 1992 John Wiley & Sons Ltd

studies are carried out [4], which are complementary to the GCRP guidelines.

SELECTION OF INVESTIGATORS AND CENTRES

The first matter to be considered in the conduct of any clinical research project is the selection of the clinical investigator(s) and the centre(s) at which the study is to be conducted. For studies sponsored by pharmaceutical companies, the company medical adviser must define a requirement for each specific study using the criteria set out in the industry guidelines which apply to the selection of investigators and centres. These criteria include the experience of the investigator; the location of any centre, be it hospital, contract laboratory or general practice; the suitability of the facilities and the availability as well as the suitability of the staff expected to be involved; the commitment or otherwise of an investigator to other studies; the availability with regard to time for an investigator actually to conduct the study within his or her normal clinical commitment; the existence of an adequate subject population from which the study subjects may be drawn; and the special need, if the study is to be a multicentre one, to identify a co-ordinator either from within the company or amongst the investigators. In the context of cancer research, certain limitations in the number of investigators competent to conduct such a study, and particularly the number of patients available for the conduct of such a study, are relevant details. Of considerable significance is the role of the local research ethics committee in this context, and this is discussed below.

THE PROTOCOL

If a study is to be sponsored by a pharmaceutical company, the medical adviser of the company, when discussing the study with any potential investigator, must have a clear idea of the objectives of the study. However, the detailed protocol should follow rather than precede initial discussions with potential investigators, and this is particularly important in the field of cancer research. In any event, the following criteria for the protocol should be met:

(1) It must meet the objectives of the study.
(2) It must be ethical and approved by a properly constituted research ethics committee.
(3) It must be capable of measuring the expected effects of the medicine under investigation.
(4) Adequate measures must be taken to determine the safety of the medicine.

(5) The study design must be practical and acceptable to the investigator.
(6) The protocol must meet all legal and regulatory requirements.
(7) The number of patients involved in the study should be stated, justified and realistic.

The regulations from Europe require that a protocol should be updated during the course of a trial with the agreement of all concerned if new data arise. However, experience in the UK suggests that the approval of a *variation* to the protocol, by the research ethics committee, and by the licensing authority, should be sought. The European proposal could be misconstrued as well as tempting to alter things as the trial progresses without seeking approval. A variation to the protocol, to which exactly the same criteria should apply as to the original, should not be undertaken lightly and the UK policy tends to act as a deterrent to introducing unjustified changes in the protocol during the context of the trial.

The European guidelines also state that the clinical trial monitor should be available at any time for consultation with the investigator. ABPI guidelines refer to the need for a contact telephone number, but appear to work well in practice. It is nevertheless essential, in the context of original research into novel therapy, specifically for cancer, that a pharmaceutical physician of the company concerned is constantly available, as the therapy may well be toxic as well as potent. There is also a European requirement for the investigator to sign off the trial report at the end of the study, whereas in the UK the guidelines only specify that a signature is necessary when the report is to be submitted to a regulatory authority—and again this appears to work well in practice.

With regard to the number of patients to be recruited by any given investigator, the particular problems arising in phase III trials on novel therapies, where only a small number of suitable patients may be available, must be recognized. However, so long as it is appreciated by all interested parties that the numbers of patients able to be recruited may be smaller than is generally considered acceptable for such trials—because of the very nature of the disease being treated—and so long as the principles of GCRP are otherwise followed appropriate allowances can be made. It is most important, however, that the possibility of moderate improvement in survival is not missed, specifically because of the small numbers involved.

RELATIONSHIPS BETWEEN INVESTIGATORS AND SPONSORING COMPANIES

It is appropriate at this stage to mention another report produced by the ABPI. This is on the relationships between the medical profession and the pharmaceutical industry, published in May 1988 [5]. Three sections in this report refer to the conduct of clinical trials—on standards, on costs and on the need for a contract. The section on standards clearly sets out what should be aimed at by both the company and the investigator in the context of clinical research and it emphasizes the need for an agreed protocol to be followed and indeed complied with. This section is linked to that on contracts or formal agreements, where it seems only right and proper that doctors who have agreed to fulfil a protocol—and, similarly, pharmaceutical companies that have agreed to meet their responsibilities set out in a protocol—should feel that this commitment is absolute, and that appropriate sanctions should be applied if there is a violation of the protocol during the conduct of the study. One obvious sanction is not to pay an errant investigator the full amount of money for taking part in the clinical trial; this is effective, and has proved workable and acceptable in the UK. It is, however, not a good enough sanction when it comes to frank misconduct or even fraud. Then it is necessary to take further appropriate action, and this will be referred to below in the section on monitoring of clinical studies.

Misconduct in the context of research is rare, but meetings between representatives of the medical royal colleges and the British Medical Association (BMA) with the pharmaceutical industry to seek agreement on the need to maintain the highest possible standards of clinical research have been welcomed. There is a strong wish on the part of the medical profession to have a formal agreement for every clinical trial which is sponsored by a pharmaceutical company, and the ABPI has recently circulated a checklist of all the headings which should be considered by a company when drawing up a formal agreement with an investigator. Agreement has also been reached with the medical profession on a conciliation procedure, should there be any insoluble dispute between an investigator and a company over the way in which a trial has been conducted. This comprises referral of the dispute to the current president of the BMA, or his or her nominee, for arbitration and conciliation. The status of the president, who is always a distinguished experienced physician, and that of the BMA, which represents the interests of all doctors including pharmaceutical physicians, has enabled this to be readily accepted by all parties. It is a good example of the way in which acceptable voluntary procedures can be devised with the confidence of all concerned.

CASE REPORT FORM DESIGN

The form on which investigators report is important, and the accuracy and completeness of clinical trial data are heavily dependent on the preparation of appropriate case report forms (CRFs) which should enable the recording of data to be easy and its analysis to be facilitated. This obviously applies to cancer research projects, as good CRFs help the progress of a study. Also to be borne in mind are the implications of the Data Protection Act in the UK with regard to patient confidentiality and patient access to data whenever the information collected is to be put onto computer. Additionally, the Patient Access to (Medical) Records Act in effect extends the provision of the Data Protection Act insofar as these provisions affect medical records, to records which are held in hard copy—written, typed or printed.

European guidelines in this regard permit computerized records, but the time does not yet appear to be ripe for research in the UK to go over to the wholesale use of computers as opposed to the use of paper. That will undoubtedly come, and private schemes are being evaluated, but it is premature to anticipate widespread computer use in this particular regard for the time being.

Given, therefore, that they will at present be in written format, the clinical report forms, when completed, must be signed by the investigator as a correct record. That fulfils UK requirements for validation of data for pivotal studies, but does not fulfil FDA requirements. Clinical trials conducted for the FDA require site audit, with the validation of original clinical data; this has been explained in detail to the leaders of hospital management and of the medical profession as well as to individual investigators in the UK, and has been accepted by them. In practice, therefore, this need present no problem, though confidentiality of patient data must be upheld. There is no justification for taking any short cuts in this particular regard for research into novel therapy or into treatment for cancer.

RESEARCH ETHICS COMMITTEES (Chapter 7)

Experience in the UK in the operation of ethics committees is considerable, but it is variable. Pharmaceutical industry guidelines state that all protocols for clinical trials must be approved by a "properly constituted independent ethics committee". This must also apply to cancer research. Although the definition of such a committee is not universally agreed throughout the UK, there are a number of benchmarks. The first (chronologically) is a report of the Royal College of Physicians on the role and practice of ethics committees for medical research in patients, originally drafted in 1967, reviewed in 1973, republished in 1984, and completely revised in 1990 [6]. The second benchmark is the circular issued by the Department of Health in 1975 and reissued in a completely new guise as a consultation document in 1989 on local research ethics committees [7] and now issued in definitive form. The third benchmark is the guidance given by the British Medical Association in the booklet entitled *The philosophy and practice of medical ethics*, produced by the Medical Ethics Committee of the BMA [8].

The current situation is that ethics committees called local ethics research committees are established by district health authorities in the UK with the responsibility of giving ethical approval or otherwise to protocols for any research conducted on patients in that district. The effectiveness of such committees is variable, and the inactivity or inappropriate activity of some of them has positively frustrated clinical research in a number of instances. However, some local research ethics committees function well, and operate efficiently and effectively. Nevertheless training is essential for members of ethics committees, and this should be provided by the Department of Health.

Both the Royal College of Physicians (RCP) 1990 report and the Department of Health consultation document recommend a revised membership. The RCP advice is as follows:

Medical members, including both those occupied chiefly with clinical care and clinical investigators; and a general practitioner, whether the committee reviews projects in general practice or not.

Non-medical workers or scientists, according to the type of work coming before the committee.

At least one nurse.

Lay members, including at least two persons not practising or trained in any medical or paramedical discipline; at least one lay member should be independent of the institution or health authority served by the committee.

Both sexes should be represented.

The committee should elect its own chairman from amongst its members.

The committee should be of manageable size—that is, not more than twelve, but a busy committee may find it useful to have alternates for some members, to ensure a quorum.

It would appear compatible with the RCP recommendations that a cancer specialist or specialists should be present as members whenever research projects for cancer therapy are being considered; alternatively, specialist needs can be met by co-option, or by formation of a subcommittee, with overlapping membership with the main committee.

There is a problem with approval of multicentre trials which must be addressed by all parties concerned. The ABPI has previously stated that ethical clearance given by one properly constituted independent ethics committee would be adequate for clearance for the whole study at all centres, always nevertheless emphasizing the right of each investigator to refer to his or her own local committee for additional approval. It is now felt essential, however, that local clearance should also be obtained, assisted if necessary by advice from a national or central ethics committee, such as that est-ablished by the Royal College of General Practitioners. Much discussion is currently taking place on this matter, involving the medical royal colleges, legislators and chairmen of ethics committees themselves (Chapter 8). The very nature of cancer research makes its ethical approval of great importance.

The situation in Europe varies a great deal. Ethics committees are virtually non-existent in some countries, but the European proposals are tough on some ethical aspects. For instance, they require that the sponsor or investigator should request the opinion of the ethics committee on any serious adverse event occurring during the trial; and that ethics committees should consider details of insurance or indemnity to cover liability of the investigator and sponsor—an aspect which is covered by the voluntary policy operating in the UK.

INFORMED CONSENT

The purpose of informed consent is to make sure that anyone who is the subject of a clinical trial is made as aware as possible of what the clinical trial involves, and of his or her own rights and responsibilities within that clinical trial. Whether the consent provided by the person concerned should be written or verbal has previously been up to the trial co-ordinator investigator to determine, but it is now felt that in virtually all circum-stances the consent should be written. Special care should be taken in the context of cancer research, where it may not always be in a patient's best interests to be told that he or she is taking part in a clinical trial into cancer therapy.

Consent, when obtained, should not be held by a sponsoring pharmaceutical company, but by the investigator, with the investigator submitting a signed declaration that the consent has been obtained, and is held on file. The full elements of informed consent should be familiar to any investigator and comprise the following:

(1) The trial is a research procedure, the nature and type of which will be explained.
(2) The scope, aims and purpose of the research should be explained, together with details of *known* and *foreseeable* risks and discomforts the subject might experience.
(3) The *known* benefits, if any, of participating in the study should be explained.
(4) Appropriate alternative therapies should be disclosed so that the patient can decide whether or not to take part.

(5) The patient should be reassured that participation in the trial is confidential, but that data and record forms might have to be disclosed to a regulatory authority; this has presented little difficulty in practice.

(6) Compensation arrangements for any medicine-induced injury or, indeed, for any harm arising to the subject from participation in the study, should be explained—and there are clear ABPI guidelines on this.

(7) The name and telephone number of appropriate persons to contact should be given to the subject.

(8) An emphatic statement should be included that participation in the study is entirely voluntary.

(9) Adequate time should be given to the subject to decide whether or not to take part.

(10) It should be explained that the subject has a right to withdraw from the study at any time without any prejudice to patient care.

(11) It must be carefully explained that any other drug use, be it of prescribed medicine or from any other source, should be revealed, and that any change in drug use during the study must be disclosed.

(12) An explanation that any significant new findings which arise during the study, which adversely affect the study, will be disclosed to the patient.

(13) How many others are expected to take part should be disclosed.

(14) The consent form should include a statement that the patient, in giving consent, understands what the study is all about.

Ethical approval should be sought and obtained if any of these elements are to be omitted for any research project into cancer therapy.

MONITORING OF CLINICAL STUDIES

The monitoring of clinical trials is important, and GCRP guidelines make it quite clear that the responsibilities of the designated study monitor are to oversee the progress of the study and ensure that it is conducted and reported in accordance with the protocol. Pre-trial visits are themselves important to check and record general and specific aspects of the trial, and to make sure that the laboratory and clinical elements that are wanted are capable of being produced. This means that the competence and experience of the relevant staff must be assessed as appropriate to undertake the measurements defined in the protocol.

An important aspect of GCRP is that primary contact should be made with the clinical investigator and that the contract which will form the agreement between the pharmaceutical company and the investigator should be held by the investigator himself, involvement of laboratory staff being effectively established by the clinical investigator. This essentially means ensuring that the clinician liaises closely with management and with his or her consultant colleagues in the appropriate pathology laboratories, and, where applicable, with the radiology department, to ensure their maximum co-operation and collaboration. Once that has been established, introductions can be made for the trial monitor to visit the laboratories or other facilities; the first person to be involved in arranging all this should nevertheless be the clinical investigator himself.

Monitoring visits have to be made during the study period, but the frequency of these depends on the nature of the study. The overall progress of the study must be assessed, including the rate of recruitment and the completeness of clinical record forms. Having conducted such a visit, it is even more important that any recommendations which might arise from that visit should be recorded and passed on to the co-ordinator of the study, and the pharmaceutical physician responsible for the study—where this is appropriate—without delay. It has transpired that because this is not always achieved as efficiently as it should be, standards may have been allowed to slip. The training of investigators is thus of great importance, and the pharmaceutical industry has collaborated with the RCP to provide a training seminar on the design, development and decline of a medicine; further initiatives are planned.

Although the standards of clinical research practice in the UK are acknowledged to be generally high, in spite of good monitoring a small number of investigators let standards slip too far, and misconduct or fraud is detected which must be dealt with by appropriate action—if necessary by referring the case to the General Medical Council, or by due legal process.

Sometimes as a result of successful clinical trials, particularly in the field of cancer therapy, but before a medicine has been given a product licence, clinicians may wish to use unlicensed medicines on a named patient basis. It is essential that such medicines are not abused, and that all clinicians choosing to use such medicines must recognize that they are wide open to litigation if things go wrong. Guidance on the supply of unlicensed medicines on a particular patient basis are currently being drafted to assist doctors who wish to provide such treatment for their individual patients.

REPORTS OF VOLUNTEER STUDIES AND CLINICAL TRIALS

Much criticism has been levelled against the pharmaceutical industry about its reluctance to publish reports of negative findings, but it is important that a report is written for every study, either as a report confidential to the company, including those needed for regulatory purposes, or as a report intended for publication in a medical journal. It must be made quite clear to the investigator that this is intended. Both types of report must present results of trials accurately, clearly and unambiguously, without bias, and provide a balanced and reasonable interpretation of the data. For regulatory purposes, reports should follow an agreed format.

STATISTICS

Statisticians tend to be forgotten although they are essential members of a research team, so involvement of the statistician who is going to analyse the data in the drafting of a protocol, and particularly in the drafting of clinical record forms, is essential at an early stage. Guidance on the statistical aspects of clinical research is given in outline in the GCRP guidelines.

SUPPLIES FOR CLINICAL TRIALS AND QUALITY ASSURANCE

All clinical trial material should be clearly packaged, labelled, coded and assayed. There is no justification for any short cuts in the provision of novel therapy intended for research on patients with cancer. From a quality-assurance point of view, the assay of clinical trial supplies, particularly of biological preparations, is important, as the clinical trial supplies may well have been prepared under conditions which are different from those applying when the product is manufactured commercially. Indeed, quality assurance must be given due emphasis, and good clinical research practice demands that clinical investigators understand why so much monitoring of what they will be doing needs to take place. Ideally, the persons undertaking quality control should be functionally independent of those conducting a study, and the principles of good clinical research practice specify certain activities which may be performed before, during and after a study.

To give some examples: before any study it is necessary to ensure that a clinical trial certificate or clinical trial exemption certificate has been obtained, and that the protocol fulfils ethical and legal requirements, with appropriate ethical clearance and an undertaking by the investigator and all involved to adhere to the Declaration of Helsinki; during the study, random checks can be made on adherence to the protocol, such as the timing of blood samples, and on adherence to the principles of GCRP; after the study, reviews and audits of the report of the study are important to ensure that it properly describes what was done and that the results accurately reflect the raw data.

ARCHIVING

It is necessary for copies of all records referring to clinical trial studies to be held for, in the UK, at least ten years from the date on which the study is submitted to a licensing authority. European legislation has made this 15 years. It should go without saying that the data must be kept in a secure place, with controlled access and be managed in such a way as to prevent loss of, or tampering with, the records.

SPECIAL DIFFICULTIES FOR NOVEL THERAPIES

It has to be noted, as mentioned previously, that smaller numbers of patients may be involved in clinical trials for novel therapies than is usually the case. Regulatory authorities are encouraged to recognize this. However, because of the smaller numbers involved many studies may be inconclusive. Understandably, specialist investigators who may have detected some benefit for their trial patient subjects may wish to continue with the novel therapy under trial, and arrangements can be made for this to happen. Such therapies may well never come to the licence application stage, and may merely remain available on a named patient basis. That, though, is an unsatisfactory state of affairs, as the prescribing doctor is more vulnerable to criticism and possible litigation if not protected by the licensed status of a medicine, or its formal approval as a trial medicine with a Clinical Trial Certificate (CTC) or Exemption Certificate (CTX or DDX). Even in the context of novel therapies, therefore, pharmaceutical companies encourage full-scale trials which confirm efficacy and which would lead ultimately to a product licence. At the same time, however, companies are reluctant to invest a great deal of money in such trials if they are likely to show inadequate efficacy, and for the product to go no further.

What in practice happens is a decision by a company to put a novel therapy into a full-scale phase III trial, based on positive evidence accumulated from the various small-scale trials already conducted. An agreed trigger mechanism could possibly improve this, whereby all the evidence from small-scale studies is reviewed, once one or more experts in the field believe this stage has been reached.

CONCLUSION

Guidance issued by the ABPI is intended to provide information for its member companies on good clinical research practice, and its use is voluntary. It has, however, been quite vociferously endorsed by the UK licensing authority and by the leaders of the medical profession. That means it has become custom and practice to follow it, and there is little justification for not doing so in the conduct of research into novel therapies. Indeed, it could be argued that the safeguards given by following these guidelines are especially important in the field of cancer research, when innovative treatment is being used.

Understandably, the guidance is orientated towards the UK, but it should in practice be compatible with what has been issued as definitive policy for the European Commission.

A great deal of effective research into novel therapies is being conducted in many countries throughout the world; and in most of these countries, including the UK, it is conducted to commendably high standards, fulfilling the principles of good clinical research practice. These principles nevertheless need reinforcing to those who may be under-aware—or even unaware—of what good clinical research practice is all about. That all our research should voluntarily be conducted to a high standard is essential if legislative procedures—which could seriously inhibit innovative research into novel therapies for serious diseases—are to be avoided.

REFERENCES

1. Guidelines on good clinical research practice (1988) Association of the British Pharmaceutical Industry, London
2. Guidelines on postmarking surveillance (1988) Br Med J 296: 399–400
3. Guidelines for medical experiments on non-patient human volunteers (1988) Association of the British Pharmaceutical Industry, London
4. Facilities for non-patient volunteer studies (1989) Association of the British Pharmaceutical Industry, London
5. Relationships between the medical profession and the pharmaceutical industry (1988) Association of the British Pharmaceutical Industry, London
6. Guidelines on the practice of ethics committees in medical research involving human subjects (1990) Royal College of Physicians of London
7. Consultation document: local research ethics committees (1989) Department of Health, London
8. Research in human subjects: controlled clinical trials (1989) In: Philosophy and practice of medical ethics. British Medical Association, London

ABOUT THE AUTHOR

A graduate of the Royal London Hospital, **Dr Frank Wells** has, since 1986, been Director of Medical Affairs of the Association of the British Pharmaceutical Industry. He is responsible for servicing the ABPI Medical Committee and associated working parties and for providing an interface between the pharmaceutical industry and the medical profession. He has a particular interest, in the context of Europe, in clinical research guidelines, the provision of patient information and pharmacovigilance.

Dr Wells was a general practitioner in Ipswich, Suffolk, for nearly twenty years, during which time he was actively involved in local and national medico-politics and in the organization of the National Health Service. For four years he was one of the general practitioner representatives associated with the Committee on Safety of Medicines.

In 1979 Dr Wells was appointed Under-Secretary of the British Medical Association (BMA), where he was responsible in turn for science and ethics, then the interests of general practitioners and finally the interests of hospital consultants, junior doctors and medical students. Throughout his service with the BMA he was responsible for the medical secretariat of the British National Formulary.

He is an elected member of the Council of the British Medical Association, and of its Medical Ethics Committee.

20 The Clinical and Registrational Strategy for Analogs

RENZO CANETTA, STEPHEN K. CARTER, CLAUDE NICAISE and MARCEL ROZENCWEIG

The clinical evaluation and the registrational strategy for analogs poses unique challenges. One of the key differences which sets analogs apart from new chemotypes, or new therapies of any kind, is that efficacy and safety, per se, do not represent a sufficient end-point for their development. What is crucial is the comparative activity and toxicity, with the comparison being to the parent compound. Because of this characteristic, the end-points for phase I, II and III clinical trials of analogs may be different than for other chemotypes. It is the purpose of this chapter to review the basic principles of clinical evaluation of analogs in cancer chemotherapy, using examples from our direct experience of the past few years.

An analog can be superior to its parent structure in several ways. Table 1 depicts some representative examples of successful analogs we have chosen among those we have been involved with. Obviously many other examples exist, virtually across every chemotherapeutic class, albeit more often with a negative rather than a positive outcome. The hoped for potential of an analog originates mainly from the experimental database. While the particular proposed advantage becomes the focal point of the clinical trial strategy, the empirical nature of cytotoxic chemotherapy, combined with the relatively poor predictability of the current experimental systems, requires that all possible advantages be fully explored.

PHASE I

The phase I study of an analog has specific decision-making end-points depending upon which of the four proposed advantages outlined in Table 1 are dominant in the development strategy. If an efficacy gain is the main goal for the analog, then not only could toxicity be compared to the parent compound but even a greater or a novel toxicity could be acceptable. Urinary bladder and central nervous system toxicity in the case of ifosfamide and, when compared to the parent compound, cyclophosphamide exemplify this concept [1]. The type of proposed pre-clinical advantage could direct, but not necessarily exclude, the selection of a particular patient population right

Introducing New Treatments for Cancer: Practical, Ethical and Legal Problems. Edited by C. J. Williams
© 1992 John Wiley & Sons Ltd

Table 1. Potential advantages for a cytotoxic analog over the parent structure

Proposed advantage	Potential end-points	Examples (ref.)
1. Superior activity in a tumor type responsive to the parent compound	a. Higher objective (or higher complete) response rate b. Longer duration of response or time to progression c. Longer survival	Ifosfamide and cyclo-phosphamide in sarcomas (1) and in testicular cancer (2)
2. Activity in a tumor type not responsive to the parent compound	a. Meaningful efficacy for the particular tumor type in question	Carboplatin and cis-platin in acute leukaemias (3)
3. Lack of cross-resistance with parent compound	a. Meaningful efficacy in "refractory" patients	? Teniposide and etoposide in acute leukaemia (4); ? carboplatin and cisplatin in ovarian cancer (5)
4. Diminished and/or different acute and/or chronic toxicity	a. Qualitative lack of a particular toxicity b. Quantitative reduction in incidence and/or severity of a particular toxicity	Carboplatin and cisplatin (6)

(1) Bramwell, V. et al. (1987) *Eur. J. Cancer Clin. Oncol.* 23: 311–321.
(2) Loehrer, P. et al. (1989) *Semin. Oncol.* (Suppl. 3) 16: 96–101.
(3) Lee, E. and Van Echo, D. (1990) In: Bunn, P. et al. (eds) *Carboplatin: current perspectives and future directions.* Saunders, Philadelphia; pp. 361–365.
(4) Canetta, R. et al. (1982) *Cancer Chemother. Pharmacol.* 7: 43–98.
(5) Evans, B. et al. (1983) *Cancer Treat. Rep.* 67: 997–1000.
(6) Canetta, R. et al. *Cancer Treat. Rer.* 12 (Suppl A): 125–136.

from the start of the clinical development of an analog, with special emphasis on diagnosis and critical pre-treatment characteristics such as prior treatment. For every other practical purpose, if a significant advantage in activity is envisioned, that would not change the usual phase I end-points. An acceptable toxicity spectrum at a reasonable maximum tolerated dose (MTD) would lead on to phase II.

If, instead, an improvement of the therapeutic index through a modification of the toxicological pattern is the main goal, then the end of the phase I study can very well represent the critical decision point for further development or discontinuation of the compound. In our own experience, the cases of carboplatin and of marcellomycin are a paradigm. An improved toxicity spectrum at a reasonable MTD supported a rapid implementation of the phase II program for the former compound; erratic and severe myelo-suppression prompted the discontinuation of the clinical development for the latter [2]. When major differences in the spectrum of toxicity do exist, relative to the parent compound, these differences could be rapidly detected and can be influential during early stages of clinical development: patients with impaired kidney function who were not suitable to receive cisplatin were admitted to the phase I clinical trials of carboplatin.

PHASE II

The phase II evaluation strategy also depends upon the targeted goal for the analog. If the goal is greater efficacy in a tumor type sensitive to the parent compound, then a classical phase II study design may not provide information sufficient to support the decision-making process. In fact, in this situation what is desired is evidence of a reasonable probability of success in a future controlled trial with clear demonstration of superior efficacy. Small numbers of patients and uncontrolled phase II studies might not satisfy that need with sufficient approximation. In addition, the usual single-institution setting of these trials may or may not be predictive for a necessarily larger, often multicenter-based subsequent comparative effort [3].

Two alternative approaches could be considered. One would be to increase the number of patients in the non-randomized phase II trials and to project the sample size according to satisfactory confidence intervals. A second approach would be to design a randomized phase II trial using the parent compound as the control. Stopping rules would be provided prospectively in order to safeguard against insufficient efficacy, and interim analyses could also be planned in order to assess the probability of success for the projected advantage (Chapter 15). If indicated, the trial could be expanded to a phase III evaluation without loss of time and resources. Although the analog was ultimately proven unsuccessful, this approach was part of the clinical development plan devised for spiroplatin. Another possible variation could be proposed if several analogs are available concomitantly. In this case, randomized phase II studies of the analogs in several tumor types may enable the identification of the most promising candidate in terms of efficacy or toxicity. Carboplatin and iproplatin have been developed along these lines by our group as well as by the US National Cancer Institute.

If activity of the analog is expected in a tumor type not sensitive to the parent compound or in tumors which developed resistance to the parent compound, then the phase II evaluation could become indistinguishable from that of any other drug. In the first case the desired level of efficacy would be the same as for any new chemotype. In the second case, the criterion of efficacy would also be similar, although the definition of refractoriness to the parent compound would play a key role in setting the efficacy goal. Thus, assessing patients with cisplatin-pretreated carcinoma of the ovary, a number of different subsets with very different prognostic characteristics could be identified. Response rate to a cisplatin analog would be the lowest in the group experiencing treatment failure while receiving cisplatin-containing therapy (primary resistance) or developing a tumor relapse while still on cisplatin (secondary resistance). No change after a prolonged treatment with cisplatin would probably result in an intermediate outcome. The best results could be achieved in the group initially responding to the parent compound and relapsing only after discontinuation of cisplatin. In our retrospective analysis of the carboplatin phase II data with more than 300 evaluable patients, the objective response rate in these three different clinical situations rose from 5% to 16% to 28% [4]. Adequacy of prior treatment with the parent compound, both in terms of dosage and duration, as well as length of prior remissions are other variables that complicate the evaluation of residual tumor chemosensitivity (Chapters 10 and 11).

A randomized phase II trial of analogs, followed by a second-line treatment with the parent compound in each arm, would add further value to the comparative design. However, in the case of variable degree of cross-resistance between first and second-line treatment options, this approach could blur the effect on survival of the initial treatment, as suggested in the case of carminomycin and doxorubicin.

If the goal is a less toxic analog, then the phase II emphasis would be on evaluation of the analog in tumors sensitive to the parent structure, as we did in the case of tallysomycin S10B, a bleomycin analog [5]. This strategy would allow prolonged treatments which could be a prerequisite for evaluating chronic toxic manifestations. The minimal requirement for efficacy would be evidence of potentially comparable activity with the parent compound. It might be unwise not to empirically test the analog in major tumor types not responsive to the parent compound, although failure to observe activity in this situation would not prevent further advancement of the analog to phase III, as long as the toxicity benefit coupled with activity in sensitive tumor types were to be observed during phase II.

PHASE III

Phase III trials can be designed with different intents. In general, the objective of phase III is elucidating the role of a drug, or a treatment, in a particular clinical situation or indication. As a result, the outcome should ideally influence the future therapy for the involved situation in the larger population-based reality. Some phase III studies could also be used to prove the efficacy and the safety of a new drug to health regulatory authorities, so as to enable access to the drug to all patients who might benefit from it. Indeed, not all phase III studies are designed in a manner which will allow them to serve the latter purpose. The clearest dissection of the particular contribution of a given drug to a successful treatment is not always possible in cancer chemotherapy. Very often, and particularly so in the USA, health authorities have maintained that registrational trials must be designed to allow for that contribution to be singled out [6]. For an analog, whether its expected advantage is superior activity in a tumor type sensitive to the parent compound or diminished toxicity in the presence of a similar efficacy, the registrational phase III study design has almost invariably been a direct comparison of the analog to the parent structure. When this comparison is between single agents, then the interpretation is relatively simple. When the comparison involves multidrug regimens and/or combined modalities of treatment, the analysis of the results becomes more complex.

In a registrational trial, a key issue is the end-point required by the regulatory authority. One such end-point could simply be a reasonable demonstration that the analog is safe and effective in comparison to the parent drug. An example of such a trial is the one performed by the Royal Marsden Hospital in the UK, in which full dosages of either carboplatin or cisplatin were administered to previously untreated patients with advanced ovarian cancer. In the study, more than 100 patients were randomly allocated to receive either drug and cross-over was allowed at the time of progression or in the presence of excessive toxicity. Similar response rates and survival were observed in both arms. Since the study population was relatively small, the lack of any statistically significant difference did not completely rule out the possibility, albeit remote, of a different therapeutic outcome, in either direction. Despite this possibility, this study was deemed acceptable by the health registrational authorities in the UK, the rest of Europe and elsewhere. Also it became widely accepted in the oncology community that carboplatin was an effective drug in ovarian cancer, with a safety profile which compared favorably with cisplatin. The limited *potential* risk of a diminished efficacy was worth accepting in view of the *actual* benefit of a reduced toxicity, and the level of comfort in this stance was raised by a very large amount of data indicating consistently high response rates for carboplatin in ovarian cancer, both in first and second-line treatment [4].

Despite the subsequent confirmation of the results of this trial by two independent groups, the Food and Drug Administration (FDA) in the USA has taken a different view of carboplatin in first-line therapy of ovarian cancer. For this regulatory agency, the demonstration of efficacy and safety alone has not been sufficient and the demonstration of no risk of loss of relative survival benefit in comparison to cisplatin has been demanded. This outcome is commonly referred to by statisticians as the "null hypothesis". Moreover, the FDA would not accept a study design like that of the Royal Marsden trial due to the presence of an established cross-over which could blur the effect of each individual drug on survival. Finally, single-agent chemotherapy is less popular in the USA as the initial modality of treatment in advanced ovarian carcinoma. Therefore, the registrational strategy for carboplatin in the USA has required the designing of two different trials. Combination chemotherapy, considered in the USA to represent the standard form of treatment, had to be chosen. The choice of the control arm required some special consideration: the combination of cyclophosphamide and cisplatin was selected because cisplatin added to cyclophosphamide had resulted in longer survival as compared to cyclophosphamide alone. At the time, no controlled clinical study had suggested that the combination of doxorubicin, cyclophosphamide and cisplatin was superior to cyclophosphamide and doxorubicin in terms of survival. The dose of cyclophosphamide had to be the same in combination with either cisplatin or carboplatin. It had to be based on the presumed contribution of each individual component to the combination and take into account the intrinsic differences existing between carboplatin and cisplatin in their respective ability to be combined with cyclophosphamide. At the Mayo Clinic, the comparison was made using their standard regimen, cyclophosphamide $1000 \, mg/m^2$ and cisplatin $60 \, mg/m^2$. When it came to designing the experimental regimen, the same dosage of cyclophosphamide was kept, which did not allow the administration of more than $150 \, mg/m^2$ of carboplatin, due to its myelosuppressive effects [7]. Despite some hints of a dose–effect relationship for carboplatin in that very pilot study, these dosages were maintained for the phase III trial which, not totally unexpectedly, showed superior efficacy in the cisplatin plus cyclophosphamide arm [8]. A different study design, whereby flexible optimal dosing of *both* components of each treatment arm had been allowed, would have been of scientific interest but of no clear-cut regulatory impact. The administration of different dosages of cyclophosphamide could have started an endless discussion about their relative merit, both in terms of efficacy and safety. If cisplatin plus cyclophosphamide resulted in superior survival versus cyclophosphamide, the same could not be shown for trials comparing cisplatin plus cyclophosphamide with cisplatin alone. Our bias is that the platinum-containing drug is the most important component of the combination with cyclophosphamide. Accordingly, for both the registrational phase III trials performed by the Canadian National Cancer Institute (NCIC) and the Southwest Oncology Group (SWOG) we decided to keep a relatively lower dosage of cyclophosphamide ($600 \, mg/m^2$) but to push *both* platinum-containing drugs as high as possible. This resulted in doses of $75–100 \, mg/m^2$ for cisplatin and of $300 \, mg/m^2$ for carboplatin. Both trials, which began in 1985, have been closed for accrual and reported. Overall, more than 700 patients have been evaluated and no statistical difference has been observed in objective response rates, pathologically documented complete response rates, time to progression or survival (Table 2). Unfortunately, 95% confidence intervals around the survival odds ratio can remain relatively wide even with these sample sizes and, in any event, there are no undisputably defined confidence intervals for demonstrating therapeutic equivalence with acceptable boundaries. The FDA has now reviewed and approved the application.

The carboplatin registrational process for first-line treatment of ovarian cancer exemplifies the difficulties of analog development when the

Table 2. Analysis of survival in two randomized trials in first-line chemotherapy of ovarian cancer [a]

Study	NCIC[b]		SWOG[c]	
Treatment arms	CDDP/CTX	CARBO/CTX	CDDP/CTX	CARBO/CTX
Patients randomized	223	224	170	172
Patients evaluated	209	208	148	137
Patients alive	106	109	70	82
Median follow-up	103 wks	101 wks	59 wks	62 wks
(range)	(0–185)	(20–192)	(12–147)	(20–168)
Median survival	99 wks	107 wks	76 wks	91 wks
p-value	0.876		0.437	
Odds ratio	1.090		0.862	
(95% confidence intervals)	(0.819, 1.447)		(0.613, 1.213)	

[a] Statistical analysis by Bristol-Myers Squibb Biostatistics/Data Management Department; p values (log-rank test) after stratification by prognostic factors.
[b] Pater, J. (1990) Cyclophosphamide/cisplatin versus cyclophosphamide/carboplatin in macroscopic residual ovarian carcinoma: initial results of a National Cancer Institute of Canada (NCIC) clinical trials group trial. *Proc. Am. Soc. Clin. Oncol.* 9: 155 (Abstract).
[c] Alberts, D. et al. (1989) Improved efficacy of carboplatin/cyclophosphamide versus cisplatin/cyclophosphamide. *Proc. Am. Soc. Clin. Oncol.* 8: 151 (Abstract).

phase III comparison is with the parent compound and the end-point is equivalence in efficacy. Similar scenarios could be hypothesized for combinations with carboplatin or cisplatin plus etoposide in small-cell lung cancer or fluorouracil in head and neck cancer. In the USA such scenarios would be even further complicated by the fact that cisplatin has not received regulatory approval in either disease and that fluorouracil is not approved to treat head and neck cancer.

The registrational evaluation of the analog would be much simpler, and similar to that of any other new drug, when the parent compound does not represent a suitable control, either because a tumor type unresponsive (or no longer responsive) is being studied, or because the clinical situation being approached would not justify the use of the parent compound. Unfortunately, in many of these instances, a regulatory approval or even a medical acceptance of an alternative standard form of treatment just does not exist. Regulatory agencies and the research community have most of the times rejected the possibility of adopting a placebo control arm.

Salvage therapy for germ cell tumors after cisplatin, vinblastine, etoposide and bleomycin or second-line treatment of ovarian cancer after cisplatin are typical examples of this dilemma. Flexibility and creativity may be needed in identifying a suitable control group for regulatory purposes. This could be selected in different ways. First, patients could be serving as their own controls, as in the case of testicular cancer patients who failed to achieve long-term survival with approved active drugs and who could achieve that goal with the same drugs plus ifosfamide. Second, the analog could be tested against another experimental treatment, as in the case of a trial in which cisplatin-pretreated ovarian cancer patients were randomized to receive carboplatin or either continuous-infusion fluorouracil or etoposide. The choice of a meaningful control arm would require, as in the latter case, a careful screening of what treatment could be considered of potential benefit to the patient. Assessment of the patient's quality of life may represent an alternative end-point of major importance in this particular setting. Finally, a comparison of different doses of the same analog could be devised. The documentation of a dose–effect relationship could be adequate to demonstrate efficacy. It is possible that the availability of biological or biochemical modulators of toxicity of anticancer agents may provide some successful examples of this strategy in the future, particularly if the regulatory agencies accept the concept.

CONCLUSIONS

Developing analogs of cytotoxic agents poses a series of questions that are relevant to various aspects of rationale drug development. Based on our past experience, success in developing analogs may be a lengthy process, and many challenges resulting from unique scientific, ethical, organizational and regulatory issues have to be faced. We believe that only the active interaction and co-operation of all the interested parties, including the sponsor, the investigator and the health authorities, can lead to an efficient developmental process.

REFERENCES

1. Sarosy G (1989) Ifosfamide: pharmacologic overview. Semin Oncol 16 (Suppl 3) 2–8
2. Rozencweig M, Nicaise C, Dodion P et al (1982) Preliminary experience with marcellomycin: preclinical and clinical aspects. In: Muggia FM, Young CW, Carter SK (eds) Anthracycline antibiotics in cancer therapy. Developments in Oncology 10, Martinus Nijhoff, The Hague, pp 549–561
3. Sylvester RJ, Pinedo HM, DePauw M et al 1981 Quality of institutional participation in multicenter clinical trials. N Engl J Med 305: 852–855
4. Canetta R, Bragman K, Smaldone L, Rozencweig M (1988) Carboplatin: current status and future prospects. Cancer Treat Rev 15 (Suppl B): 17–32
5. Nicaise C, Hong WK, Dimery W, Usakewicz J, Rozencweig M, Krakoff I (1990) Phase II study of tallysomycin S10B in patients with advanced head and neck cancer. Invest New Drugs 8: 325–328
6. Wittes RE (1987) Antineoplastic agents and FDA regulations: square pegs for round holes? Cancer Treat Rep 9: 795–806
7. Edmonson JH, McCormack GW, Krook JE, Long HJ, Jefferies JA, Richardson RL (1987) Pilot study of cyclophosphamide plus carboplatin in advanced ovarian carcinoma. Cancer Treat Rep 71: 199–200

8. Edmonson JH, McCormack GM, Wieand HS et al (1989) Cyclophosphamide–cisplatin versus cyclophosphamide–carboplatin in stage III–IV ovarian carcinoma: a comparison of equally myelosuppressive regimens. J Natl Cancer Inst 81: 1500–1504

ABOUT THE AUTHORS

Dr Renzo M. Canetta was born in Milan, Italy, on 3 May 1951. He was trained at the Istituto Nazionale Tumori in Milan under Dr Gianni Bonadonna, where he worked from 1976 to 1980. He has since joined the Bristol-Myers Squibb Pharmaceutical Research Institute, first in New York, and then in Wallingford, Connecticut, where he is Director of Clinical Cancer Research.

Dr Canetta's career has focused on clinical trials and new drug development, including anthracyclines, podophyllotoxins, platinum co-ordination compounds and, more recently, nucleosides for the treatment of HIV-related disease and taxanes for the treatment of cancer. Dr Canetta holds academic appointments at New York University School of Medicine, as well as at Yale University School of Medicine, New Haven, Connecticut.

Stephen Carter, a New Yorker by birth, graduated from the New York Medical College in 1963. Following internship and residency at Lenox Hill Hospital, New York, he moved to the National Cancer Institute in 1967. During his decade at the NCI he rose to be Deputy Director of the Division of Cancer Treatment, subsequently moving to the west coast to be Director of the Northern California Cancer Program from 1976 to 1982. He then became Vice President of Anti-Cancer Research for Bristol-Myers, New York, subsequently rising to be Senior Vice President, Worldwide Clinical Research and Development for Bristol-Myers Squibb Pharmaceutical Research Institute, Lawrenceville, New Jersey.

Dr Marcel Rozencweig was born in Brussels, Belgium, on 7 December 1945. He trained in medical oncology at the Institute Jules Bordet in Brussels and at the National Cancer Institute in Bethesda, Maryland, USA. He subsequently became head of the New Drug Section at the Institute Jules Bordet and was also very involved in drug development within the European Organization for Research and Treatment for Cancer. In 1983 he joined the Bristol-Myers Squibb Company where he is presently directing, as Vice President, the worldwide clinical development of new anticancer agents. He also holds an academic appointment at the New York University School of Medicine.

Dr Claude Nicaise was born in Belgium on 1 September 1952. He trained in internal medicine and oncology at the Institute Jules Bordet in Brussels, where he held an appointment until 1983. Since then he joined the Bristol-Myers Squibb Company as Medical Advisor of Clinical Oncology with the Belgium subsidiary and subsequently as Director of Clinical Cancer Research.

Dr Nicaise has been involved in the development of new anticancer agents as well as in the area of biological therapy of cancer. He has also participated in the development of new antiretroviral agents for the treatment of AIDS. He holds an academic appointment at Yale University School of Medicine, New Haven, Connecticut.

21 Oncology in the 1990s: Economic and Legislative Issues

Health care providers have become increasingly aware of disturbing changes in medical practice. Escalating costs of health care delivery and the current budgetary constraints in many countries threaten to seriously compromise patient care and innovative biomedical research. In a recent Harris poll of Americans, Canadians and the British, 89% of Americans and 69% of Britons stated that their health care system required fundamental changes. In fact, 61% of Americans stated they would prefer a Canadian system [1]. In contrast, the majority of Canadians (56%) expressed general satisfaction. Governments, and industry as well, are examining various models of health care delivery [2–9].

THE PROBLEMS

RISING HEALTH CARE COSTS

Much has been made of the rising costs of medical care. The USA currently spends approximately 12% of gross national product (GNP) on medical care, in contrast to approximately 9% for Canada and 7% for Great Britain (6.1% for the National Health Service and the remainder privately funded) [10]. For comparison, Americans spend approximately 15% of the GNP on recreation. While health care policy makers are alarmed by rapidly increasing health care costs, the American people have repeatedly responded in surveys that they want more and better health care services. The American people, through Congress and the National Cancer Institute (NCI), have also consistently given high priority to clinical cancer research. Blendon has found that when health care experts recommend policies not supported by public opinion, their advice may not be implementable [11]. One large component of American health care expenses that patients and physicians both would cheerfully do without is the 20% spent on administration, compared to 2% in Canada [12]. Micromanagement of clinical practice by non-physicians is a large and growing US industry [4]. A substantial component is determining whether an individual patient is eligible for an itemized service rendered. There are hundreds of health plans each with its own set of forms.

Introducing New Treatments for Cancer: Practical, Ethical and Legal Problems. Edited by C. J. Williams
© 1992 John Wiley & Sons Ltd

Additional hidden costs are the physician office's time filling out and submitting innumerable forms [13].

ACCESS

During the Reagan administration in the USA, emphasis was to be on health care as a cost-effective business rather than a profession [14]. However, when hospital costs of non-paying patients could no longer be cost shifted to patients with insurance, access to care for the 37 million uninsured (and millions more who are under-insured) developed into a major issue [2, 15–17]. These are often the working poor since the unemployed are sometimes covered by Medicaid. Americans perceive a moral obligation to provide basic care of life-threatening illness such as cancer [18]. While many physicians may be willing to provide *pro bono* care for poor patients, who will pay for expensive medications or for in-patient admissions? A recent editorial, "Health care tickets for the uninsured: first class, coach or standby?", suggested that "standby" care for life-threatening illness is unacceptable to the American public and that the uninsured were entitled to basic services [18]. Also disturbing are statistics documenting that minority Americans, *even those with insurance*, have less access to health care and higher death rates for most cancers [15, 19, 20].

Congress has been attempting to ensure access while controlling costs. When Medicare costs for in-patient services were capped, out-patient costs soared [14, 21]. Congressional planners have also observed that when the cost of a service is capped, physicians merely do more of them [22–24]. Congressional aides sometimes attribute the additional volume to physicians doing unnecessary procedures, but a significant factor is also an increasing demand for entitled services [2]. Congress has recently enacted physician payment reform based on the Harvard Relative Value Scale (HRVS). With the inception of insurance coverage, the costs of in-patient procedures which were covered increased faster than out-patient services which were out of pocket. The differences between subspecialty incomes has now become so substantial that recent medical school graduates have increasingly chosen procedure-oriented subspecialties rather than primary care specialties such as internal medicine and pediatrics. Thus the pool of candidates for oncology–hematology training is shrinking. Furthermore, tight grant funding is discouraging those who pursue oncology training from continuing in academic medicine [25]. Increasing reimbursement for cognitive skills should allow physicians to spend more time with patients and encourage more graduating medical students to pursue careers in primary care specialties. The medical oncology section of the HRVS is currently under review. As part of the general review of billing practices, customary, prevailing and reasonable charges are being revised to reflect costs incurred by efficient physicians providing it [23, 26]. The Common Procedural

Terminology (CPT-4) codes do not presently recognize explicitly a professional component for developing a treatment plan and ordering chemotherapy administration for cancer patients. The chemotherapy administration codes should ideally reflect both components of chemotherapy administration, cognitive and technical.

QUALITY OF CARE

Non-government health care insurers are also under great financial pressure, and are understandably committed to reducing the costs of health care. Private third-party payers' efforts to contain costs have included the development of health maintenance organizations (HMOs) and managed care systems. Indeed Congress has been concerned that there continue to be incentives to provide quality care in settings with a major emphasis on cost containment [27]. Some third-party insurers are moving to preferred providers for high-cost procedures such as bone marrow transplant. In some managed care settings, patients may not be offered investigational therapy or even expensive state-of-the-art therapies.

THE ISSUES

INVESTIGATIONAL CARE

Over the past two to three years there has been considerable discussion of the impact of recent third-party refusal to cover some patients treated on investigational protocols [25, 28–32]. Reimbursement for standard care has also sometimes been refused if delivered as part of a study (eg MOPP versus ABVD) or for an indication which is not specifically cited on the Food and Drug Administration (FDA) label. In these settings particularly, the argument that such a treatment is research merely because data are being collected is untenable. HCFA is currently moving to collect exactly such data on Medicare patients as part of a program to determine outcome assessment [33]. Incentives to avoid expensive care can be subtle. A physician who spends considerable time attempting to obtain coverage for a patient for medically appropriate investigational therapy or a non-FDA-approved indication may think twice before recommending such a treatment to other patients [34].

Who should cover the patient care costs of patients participating in clinical trials [30]? One approach would have patients cover these costs themselves [35]. This would create a policy guaranteeing that new, experimental therapies would be available only to the affluent members of society [29].

A second approach is the reinstitution of *patient care costs* into research grants. Current research grant budgets generally cover the costs of collecting data, sending slides for histological review, and laboratory tests not otherwise required for patient care. The *research* cost per patient for a phase I or II trial is generally in the range of $1000–2000. The assumption of patient care costs would further compromise a National Institutes of Health (NIH) budget that is already under significant constraints. Furthermore, patients with advanced cancer require hospitalization for complications coincident with but unrelated to administration of investigational therapy. These costs are properly assumed by their insurance coverage [28].

A third possibility is that the pharmaceutical industry support patient care costs of clinical research. Pharmaceutical firms have already invested substantially in drug development, frequently provide drugs without cost and often cover laboratory tests associated with clinical trials. Complete coverage of hospitalization expenses would be a financial disincentive to drug development and, furthermore, pharmaceutical firms should not be responsible for the patient care costs of treating the complications of the underlying malignancy [28]. There would be the additional problem of real and perceived conflicts of interests in the reporting and interpretation of the data. Would other physicians (and government and private insurance carriers) implicitly trust the results of pharmaceutical industry sponsored research? While it is less likely that fraudulent data would be manufactured, there would be a substantial risk of exacerbating already existing reporting biases. (Positive studies are most likely to be reported.) Many multi-institutional trials could be initiated. Since no one institution has control over the data, negative data can efficiently be buried and never published.

Historically, hospital expenses of patients participating in phase I and II studies have been paid by the health insurance policies to which they and their employers have contributed. Whether this is appropriate depends on a determination of the best available medical treatment. In the absence of a research trial, many patients would be treated with FDA-approved therapies despite a lack of demonstrated benefit [28]. Standard therapy for metastatic lung cancer, for example, produces partial tumor regression in a minority of patients with no improvement in survival [15]. Such marginal treatments are routinely compensated by third-party payers. Thus participation in scientifically and ethically sound therapeutic trials by patients with advanced, incurable cancers is the *best available form of medical care* and thus should be covered by third-party payers [28]. While ineffective standard treatments may not warrant reimbursement, adopting such a position need not inhibit research on better modes of treatment [36].

A modest improvement in survival of patients treated with the investigational treatment protocols proved cost effective in two NCI Canada trials, with the cyclophosphamide, adriamycin and cisplatin (CAP) chemotherapy arm less expensive than the supportive care-only standard therapy in non small-cell lung cancer [37–39]. While investigational treatment may increase medical costs in the short run, where they evolve into curative therapy, the costs of an illness to society in terms of medical costs and lost productivity are decreased [40]. The costs are ultimately paid by health care consumers who are the ultimate beneficiaries of any improvements resulting from the clinical trial.

Patients with advanced cancer often ask for investigational therapy even if their physician indicates that supportive care is a reasonable option. Patients typically assume that they are covered for investigational therapy if no effective standard therapy exists for a lethal disease. They are frequently surprised and angry when their insurer does not cover these costs [28]. There is a growing discrepancy between patients who believe they are buying coverage of state-of-the-art medical care as determined by their physician, and insurers who perceive insurance as a legal contract with stated limitations. By refusing to reimburse the patient care costs of investigational therapy, third-party carriers are *de facto* making medical decisions [4, 28]. Patients in any health care system should be informed of third-party influence on medical decision making [41]. The current system of refusing to pay for hospitalization costs for investigational therapy is expensive to monitor, arbitrary, and thus unfair to specific patients.

Requested by the NIH to assess of the availability of appropriate resources for patient-related research, the Institute of Medicine released a report on resources for clinical investigation [25] which concluded that clinical investigation in the USA is currently threatened by fundamental changes in the organization of health care, major efforts at cost containment in clinical medicine, rapidly escalating expenses associated with drug development, and a reduction in the number of individuals pursuing a career in clinical investigation. The committee unanimously agreed that these issues must be "thoughtfully and vigorously addressed to prevent serious deterioration in clinical investigation" in the USA.

A major impediment to assessing the existing problem is the current lack of even baseline data on clinical research costs. Grants which merely involve the use of human tissue are considered "clinical investigation" by the NIH while some dose finding and early efficacy studies are not currently included under the designation clinical investigation. Thus actual NIH funding for studies that involve patient–investigator contact cannot currently be determined. The report concludes that failure to appropriately define clinical trials "could lead to inappropiate conclusions as to the requirements for trained investigators, the needed financial resources, the type of organization required to pursue clinical trials and the availability of patients". Recognizing the increasing reluctance of third-party payers to cover the patient care costs of patients participating in clinical trials, the committee concluded that:

> it is wholly inappropriate for third party payers to deny reimbursement for all appropriate and necessary patient care costs (not marginal costs owing to investigational intervention) that would have been incurred in any case simply

because a patient is on an investigational protocol. Such denial would be tantamount to an abrogation of contractual obligation . . . These policies interfere with the patient–doctor relationship and patient free choice. They also add a potential burden to the NIH in funding clinical investigation because of the absence of funding of necessary and appropriate patient care costs and by limiting patient access to investigational protocols . . . Finally, they limit the hospital's ability to continue to support early clinical investigation which is a significant portion of the costs of clinical investigation . . . This requires a clarification in current Medicare regulations involving definitions of medically necessary care. State regulatory agencies should require conforming changes by all other third party payer policies. [25]

Clinical trials have proven particularly vulnerable to cost-cutting by both the federal government and third-party insurers, despite a proven track record in the development of curative therapy for childhood leukaemia, Hodgkin's disease, non-Hodgkin's lymphoma, testis cancer and many pediatric solid tumors, and a decreased mortality in pre-menopausal women with breast cancer—although these advances have been disputed by the General Accounting Office study [42]. There is growing and legitimate concern that the pace of clinical research will be significantly impeded at a time when many exciting developments will soon be ready for clinical trials [30, 43]. The molecular steps in carcinogenesis are being rapidly documented for common malignancies such as colon cancer. Immunological, biological and hormonal approaches, surgical trials of organ preservation (such as breast, limb and bladder preservation), and emerging technologies such as bone marrow transplantation or antibody toxin conjugates are already under study in the clinic. The Institute of Medicine study specifically noted (and recommended that the NIH and FDA further examine) why larger numbers of large-scale clinical trials are now completed in Europe than in the USA and whether children, women, minorities and the elderly may be inappropriately excluded from participation in clinical trials in the USA. Finally they strongly recommended outcome assessment as an integral part of clinical trials [25].

FEDERAL APPROPRIATIONS FOR RESEARCH

An additional factor in changing conditions in medical practice is the constrained federal budget. Particular policy issues that will require comment in 1991 are the reauthorization of the NCI, and appropriations for bio-medical research. The NCI budget for 1989 is $1.57 billion (minus an estimated $86 million lost in the Gramm–Rudman sequestration of one-third of the year's budget). Adequate federal appropriation levels are required to avoid the loss of cancer centers, decreased funding of co-operative clinical trials, and unprecedented level of competition for grants [44]. Young laboratory and clinical investigators may think twice before choosing a career in academic medicine, an issue also addressed by the Institute of Medicine study [25]. The large educational debt incurred by recent graduate physicians, the discrepancy between incomes of clinical investigators and colleagues in private practice, increasing difficulty in funding clinical research from the NIH and other sources, and particularly difficulties in advancement in the academic community were recognized as discouraging the recruitment of clinical investigators [25, 45]. An estimated 1000 new clinical investigators are necessary per year merely to replace existing faculty who retire or who enter private practice [25].

Training

To adequately train independent clinical investigators, the committee recommended a five-year training program (following a standard clinical residency). An appended report, by Dr David Nathan (Children's Hospital, Boston) observed that "recently, the NIH has developed five year physician–scientist, clinical investigator and academic investigator awards to complement the traditional research career medical awards for medical school graduates, but the funding for these awards is limited" [25]. The committee concluded that the NIH should expand funding for clinical research training grants to support the first three years of training. The final two years should be competitively funded by a mechanism similar to the NIH Career Development Awards. The committee further recommends that the trainee be supported by a "national system that provides career stabilization and secures ultimate entry onto a tenured academic track" [25].

That the majority of advanced cancers remain incurable underscores the importance of safeguarding the mechanisms for new technology transfer from the laboratory bench to the bedside, and also the value of investing in prevention of cancer. Dr Sullivan, Secretary of Health and Human Services in the USA, estimates that we could eliminate 23% of deaths from cancer with early detection, intervention and behavioral changes [19].

The American Society of Clinical Oncology (ASCO) has adopted the following positions on the issues of third-party reimbursement for patients treated on investigational protocols or with a medically indicated, commercially available agent for a malignancy which is not specifically listed as an indication for that drug:

(1) Patients with serious and immediately life-threatening diseases should not be denied coverage for best available therapy because they are on a clinical trial providing that the trial is approved by the IRB and the drug(s) used in the trial are either approved by the FDA for marketing or have received an IND exemption.

(2) A drug approved for marketing by the FDA should be reimbursed for a use not included in the labeling if such use is referenced in

the standard medical compendia* or otherwise recognized in medical literature.

Recent statements by the Health Insurance Association of America and Blue Cross have recognized the legitimacy of coverage for off-FDA label indications.

Health policy legislation and decisions by the insurance industry directly impact on physicians, facilitating (or often impeding) the care physicians are able to provide. Who makes health policy decisions? Increasingly not physicians [4]: experts in public health, economists and, more recently, large industries grappling with the cost of providing insurance coverage and its effects on competitive pricing in a world market. How have physicians responded?—generally reactively (analyzing and reacting to legislation as it arises). If physicians do not do their part in developing creative solutions for current problems, solutions will be imposed by administrators. Physicians must begin to develop, not react to policy. Within our profession we have the expertise to address issues of cancer prevention, appropriations for biomedical research and the delivery of cost-effective cancer therapy. The alternative is health care policy designed by government and big business interests without practical experience in the field of biomedical research or patient care. Achieving this end is currently complicated by congressional perceptions of physician interest groups. Congress does distinguish between recommendations for public policy by educational or non-profit organizations (such as ASCO and the American Cancer Society) when requesting testimony and groups perceived as having lobbying interests. Thus, physician organizations need to best position themselves to influence the development of medical policy particularly as it relates to the prevention, diagnosis and treatment of patients with cancer over the coming decades.

REFERENCES

1. Blendon RJ, Taylor H (1989) View on health care: public opinion in three nations. Health Affairs (Millwood) 8: 150–7
2. Levey S, Hill J (1989) National health insurance: the triumph of equivocation. N Engl J Med 321: 1750–1754
3. Dickman RL, Ford AB, Liebman J, Milligan S, Schorr A (1987) Sounding board: an end to patchwork reform of health care. N Engl J Med 317: 1086–1088
4. Caper P (1988) Solving the medical care dilemma. N Engl J Med 318: 1535–1536
5. Inglehart JK (1986) Canada's health care system. N Engl J Med 315: 202–208
6. Inglehart JK (1988) Japan's medical care system (part 2). N Engl J Med 319: 1166–1172
7. Inglehart JK (1988) Japan's medical care system. N Engl J Med 319: 807–812
8. Inglehart JK (1989) The United States looks at Canadian health care. N Engl J Med 321: 1767–1772

---

*Standard medical compendia: USP DI—*United States Pharmacopoea: Drug Information* (updated every two months); AMA DE—*American Medical Association Drug Evaluation; Hospital Formulary.*

9. Rusthoven JJ, Wodinsky H, Osoba D (1986) Canadian cancer care: organizational models. Ann Intern Med 105: 932–936
10. Lister J (1988) Occasional notes: prospects for the National Health Service. N Engl J Med 318: 1473–1476.
11. Blendon RJ (1985) Policy changes for the 1990's: an uncertain look into America's future. In: Ginsberg E (ed). The US health care system: a look to the 1990's. Rowman & Allanheld, Totowa, New Jersey.
12. Himmelstein DU, Woolhandler S (1986) Cost without benefit: administrative waste in U.S. health care. N Engl J Med 314: 441–445
13. Antman K, Aledort LM, Yarbro J et al (1989) Cost-effectiveness and reimbursement in patient care. Semin Hematol 26: 32–45
14. Ginsberg E (1987) A hard look at cost containment. N Engl J Med 316: 1151–1154
15. Greenberg ER, Chute CG, Stukel T et al (1988) Social and economic factors in the choice of lung cancer treatment. N Engl J Med 318: 612–616
16. Mayer RJ, Patterson WB (1988) How is cancer treatment chosen? N Engl J Med 318: 636–638
17. Nutter DO (1987) Medical indigency and the public health care crisis. N Engl J Med 316: 1156–1158
18. Welch HG (1989) Health care tickets for the uninsured: first class, coach or standby? N Engl J Med 321: 1261–1264
19. Sullivan LW (1989) The health care priorities of the Bush administration. N Engl J Med 321: 125–128
20. Hayward RA, Shapiro MF, Freeman HE, Corey CR (1988) Inequities in health services among insured Americans: do working-age adults have less access to medical care than the elderly? N Engl J Med 318: 1507–1512
21. Vladeck BC (1988) Hospital prospective payment and the quality of care. N Engl J Med 319: 1411–1413
22. Roper WL (1988) Perspectives on physician-payment reform: the resource-based relative value scale in context. N Engl J Med 319: 865–867
23. Inglehart JK (1989) The recommendations of the physician payment review commission. N Engl J Med 320: 1156–1160
24. Relman AS (1988) Assessment and accountability the third revolution in medical care. N Engl J Med 319: 1220–1222
25. Marks PA, Bennett JC, Hanft RS et al (1988) Institute of Medicine: resources for clinical investigation. National Academy Press, Washington, DC
26. Hsiao WC, Braun P, Dunn D, Becker ER, Denicola M, Ketcham TR (1988) Results and policy implications of the resource-based relative-value study. N Engl J Med 319: 881–888
27. Inglehart JK (1987) Second thoughts about HMOs for medicare patients. N Engl J Med 316: 1487–1492
28. Antman K, Schnipper L, Frei E III (1988) The crisis in clinical cancer research: third-party insurance and investigational therapy. N Engl J Med 319: 46–48
29. Monaco G, Gottlieb M (1987) Treatment INDs: research for hire? JAMA 258 3296–3297
30. Wittes RE (1987) Paying for patient care in treatment research: who is responsible? Cancer Treat Rep 71: 107–113
31. Wittes RE (1987) Antineoplastic agents and FDA regulations: square pegs for round holes? Cancer Treat Rep 71: 795–806
32. Wittes RE (1988) From research to approved treatment: overcoming the obstacles. Semin Oncol 25: 38–42
33. Roper WL, Winkenwerder W, Hackbarth GM, Krakauer H (1988) Effectiveness in health care: an initiative to evaluate and improve medical practice. N Engl J Med 319: 1197–1202

34. Grumet GW (1989) Health care rationing through inconvenience. N Engl J Med 321: 607–611
35. Oldham R (1987) Whose life is it anyway? Wall Street J 24 April
36. Leaf A (1989) Cost effectiveness as a criterion for medicare coverage. N Engl J Med 321: 898–900
37. Jaakkimainen L, Goodwin PJ, Peter J, Warde P, Rapp E (1989) Counting the costs of chemotherapy in a randomized trial in non-small cell lung cancer. Proc Am Soc Clin Oncol 8 (Abstract 858): 221
38. Goodwin PJ, Feld R, Evans WK, Pater J (1988) Cost-effectiveness of cancer chemotherapy: an economic evaluation of a randomized trial in small-cell lung cancer. J Clin Oncol 6: 1537–1547
39. McVie JG (1988) Counting costs of care. J Clin Oncol 6: 1529–1531
40. Detsky AS (1989) Are clinical trials cost effective? JAMA 262: 1795–1800
41. Englehardt HT, Rie MA (1988) Morality for the medical–industrial complex: a code of ethics for the mass marketing of health care. N Engl J Med 319: 1086–1089
42. Boffey PM (1987) Gains against cancer since 1950 are overstated, Congress is told. New York Times 16 April: 1–2
43. Markman M (1988) An argument in support of cost-effectiveness analysis in oncology. J Clin Oncol 6: 937–939
44. Palca J (1989) Hard times at the NIH. Science 246: 988–990
45. Healy B (1988) Innovators for the 21st century: will we face a crisis in biomedical-research brainpower? N Engl J Med 319: 1058–1064

ABOUT THE AUTHOR

Karen Antman completed her medical education at Columbia University, College of Physicians and Surgeons, and did a residency in internal medicine at Columbia Presbyterian Medical Center. She then became a fellow at the Dana-Farber Cancer Institute and upon completion of her fellowship joined the faculty. Her major research interests include pharmacology of dose-intensive treatment, hematopoietic stem cells and growth factors as well as the treatment of sarcomas and mesotheliomas. She is currently an Associate Professor of Medicine at Harvard Medical School.

Section IV

TREATMENT OF PRE-MALIGNANT LESIONS AND CANCER CHEMOPREVENTION

Notes on Section IV

This section consists of three chapters devoted to the pros and cons of methods of preventing cancer developing. In Chapter 22 **Charles Hamilton** discusses a situation that has recently become topical—that of carcinoma in situ in the breast. Although not a new diagnosis we have become increasingly aware that women with an invasive intraductal carcinoma often have concurrent non-invasive intraduct carcinoma. This is often extensive in nature and there has been much debate about the most appropriate therapy. Screening programmes are also revealing more cases of this pre-malignant condition. The possible treatments—observation and treatment as required, mastectomy or radiotherapy—are all likely to be successful in the great majority of patients but each has its disadvantages. The permutations of advantages and disadvantages, both short and long term, are complicated, and sophisticated long-term trials are needed to sort out the situation. Decisions may still need to be individualized to suit the particular patients needs; the problem at present is that one cannot quantify the pluses and minuses. Hamilton is clearly unhappy with some potential dangers inherent in the use of radiation and of the emotional consequences of withholding immediate treatment and of close observation. He underlines that this condition, in screen-detected patients, is what he describes as an iatrogenic disorder—we are now contemplating radical therapy or observation bound to cause anxiety in patients who are perfectly well and who may or may *not* develop breast cancer. Though such a situation is fraught with ethical dilemmas, it seems to me that it would be reverting to an unwanted form of paternalism not to mention the situation and to ignore the disorder. If we have to take note of the diagnosis I can only see that a properly controlled trial is the best solution. Consent is a major difficulty since the balance of advantages and disadvantages is so complex. Large numbers are essential, making such a difficult study more difficult to complete successfully. The use of the pre-consent randomization technique (Chapter 14) is an interesting possibility in this situation, though it is far from clear whether the extra patients accrued would really outweigh the disadvantages of refusal of the allocated treatment.

Chapters 23 (**Alison Jones** and **Trevor Powles**) and 24 (**Richard Love**) report on the development of two important trials of tamoxifen as a chemo-prevention agent in breast cancer. Jones and Powles discuss chemoprevention in general and the design of prevention trials, with a special emphasis on the need for large numbers of subjects (even breast cancer is relatively

Introducing New Treatments for Cancer: Practical, Ethical and Legal Problems. Edited by C. J. Williams
© 1992 John Wiley & Sons Ltd

uncommon in a healthy population, 1.75 per thousand women per year).
Compliance needs to be high or even larger numbers are needed. They make
a plea for randomized trials since case–control studies can be confounded
by a variety of factors. They then discuss their own pilot study of tamoxifen
versus placebo in women with a high family risk of breast cancer. This
concentrated on examining the potential toxicities of tamoxifen and
compliance rates. So far the feared increased risk of cardiovascular disease,
osteoporosis, liver and uterine tumours has not occurred. Indeed, if anything
tamoxifen may substantially reduce the risk of cardiovascular disease. They
conclude that a large-scale study is possible and should be undertaken. The
UK Cancer Co-ordinating Committee is currently in the final stages of
designing a protocol for a placebo-controlled trial in 15 000 women at high
risk of breast cancer. This will also examine the effects of such an intervention
on other health issues such as cardiovascular disease and osteoporosis.

Love, in his chapter, also tackles similar issues, but prefers to regard the
trial he proposes as a "tamoxifen health trial" (Chapter 24), stressing the
overall effect of this intervention rather than its possible cancer prevention
effects. The Wisconsin group have also carried out an extensive pre-trial
evaluation of the known possible toxic effects of tamoxifen. They concur
that there may be protective effects which reduce the risk of coronary heart
disease. These may be as useful or more useful than the anticipated reduction
in breast cancer risk and for this reason their aim is to assess the impact
of tamoxifen on general health. They have systematically examined critical
issues in design of such a study and conclude that it is both realistic and
desirable. They estimate the cost of such preventive trials as $60–100 million,
with up to 20 000 subjects being followed for ten years. This is an enormous
sum of money and such projects will have to compete with other avenues
of research. However, in cancer, there seems little chance that current
therapies will have the sort of impact that preliminary studies of tamoxifen
as a prevention agent in breast cancer could achieve. If in consequence of
such treatment there is a similar major reduction in risk of coronary heart
disease this may turn out to be a highly cost-effective trial. The major concern
in planning such trials is the anxiety that they may cause by especially
selecting women considered to be at high risk. Against this is the increasingly
sophisticated attitude on the part of women, many of whom already
acknowledge themselves as being at high risk because of their family history.
An alternative to targeting high-risk women, with possible increased anxiety,
is to open the study to all women (a possibility discussed by Love). The
disadvantage of this is that were an unexpected series long-term side-effect
to occur this would be less offset by the lower risk of breast cancer—in
addition, the trial would need to be larger.

22 Ethical and Practical Problems in Trials Testing Treatment for Pre-malignant Conditions: Breast Cancer as a Model

CHARLES HAMILTON

In the UK approximately 24 000 new cases of breast cancer are diagnosed each year. It is the commonest cancer among women, killing 15 000 people annually. More aggressive local treatment has not improved survival, suggesting metastases occur early in the course of the illness. Recent research has led to three major advances, two of which provide a survival benefit for the patient. First was the realization that, in appropriate cases, wide local excision and radiotherapy is as good a treatment for local disease as mastectomy but which allows for breast conservation. Second was the use of adjuvant hormone or chemotherapy which acknowledges the potential for early spread of disease and treats it at a time when the tumour burden is sufficiently small and sensitive to be eradicated. Third was earlier diagnosis by screening which might allow for excision before dissemination has occurred.

In July 1985 Mr Kenneth Clark, then Minister for Health, appointed a committee under the chairmanship of Professor Sir Patrick Forrest [1] to consider the information available on breast screening and suggest a range of policy options (report of the Department of Health and Social Security). Two randomized trials indicated that women offered screening had a breast cancer mortality reduced by 30% for up to ten years and that a significant benefit persisted for at least 18 years. These data were supported by case–control studies.

The World Health Organization (WHO) principles of screening were tabled by the committee and each principle was applied in turn to breast cancer. One principle was that the chance of physical or psychological harm to the screened population should be less than the chance of benefit. Under this heading the committee cautioned "that women might undergo unnecessary procedures for the diagnosis and treatment of cancer which might not have entered an invasive phase during their lifetime". On balance the benefits of screening were considered greater than the cost and recommendations that women aged 50–64 years should have

Introducing New Treatments for Cancer: Practical, Ethical and Legal Problems. Edited by C. J. Williams
© 1992 John Wiley & Sons Ltd

three-yearly mammography were made. This resulted in a national screening programme for breast cancer.

This national screening programme for breast cancer has led to asymptomatic women with screen-detected ductal carcinoma in situ (DCIS) being referred for further management. Broders in 1932 defined carcinoma in situ as "a condition in which malignant epithelial cells and their progeny are found in or near positions occupied by their ancestors before the ancestors underwent malignant transformation". In practice, under the light microscope DCIS is carcinoma of the mammary ducts without evidence of invasion through the basement membrane into surrounding stroma.

A UK trial [2] has commenced in which patients with screen-detected DCIS that has been completely excised will be randomized into four different treatment groups. These include complete excision only, complete excision and tamoxifen, complete excision and radiotherapy and complete excision with irradiation and tamoxifen. The study design allows for evaluation of each treatment, and participating clinicians are not bound to enter patients into treatment options with which they disagree, e.g. radiotherapy or tamoxifen (Figure 1).

This trial already raises several issues:

(1) Is the natural history of screen-detected completely excised DCIS known?
(2) Does the evidence exist that tamoxifen and/or radiotherapy may be beneficial?
(3) Is there any risk associated with tamoxifen or radiotherapy?

Apart from these factual questions it has to be asked whether or not this study contravenes the Forrest report by over-treating non-invasive cancer.

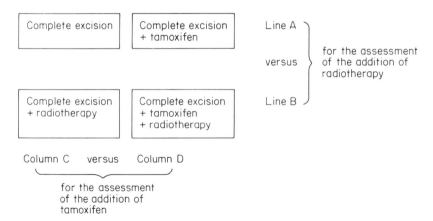

Figure 1. Trial design. Following complete excision, patients are randomized to one of four options (see boxes above). Clinicians may, if they wish, choose only to enter part of the study, e.g. avoiding all arms including radiotherapy or tamoxifen

IS THE NATURAL HISTORY OF DCIS KNOWN?

We have very little information on the natural history of screen-detected completely excised DCIS and our inferences are drawn from patients presenting with DCIS as a breast mass. Mastectomy has been the favoured approach based on the finding of a 60% incidence of residual disease and a 10–15% incidence of invasive cancer in the mastectomy specimen [3, 4]. Following radical surgery the cure rate approaches 100%.

When incomplete excision was undertaken [5] 28% of patients developed invasive cancer over a three to ten-year period. Recurrence tended to occur at the primary site and did not prejudice survival; this latter point is crucial and was the subject of a report by the American College of Surgeons [6], who found no statistical difference in survival when comparing DCIS patients managed either by mastectomy or by lesser procedures. It would appear therefore that the natural history of screen-detected DCIS is unknown but given that it has been completely excised the prognosis is probably excellent, and should the condition recur it can be safely managed at relapse—this may, however, depend on close attention to follow-up.

CAN TAMOXIFEN AND RADIOTHERAPY PREVENT RECURRENCE OF DCIS?

Since survival has been so good following a policy of initial mastectomy or mastectomy on recurrence, additional treatments are aimed at preventing recurrence and avoiding mastectomy rather than improving survival. Given that adjuvant tamoxifen reduces the risk of breast cancer occurring in the contralateral breast in patients treated for breast cancer it seems likely that this aim would be achieved. Similarly, there is evidence that radiotherapy reduces the likelihood of local recurrence of DCIS. In the National Surgical Adjuvant Breast Project (Protocol BO6), 78 cases of DCIS were identified, 51 were managed by lumpectomy with or without irradiation and 7 (14%) developed local recurrence close to the primary site [7]. Two of the 29 irradiated after local excision (7%) versus 5 out of 22 (32%) treated by lumpectomy alone recurred. Strong indirect evidence does exist that tamoxifen and irradiation may prevent DCIS progressing to invasive breast cancer.

IS THERE ANY HARM FROM RADIOTHERAPY OR TAMOXIFEN?

Following Röntgen's discovery of X-rays in 1895 they were used to treat a wide range of disorders, but as the potentially harmful late effects of irradiation became apparent so the use of ionizing radiation became restricted to the palliation of advanced malignancy and the cure of patients with potentially lethal conditions for which other treatment either did not exist or was more toxic.

This trial recommends a four to five-week course of irradiation to the breast, which will be associated with a moderate incidence of skin erythema and breast discomfort and occasional radiation pneumonitis. Much more worrying, however, are the late effects of myocardial damage and radiation-induced neoplasia which can compromise survival. There is good evidence to show that women treated with adjuvant radiotherapy after mastectomy have a survival disadvantage [8, 9] which only becomes apparent after ten years of follow-up. Figure 2 illustrates a computed tomographic scan through the central axis of a patient destined to receive radiotherapy to the left breast. A line has been drawn to connect the field edges and it is apparent that the myocardium will receive a radiation dose. This dose can be lessened by appropriate beam direction and is increased by moving the lateral border posteriorly. Not all radiotherapy centres can plan breast patients using sophisticated imaging techniques and field sizes and arrangements vary according to the practitioner. Many will try to encompass drain sites which because of their position often make the lateral border more posterior than is desirable.

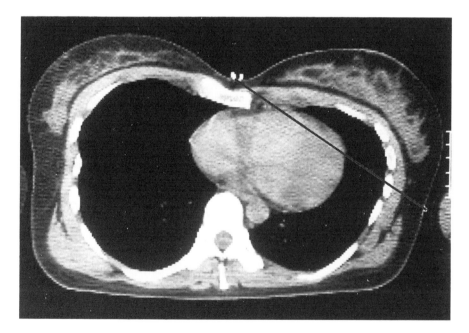

Figure 2. Scan of mid-plane section of patient destined to receive radiation to the left breast. Note how the myocardium falls into the field

Because of the good prognosis of DCIS these patients will live long enough to manifest late radiation effects. At present the evidence suggests that the risk of late effects increases with time and does not reach a plateau.

Adjuvant tamoxifen reduces the risk of death from breast cancer and its use in DCIS gives less concern than irradiation. Patients, however, have to take the medication at least for some years and a proportion will experience modest unwanted effects. In the long term endometrial carcinoma represents a theoretical concern which has not so far been a major problem. The financial cost of several years' therapy with tamoxifen in a large group of women is not insubstantial and at a personal level continued medication may maintain anxiety at an abormally high level.

In answer to the three questions posed above:

(1) The natural history of completely excised DCIS is unknown, but the prognosis is probably excellent.
(2) The evidence suggests that tamoxifen and radiotherapy either delay or prevent recurrence.
(3) Radiotherapy is associated with potentially harmful late effects.

The woman presenting for breast screening is very different from the patient with a breast lump. The former is, in my experience, an individual who expects nothing abnormal to be found and is only looking for confirmation that all is well, whereas the patient with a breast lump is extremely concerned and is seeking help. The patient with a screen-detected abnormality crosses the dividing line from non-patient to patient very quickly and frequently suffers mixed emotions. Anxiety can be kept to a minimum by good patient handling and fast referral for diagnosis. In the case of DCIS that has been excised, can one justify entering patients into any randomized study when the natural history of the disease is poorly understood and survival does not seem to be in question? It can certainly be argued that it is wrong to follow up an operation that might not even have been needed with a five-week course of radiotherapy that is potentially harmful.

This is a very new area of medicine in which practitioners have set out to improve the outlook of patients with a particular beast—breast cancer—and have brought home a different animal—DCIS. Admittedly it bears a close morphological similarity to breast cancer but its natural history is not known. Screen-detected DCIS can be regarded as an iatrogenic diagnosis and there is a risk of labelling these patients as being at risk of invasive cancer and by over-treatment inducing further iatrogenic disorders. The ethical considerations here are different from patients presenting with a known disease entity. Is it ethical to screen a population and to subject those who are found incidentally to have a benign or pre-malignant condition to a prospective randomized trial, or is this medical interference—study for the sake of study?

It could be argued that by preventing recurrence or progression of DCIS fewer out-patient attendances and fewer re-operations would be needed, leading to less anxiety and a better quality of life, but these points are not addressed in this study. What is the level of anxiety and what are the expectations of a patient attending for screening and what happens to this subsequently? We know little about these important areas.

Since informed consent is a requirement for entry into this study, surely patients will be free to choose if they enter or not. This, however, depends on whether consent can ever be truly informed. In the UK no legal precedent exists to ensure that patients receive full information about procedures they are to undergo. The amount of information given rests with the doctor and if litigation follows he is judged by the behaviour of his colleagues in similar circumstances. One can easily understand patients consenting to a study that seems likely to reduce the risk of invasive cancer, but if they were told their survival was not at risk and that recurrence if it occurred could be treated and that the radiotherapy might cause cancer and heart damage, consent would seem very much less likely.

This trial is already breaking new ground and yet it has received local ethical committee approval up and down the country. I have been unaware of any ethical committee raising the above points. In particular, no one has questioned the Forrest report comments, based on the WHO recommendations, cautioning against the over-treatment of patients who might have been found to harbour cancer never destined to be invasive during their lifetime. Similarly no one has questioned the potentially harmful effects of irradiation. Surely, the unquestioning blanket approval of this study undermines the very foundation of local ethical committees with regard to their structure and their expert guidance.

The state of the nation's health is everyone's concern. Breast cancer screening is essential; it encourages us to realize we are all human and that we too may cross the dividing line from non-patient to patient. Early diagnosis is important for most cancers and people must not be discouraged from coming forward if they have worries. This study runs the risk of jeopardizing public confidence by over-treating individuals with DCIS that has been completely excised. A simple alternative to a potentially destructive trial lies in careful documentation of individual patients and their pathology and close observation; in that way the natural history of the disorder will be learnt, high-risk groups identified and public confidence maintained.

REFERENCES

1. Breast cancer screening (1986) Chaired by Sir Patrick Forrest. DHSS. HMSO, London

2. Protocol of the randomised trial for the management of screen-detected ductal carcinoma in situ of the breast (1989). CRC Clinical Trials Centre, Rayon Institute, London
3. Rosen PP, Servie R, Schottenfield D, Ashikari R (1979) Non invasive breast cancer: frequency of unsuspected invasion and implications for treatment. Ann Surg 189: 377–382
4. Carter D, Smith RRL (1977) Carcinoma in situ of the breast. Cancer 40: 1189–1193
5. Page DL, Dupont WD, Roger L, Landenburger M (1982) Intraductal carcinoma of the breast follow up after biopsy only. Cancer 49: 731–738
6. Rosner D (1980) Non invasive breast cancer: results of a national survey by the American College of Surgeons. Ann Surg 192: 139–147
7. Fisher ER, Sass R, Fisher B, Wickerham L, Paik SM (1986) Pathologic findings from the National Surgical Adjuvant Breast Project (Protocol 6) 1. Intraduct carcinoma (DCIS). Cancer 57: 197–208
8. Cuzick J, Stewart HJ, Peto et al (1988) Overview of randomised trials of post-operative adjuvant radiotherapy in breast cancer. Recent Results Cancer Res 111: 105–129
9. Haybittle JL, Brinkley D, Houghton J, A'Hern RP, Baum M (1989) Postoperative radiotherapy and late morbidity: evidence from the Cancer Research Campaign trial for early breast cancer. Br Med J 298: 1611–1614

ABOUT THE AUTHOR

Charles Hamilton MRCP FRCR qualified from St Bartholomew's Hospital in 1977 and worked there in the Department of Medical Oncology for the Imperial Cancer Research Fund prior to entering the hospital's radiotherapy training programme. He was appointed Lecturer to the Academic Unit of Radiotherapy at the Royal Marsden Hospital in 1983, where apart from one year as Leon v Goldberg travelling fellow at the Princess Margaret Hospital, Toronto, he remained until June 1989. Since that time he has been Consultant in Radiotherapy and Oncology at the Wessex Regional Radiotherapy Centre.

His research interests have been in normal tissue damage from radiotherapy and chemotherapy and in the use of radiolabelled monoclonal antibodies. His present major areas of clinical interest are the lymphomas and breast cancer.

23 The Development of Cancer Chemoprevention Trials

ALISON L. JONES and TREVOR J. POWLES

Despite advances in therapy, the treatment of many established cancers are ineffective, and cancer remains a major cause of morbidity and mortality. Epidemiological evidence has suggested that diet and other environmental factors are important determinants of cancer and attempts at prevention of cancer have focused on elimination of suspected carcinogens. Laboratory research has increased our understanding of the biological processes underlying the development of many cancers and it may be possible to use drugs or dietary additives with anticarcinogenic activity to interrupt this process. Prospective studies using these agents will test our theories concerning carcinogenesis and are essential to assess the likely cost–benefit ratio of wide-scale chemoprevention for a given cancer.

CHEMOPREVENTIVE STRATEGIES

The chemoprevention of cancer could be achieved by limiting the exposure to an identified carcinogen or, after exposure, using positive intervention with a drug or other agent which may interrupt the process of carcinogenesis. Epidemiological data have identified environmental and dietary carcinogens, a reduction in which may affect the incidence of some cancers. A clear example of this approach is the aetiological link established between smoking and lung cancer which provides a rationale for prevention of lung cancer. This type of strategy depends on well-defined risk factors which may be identified through the use of population-based cancer registration data and is implemented through education of the population and in some cases, for example industrial carcinogens, through legislation. For dietary components, the aetiological links with individual cancers are less well established although a low-fat, high-vegetable diet may have a general protective effect against most cancers. A reduction in dietary components thought to contribute to carcinogenesis may be achievable through education of the population but the success of this approach is limited by "consumer" acceptability and hence compliance.

Positive intervention using drugs or dietary supplements may also be aimed at the general population or may be targeted against a subset of the

Introducing New Treatments for Cancer: Practical, Ethical and Legal Problems. Edited by C. J. Williams
© 1992 John Wiley & Sons Ltd

population deemed to be a higher than average risk for a specific cancer. This approach depends on sound epidemiological data concerning the aetiology of cancers, and also on laboratory research which has increased our understanding of the mechanisms involved in carcinogenesis. A number of substances which have antioxidant activity may exert a chemopreventive effect through inactivation of carcinogens. Examples include β-carotene, vitamin E and ascorbic acid, the former of which is being tested as a chemopreventive agent for lung cancer. Other candidate agents for chemoprevention may interfere with tumour growth factors or their receptors.

The process of transformation to malignancy is not a single step but rather a series of multiple stepwise changes with accumulation of chromosomal abnormalities (Figure 1). The initiating event causes an irreversible genetic change within a cell, after which there is usually a latent period before promoting events lead to progressive change into a malignant clone. Both initiation and promotion may involve exposure to carcinogens. This process may involve the generation of abnormal oncogenes or deletion of tumour suppressor genes. In theory carcinogenesis could be interrupted anywhere in this process and it is likely that substances used in chemoprevention exert an effect at more than one step.

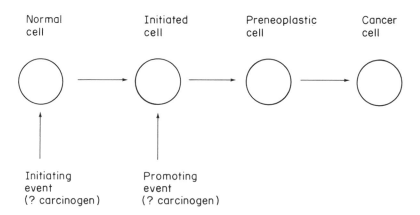

Figure 1. Process of carcinogenesis

A chemoprevention programme has been under way at the National Cancer Institute (NCI) since 1982 to develop and evaluate new agents for chemoprevention of cancer. A closely allied programme is investigating the effect of various nutrients on cancer. Many clinical trials are now in progress in the USA and in Europe which should contribute further to our understanding.

CHARACTERISTICS OF A PREVENTION TRIAL

Some chemopreventive strategies could have wide-scale application with major cost implications. Before such wide-scale use, the proposed intervention should be subject to a rigorous prospective research protocol, of similar design to protocols investigating any new treatment regimen. This includes a sound scientific basis for the intervention, use of randomization techniques with untreated control groups and careful statistical analysis. Although the general population may be the subject of such a trial, feasibility and pilot trials are best conducted on a population who are at high risk of developing the cancer concerned. This will allow design of a trial with smaller numbers of patients.

Although prevention trials have certain characteristics in common with trials comparing treatments for established disease, there are some important differences. In a prevention trial the study population will comprise healthy subjects, rather than patients in need of treatment, and consequently it is essential that the intervention used is simple and acceptable, with low subjective and objective toxicity. However, in a very high risk group some short-term side-effects may be acceptable. The appropriate age to start the intervention and the duration of treatment need to be defined. It is likely that treatment will have to be continued over a prolonged time course, maybe many years, although the optimum duration may be difficult to define at the start of the trial, as the benefit of intervention may increase with time. Unlike drug trials in established disease in which the end-points relate to remission of disease, the end objectives of an intervention trial are alterations in the incidence and natural history of the cancer concerned. These objectives may involve the use of validated screening procedures for early detection of cancer and also imply long-term follow-up to establish whether cancers in subjects receiving active intervention have different characteristics or drug sensitivity from those in the control group.

STATISTICAL CONSIDERATIONS

The number of subjects required in a prevention trial is determined by the number of cancers which are expected to develop in the untreated population. This is a function of the relative risk for the cancer concerned, the efficacy of the prevention measure, the compliance of participants and duration of follow-up. As even common cancers have a relatively low incidence (e.g. approximately 1.75 per thousand women per year for breast cancer), the size of the study population is likely to be large, involving thousands of subjects, but the number may be reduced by initially restricting the trial to a high-risk group.

If the level of compliance is low, then the number of participants in the study population has to be increased. It is possible to assess the level of compliance objectively for some chemopreventive interventions in pilot studies by monitoring drug levels in blood or urine in the study population. This could be carried out intermittently over a protracted period to monitor long-term compliance. A "run-in" period before randomization when both groups receive placebo may be useful to eliminate likely non-compliers who opt to drop out of the study and thereby strengthen statistical analysis, although this approach may give a falsely high estimate of compliance from pilot studies which would not be maintained in a larger trial. It is therefore important to have an acceptable and convenient programme to encourage compliance from pilot studies, and an analysis of expected compliance may give an estimate of the numbers of subjects required.

Increasing public awareness of risk factors for different cancers may cause the study population to modify their lifestyle, for example in terms of diet and smoking, thereby altering their relative risk. This can make analysis of a prevention study difficult and emphasizes the need for a control group. Another potential problem could occur if the subjects randomized to the control population can easily distinguish treatment from placebo and demand active intervention.

The study may be simple, consisting of a treatment group versus a control placebo group or employ a factorial design (Figure 2) which allows the testing of more than one hypothesis in the study. A combination of intervention is usually possible because of the low individual toxicities of the treatments used, but the number of agents in a factorial study may be limited by the logistic problems of managing the study. With a factorial design there may also be interactions between the different treatments and this has to be taken into account in the statistical analysis.

Breast cancer provides a model of a tumour type for which chemoprevention may be possible and appropriate. In this chapter we will discuss the scientific and statistical basis for the prevention of breast cancer, the possible approaches and the ethical and practical difficulties of introducing prophylactic treatment to normal healthy women with particular reference to a feasibility and pilot trial at present under way at the Royal Marsden Hospital, London.

		Treatment A	
		Yes	No
Treatment B	Yes	1	2
	No	3	4

Figure 2. Example of a 2×2 factorial design: 1=treatment A+treatment B; 2=treatment B only; 3=treatment A only; 4=placebo

PREVENTION OF BREAST CANCER

POPULATION AT RISK

There is a one in fourteen life-time risk of developing breast cancer for women in the UK. The incidence of the disease rises with age between 30 and 60 years and breast cancer is the most common single cause of death in women aged 35–54 years. As discussed, the introduction of a prophylactic measure should initially be conducted in a clinical trial setting to assess feasibility and potential toxicity. The selection of a high-risk group allows the trial to be smaller as a relatively high proportion of the women concerned would develop cancer. For breast cancer a number of well-defined risk factors have been identified allowing such selection (Table 1).

A positive family history of breast cancer on the maternal side is a well-defined risk factor. With one first-degree relative affected the relative risk of developing the disease is twofold. With two first-degree relatives the relative risk is increased to about four. The relative risk is further increased if the relative concerned had bilateral breast cancer (about fivefold) or if diagnosis was made when aged less than 40 years (about threefold). The increased risk incurred by a positive family history of breast cancer may be further increased by the presence of other known risk factors. These include nulliparity or late age at first childbirth although the relative risk for nulliparity or age greater than 30 years at first childbirth is only about 1.5. There is also an association between breast cancer and early menarche with rapid onset of ovulatory cycles, and late menopause and obesity in

Table 1. Agents under investigation for chemoprevention and target cancers

Agent	Target cancer for chemoprevention
Tamoxifen	Breast cancer in high-risk women
Vitamin A and retinoids (13-*cis*-retinoic acid: isotretinoin)	Recurrent basal cell carcinoma Second primary breast cancer Skin cancer (in genetically predisposed individuals) Recurrent head and neck cancer Recurrent lung cancer Lung cancer (in smokers)
β-Carotene	Lung cancer (in smokers) Recurrent basal cell carcinoma Recurrent colonic adenomas
ω-3 Fatty acids	Breast cancer
N-Acetyl cysteine	Recurrent head and neck cancer Recurrent lung cancer

post-menopausal women. These factors emphasize the likely importance of ovarian function, especially prolonged exposure to oestrogens, in the promotion of breast cancer.

An association has been recognized between benign breast disease and breast cancer, although variation in the types of benign breast disease makes assignment of risks difficult. A clinical syndrome of benign mammary dysplasia with tender, painful nodularity, especially in the upper outer quadrant of the breast, either unilaterally or bilaterally with pre-menstrual accentuation of symptoms, occurs in approximately 10–15% of women mainly from age 35 years to the menopause. This is 10–15 years before the peak age incidence curve for carcinoma of the breast. This benign syndrome may be related to relatively low pre-menstrual (luteal phase) progesterone levels allowing unopposed excessive oestrogenic activity on the breast, and such oestrogenic activity may be important in the initiation or promotion of breast cancer. Such luteal phase insufficiency may also account for the association of breast cancer with anovular cycles and infertility.

Histologically, certain subtypes of benign breast disease, in particular atypical epithelial hyperplasia and lobular hyperplasia, have been associated with an increased risk of breast cancer. The overall relative risk of breast cancer for women who have had a biopsy for benign breast disease is about twofold for women who have undergone a biopsy, with increase to a relative risk of about four in the subgroup with atypical hyperplasia. Another relatively rare variant non-invasive type of breast disease, lobular carcinoma in situ (LCIS), carries a one in three risk of subsequent development of infiltrating carcinoma. On mammography, radiological grading can identify two categories, dysplasia (DY) and prominent-duct (P2), which are associated with an increased relative risk of about 1.5 of breast cancer.

Despite the number of risk factors, a family history of breast cancer is the most consistent and easy to define. Although the relative risk with one family member is low (twofold), about 10% of all women over 50 years old have a family history, providing a large target population for prophylaxis.

SCIENTIFIC BASIS

The role of biologically active oestrogens in the aetiology of breast cancer in humans can be inferred from epidemiological data and has been established experimentally in laboratory animals. Intact ovarian function is necessary for the development of carcinogen-induced mouse mammary tumours. Such tumours can be induced by the hormone oestradiol, and prevented by ovariectomy or anti-oestrogen treatment. These data together with epidemiological data have resulted in proposals for the chemoprevention of breast cancer by the reduction of circulating oestrogen levels.

The association of early menarche, late menopause and nulliparity with increased risk of breast cancer support the hypothesis that intact ovarian function is necessary to promote breast cancers. Following the nuclear explosions in Japan in 1945, the individual radiation dose for all members of the population could be determined and subsequent epidemiological data indicate that intact ovarian function is required in order to develop radiation-induced cancers. Women who were post-menopausal at the time of radiation have not shown an increased incidence of breast cancer. Women aged 10–39 years old at the time of radiation showed an increased incidence of breast cancer after 1958, i.e. 14 years later, and this trend continues. The increase in breast cancer in women who were pre-pubertal (under 10 years old) at the time of radiation did not occur until 1965. This seven-year delay indicates that the development of ovarian function with puberty was required for the promotion of cancer. The requirement of intact ovarian function in the promotion of breast cancer is also indicated by the observation of a reduction, of about 75%, in the incidence of breast cancer in women who have undergone an early menopause. This reduction in risk is directly related to age at the time of menopause.

Although this evidence suggests that intact ovarian function is important in promotion of breast cancer, the investigation of circulating oestrogen levels in women has yielded inconclusive results. This is in part related to the cyclical variability of oestrogen levels in pre-menopausal women, and to the low levels found post-menopausally which, until recently, were at the lower limits of assay sensitivity. The percentage of free oestradiol, i.e. biologically active hormone, may be a more reliable marker than the total levels of protein-bound hormones. Most circulating oestrogen is bound to sex-hormone-binding globulin (SHBG) and the levels of SHBG are inversely correlated with breast cancer, perhaps reflecting increased free levels of oestrogen.

Anti-oestrogenic manoeuvres are effective in some patients with advanced breast cancer. For example, in pre-menopausal women oophorectomy or radiation-induced menopause results in remission in about 30% of patients. In post-menopausal women the anti-oestrogen tamoxifen and other drugs such as aminoglutethimide and 4-hydroxyandrostenedione which inhibit oestrogen synthesis may cause regression of metastatic breast cancer.

This evidence would suggest that anti-oestrogenic manoeuvres may therefore be effective in the prevention of breast cancer. It is unlikely that further epidemiological studies will clarify the hypothesis that oestrogen is involved in the endocrine promotion of breast cancer. Further progress probably now depends on well-designed endocrine prevention trials using an anti-oestrogenic intervention.

POSSIBLE PROPHYLACTIC INTERVENTIONS

Tamoxifen

The anti-oestrogenic drug tamoxifen is cytostatic to breast cancer cells in vitro and prevents the development of mammary tumours in mice.

Approximately 30–60% of patients with metastatic breast cancer respond to tamoxifen treatment and in primary breast cancer the use of tamoxifen as adjuvant therapy prolongs the disease-free interval and may affect overall survival. Patient acceptability is high, with only 4% of patients who received tamoxifen discontinuing the drug. The main symptomatic problems are nausea, vasomotor instability with hot flushes, minor weight gain, vaginal mucosal changes, headaches and depression. However, most of these side-effects, apart from hot flushes, occur at a similar frequency in the control groups receiving placebo.

Although short-term side-effects are minimal, the possibility of long-term toxicity is particularly important if the drug is to be used in well women. Effects on coagulation, bone density, lipid metabolism and possible carcinogenesis merit particular consideration. Tamoxifen has partial oestrogen agonist activity and, in patients with advanced breast cancer, may be associated with an increase in arterial and venous thrombosis. However, this may be related to the disease status itself or to concomitant chemotherapy, as an increased incidence of thromboembolism has not been seen with tamoxifen used as single-agent therapy compared with placebo. In contrast, in post-menopausal women with breast cancer treated with tamoxifen both total and low-density lipoprotein cholesterol were reduced. This reduction may have a beneficial effect against coronary heart disease but this would need to be confirmed by prospective cardiac trials.

Unopposed oestrogen is an aetiological factor for carcinoma of the endometrium and hence the partial agonist activity of tamoxifen could represent a theoretical problem for women who had not had a hysterectomy. There are some experimental data in rodents to support this but the data for tamoxifen in relation to endometrial cancer in women are inconclusive. A Scottish trial, with tamoxifen 20 mg daily as adjuvant therapy in breast cancer, did not show any increase in endometrial cancer after four to ten years follow-up, although a Swedish study, using a higher dose of 40 mg daily, demonstrated an increase in endometrial cancer in the treated group (1.4%) compared with controls (0.2%) after a median follow-up of 4.5 years. This could be a dose-dependent effect of tamoxifen and would need to be monitored in a prevention trial.

There has also been concern about the risk of accelerated bone loss and osteoporosis in women taking tamoxifen if the anti-oestrogenic activity was predominant. However, studies of adjuvant tamoxifen in both pre- and post-menopausal women have failed to show any significant loss in bone mass. Indeed, in one study, a (non-significant) gain in bone density has been reported in patients on tamoxifen. These studies investigating bone mass and tamoxifen are small and mainly retrospective with short follow-up periods, so the question of bone density changes with long-term therapy remains unresolved.

For pre-menopausal women there are other areas for concern, especially as the potential risk of teratogenicity by tamoxifen has not been adequately tested in animals. There are, however, 85 normal babies recorded for women who received tamoxifen during pregnancy, with no reports of fetal abnormalities in many thousands of other women at risk. However, if the drug is to be used in pre-menopausal women the importance of adequate contraception should be stressed.

Studies on the development of breast cancer in women taking the contraceptive pill show conflicting results, although there may be an increased risk in younger women with prolonged use of a high-oestrogen pill. The risk for low-oestrogen pills has not been established although this may reflect a relatively short period of follow-up for the women concerned and such a risk may become apparent with prolonged follow-up. Progestogen-only pills may have a protective effect, which raises the possibility of developing a progestogen-based oral contraceptive which also has a prophylactic effect against breast cancer. A prototype agent is gestodene, a synthetic progestogen, which displaces oestradiol binding in malignant breast tissue, although further research is necessary to define its activity in breast cancer, as the evidence for progestins having a potential prophylactic role is controversial.

Ablation of ovarian function by surgery or radiotherapy might be effective as chemoprevention but would neither be practical nor acceptable on a large scale. However, the endocrine ablation of ovarian function using a luteinizing hormone releasing hormone agonist may be a treatment possibility, especially if combined with selective replacement of oestrogen and progestin. This would be a complex and costly approach and the long-term toxicity of the different components is difficult to predict.

Overall, tamoxifen would appear to offer a simple, cheap and acceptable agent for the prophylaxis of breast cancer. It has proven antiproliferative activity on established breast cancer and its use in patients indicates that compliance is likely to be high. However, both short and long-term toxicity would require careful monitoring in a prospective trial before widespread use could be recommended.

Diet

Data from animal experiments have shown increased tumour growth in chemically induced mammary tumours in association with a high-fat diet. This increase is probably related to the high fatty acid composition rather than total fat content. Both ovarian-dependent and independent animal mammary tumours are promoted by a high-fat diet, which would indicate that tumour growth stimulated by fatty acids is independent of ovarian oestrogen synthesis.

The correlation between average per capita fat consumption and breast cancer incidence in different countries, and migrant data between countries, also support the influence of environmental factors. In contrast most studies investigating the influence of reduced dietary fat on breast cancer incidence have been inconclusive, with only a weak correlation if any. Dietary fat content can be difficult to assess and the quantitative reduction in fat intake required to alter the incidence of breast cancer is uncertain.

It has been estimated that 40% of circulating oestrogens may be of dietary origin. The major source is from dairy produce, with subsequent synthesis of oestrogens from cholesterol and bile acids, by bacteria present in the gastrointestinal flora. In clinical studies, reduction of fat intake from an average diet with 40% of the calories coming from fat, to a low-fat diet (20% of calories from fat), resulted in lowering of luteal phase oestrogens and a decrease in the percentage of free oestradiol. This decrease may be partly related to the increase in SHBG which has been observed in patients on a low-fat diet.

The available evidence suggests that reduction in dietary fat may be a possible area to explore in the prevention of breast cancer. However, migrant studies suggest that fat restriction would be necessary from a very young age and this implies long-term trials. The percentage reduction in fat intake required is unknown but would probably involve major dietary restriction and consequently little hope of long-term compliance.

An alternative method of dietary intervention could be by the administration of essential fatty acids which in vitro has shown inhibition of breast cancer cell lines; omega-3 fatty acids are non-toxic and early results show and cause a reduction in the production of 16α-hydroxysterone, an experimental promoter of breast cancer. A double-blind controlled trial is now under way at the Memorial Sloane-Kettering Center in the USA, designed to evaluate this agent.

Intracellular processes which generate toxic lipid peroxides through free radical formation may cause genetic damage. Antioxidants such as vitamin C and E, β-carotene and the trace elements selenium and copper may have a protective effect. These elements can be measured in blood and tissue samples, but to date there are little data to suggest a role for them in the prevention of breast cancer.

Retinoids

Retinoids are derivatives or synthetic analogues of vitamin A and its isomers. They have been shown to halt differentiation and inhibit malignant transformation in a variety of tumour types, including breast cancer, in vitro and also xerografts in experimental animals. Retinoids are of particular interest as they may halt malignant transformation in cells which have already undergone a degree of de-differentiation to the malignant phenotype. Their activity may be mediated through inhibition of enzymes involved in tumour protein synthesis, or through an increase in activity of endogenous growth inhibitory polypeptides such as transforming growth factor beta (TGFβ). A number of synthetic retinoids have been developed and are generally well tolerated. Their activity in the adjuvant treatment of patients with breast cancer is under exploration and they are also candidate agents for a prevention study.

RECRUITMENT

Before any prophylactic measure is adopted on a wide scale it is essential to conduct prospective clinical trials to test the hypothesis. The overall risk of breast cancer is approximately 1.75 per thousand women per year, but in women aged 50–60 with a family history of breast cancer the risk is increased to 5–6 per thousand per year. In a control group of 5000 of these high-risk women, approximately 250–300 cancers would be expected over a ten-year period. This number would be sufficient to detect a reduction in incidence of 25% with a 95% probability of being correct. However, if compliance is poor then an increased number of patients would be necessary. This emphasizes the need for a simple, inexpensive, well-tolerated method of intervention in a high-risk group. Using a combination of risk factors it is possible to define groups of women with relative risks of up to 11 although this group would represent a very small percentage of the population and would be difficult to identify. A more realistic aim is to select women with an easily defined risk factor such as family history. Although this alone only gives an increased risk of about twofold, the risk would be increased by the presence of a further factor such as symptomatic benign breast disease or nulliparity (Table 2). An estimated 5–10% of the female population aged 50–60 would be eligible using these criteria. Volunteers may be found in the screening clinics which have been set up for women aged over 50 years or from breast clinics amongst women presenting with benign breast disease.

In practice increasing awareness of risk factors, in particular family history, has resulted in many women requesting referral to specialist breast clinics for this reason. Although a feasibility and pilot trial has been started at the

Table 2. Risk factors for breast cancer

Risk factor	Relative risk
First-degree relative (maternal) with breast cancer	2
First-degree relative diagnosed <40 years	3
Two first-degree relatives	4
First-degree relative with bilateral breast cancer	4
Nulliparity/first child at >30 years	1.5
Benign breast disease (biopsied)	2
Atypical hyperplasia	4
Mammographic change (dysplasia/prominent ducts)	1.5
Lobular carcinoma in situ	10

Royal Marsden Hospital, it is likely that a larger multicentre study will be required in order to detect a reduction in incidence of breast cancer of 25% or less. The risk factors required for inclusion in a multicentre trial may vary between centres but should give a relative risk of about three.

FEASIBILITY AND PILOT TRIAL OF TAMOXIFEN

STUDY DESIGN

We have conducted a double-blind placebo-controlled feasibility trial at the Royal Marsden Hospital with 200 women in order to assess the logistics and ethical problems of using tamoxifen in high-risk women for the prophylaxis of breast cancer. Patients between 35 and 65 with at least one first-degree relative with breast cancer were included. The placebo arm was considered essential in a feasibility study in order to define acute and chronic toxicity. Many patients had symptomatic benign breast disease but none was at risk of pregnancy. Patients were psychologically, physically and geographically suitable for long-term follow-up.

The ethical problems posed by any chemoprevention trial are different from those posed by chemotherapy trials in patients with disease. The trial involves a large number of healthy women of whom only a small number can gain potential benefit but for all of whom there is unknown long-term toxicity, however rare. The tamoxifen prevention trial took a year to pass through the Royal Marsden Hospital Ethics Committee and was also subject to approval through family practitioner presentation, the British Breast Group and the UK Clinical Trial Co-ordinating Committee before starting the trial. The women recruited were subject to written and witnessed informed consent. The information given to these women included the rate toxicity data relating to the theoretical possibility of hepatocellular carcinoma, but this information did not affect accrual adversely.

Eligible women were told that this was an experimental trial and were offered regular follow-up and screening. Participation was based on fully informed, written and witnessed consent. Patients were aware that they could withdraw from the trial at any time for any reason. After clinical examination and mammography to exclude breast cancer patients were prescribed "tamoplac" and were randomized to receive tamoxifen 20 mg/day or placebo for two years. Various parameters including acute toxicity, acceptability and compliance were monitored. In addition serum lipids and lipoproteins, the coagulation factors fibrinogen and antithrombin III, oestradiol and SHBG, bone density (using a single-photon absorption bone densitometer) and pelvic ultrasounds were monitored serially. Patients had regular clinical follow-up and annual mammography. Surgical or other intervention were readily available if required. From two breast clinics we were able to identify about seven eligible women per week and after full discussion approximately 50% of these women consented to randomization into the trial. From October 1986, 124 patients were randomized until July 1987, when accrual was temporarily suspended following the release of rat toxicity data which indicated hepatocellular carcinoma in rats fed tamoxifen at 50–100 times the dosage used in women. Hepatocellular carcinoma has not been reported in patients on tamoxifen and after review of the data regarding the use of tamoxifen in benign conductions, the ethical committee allowed continuation of the study subject to rewriting of the protocol and consent forms. Accrual therefore continued until the total of 200 women had been reached for this feasibility trial.

INTERIM RESULTS

Generally there was little difference in acute toxicity between the tamoxifen and placebo groups. Hot flushes did occur in significantly more women on tamoxifen ($p < 0.005$) but were generally mild. There were no significant differences in nausea, headaches, weight gain, depression or menstrual changes including amenorrhoea between the two groups. Compliance after one year was high (greater than 80%) for both groups and reflects the relatively low toxicity for tamoxifen versus placebo. This may approach the maximum achievable compliance with any endocrine intervention.

Identification of any long-term toxicity will require longer follow-up. However, no adverse effects on coagulation (fibrinogen/antithrombin III ratio) and lipid profiles have yet been detected. In our study total cholesterol and low-density lipoprotein cholesterol were significantly lowered in both pre- and post-menopausal women. Apolipoprotein B was also lowered but only in post-menopausal women. The reduction in cholesterol represented a fall of 15% of pretreatment values and the reduction was most marked in women with high pretreatment values (> 6.5 mmol/l). These changes are compatible with oestrogen agonist activity of tamoxifen and are similar to those seen in women taking oral contraceptives or oestrogen replacement therapy. Any beneficial effect that these changes may have on the incidence of coronary artery or cerebrovascular disease is difficult to predict at this time, although in two large adjuvant tamoxifen trials the incidence of non-cancer deaths is lower in the tamoxifen versus the control arms. Serial external pelvic ultrasound examination has failed to detect any adverse ovarian or uterine changes and there is no evidence of accelerated loss of bone mass at this early stage in follow-up. To date no breast cancers have occurred in either group.

This study has suggested that a prevention trial using tamoxifen is feasible and safe, with an adequate level of compliance. Our feasibility study has now extended to a pilot trial with ethical approval for up to 1000 women taking tamoxifen or placebo for up to 5 years; continued surveillance of potential short and long term toxicity is essential. To date we have accrued over 400 women and with the present rate of recruitment we should achieve our planned accrual within the next two to three years. This trial alone would be sufficient to detect a 75% prevention within a mean follow-up time of five years. Smaller effects will require larger numbers with longer follow-up. For a larger trial identification of high-risk women could be achieved through the national screening programme and from assessment and symptomatic breast clinics. The potential workload and staffing for a larger trial of about 10 000 women is considerable although the actual cost of tamoxifen is relatively low (approximately £30 per woman per year of treatment).

FURTHER CONSIDERATIONS FOR A LARGER TRIAL

The encouraging data from our feasibility and pilot trial suggest that a large prevention trial is possible and that about 10 000 women would be required in order to detect a 25% prevention effect. There are other issues to consider in the design of a large trial. Screening may alter the stage at which breast cancer is detected and hence may alter the incidence and natural history of invasive cancer. Similarly, awareness of breast cancer may modify the behaviour of women in terms of diet and self-examination. These factors may also affect the incidence of cancers and make the use of a control group in a prospective trial essential. Another potential problem is non-compliance, which dictates the sample size. In our pilot study the compliance was high (approximately 80% at 12 months) and we estimate that it should remain above 50% at five years for a larger trial. This high level of compliance probably reflects several features, including the motivation of high-risk women, the regular contact with a doctor and screening service offered including ovarian ultrasound and bone density measurement. Although this additional monitoring (other than mammographic) has been important in a feasibility study, the cost implications of this for a larger programme are considerable and it remains to be seen if the level of compliance falls without these additional incentives. The optimum duration of therapy remains uncertain. Data from adjuvant trials suggest that longer treatment periods are associated with greater benefit in terms of the reduction in the development of contralateral disease and other recurrent disease. It is likely that a ten-year treatment period may be necessary in a prevention trial. This necessitates continued monitoring of toxicity as most of the data so far on tamoxifen reflects relatively short periods of treatment. Further data from long-term adjuvant trials may give some indication of late problems with prolonged hormone treatment.

Many post-menopausal women request or require hormone replacement therapy (HRT). The effect of HRT on the incidence of breast cancer is unclear although it seems likely that the use of natural as opposed to synthetic oestrogens with a progestin is not associated with increased risk. Unfortunately, in spite of the huge number of women who have had HRT, no prospective studies similar to those planned for tamoxifen have been conducted to assess the benefits and toxicity of such treatment. The possibility of using tamoxifen in combination with HRT in women who are at increased risk of breast cancer and have menopausal symptoms requiring intervention remains to be explored.

The question of prevention in pre-menopausal women has yet to be resolved. Although tamoxifen may be suitable for older women who have completed a family it is probably not appropriate for younger women at pregnancy risk. The design of oral contraceptives with the additional benefit of breast cancer prevention may be of interest. This aim and that of "designer" HRT with a prophylactic benefit stress the fact that we must consider breast prophylaxis in the context of the general health and well-being of the patients concerned.

CHEMOPREVENTION IN OTHER CANCERS

Epidemiological research suggests that various components of diet are associated with increased incidence of all or specific cancers. This has encouraged attention on dietary intervention as a means of cancer chemo-prevention. However, the identification of specific dietary carcinogens is difficult and dietary regimens involving elimination of individual components are difficult to control and maintain in prospective controlled trials. Hence the focus of attention has shifted to prevention studies using dietary factors which may have inhibitory effects on carcinogenesis.

The possible use of retinoids in the chemoprevention of breast cancer has already been discussed and synthetic analogues with greater potency and less toxicity than the parent compound are under investigation as preventative agents for several different cancers (Table 1). Unless there is a genetic predisposition towards, or histological change associated with, a specific cancer, the identification of high-risk groups can be difficult and very large numbers of patients would be necessary to detect a change in cancer incidence. To circumvent this problem some trials have concentrated on prevention of second cancers (of the same histological type) in a population who have already been treated for cancer and are therefore at high risk of a second primary. An example of this approach is a study of the synthetic retinoid isotretinoin, which is being used at low dosage for the chemo-prevention of basal cell carcinomas (BCC) in patients who have previously had two or more BCC. Similarly a variety of drugs including piroxicam (a prostaglandin synthetase inhibitor), β-carotene, and vitamins C and E are being investigated for prevention of further colon adenomas in patients who have already been treated for one or more adenomas.

CONCLUSION

The possibility of the prevention of various cancers has existed since epidemiologists established aetiological links between environmental and/or dietary factors and cancers. The maintenance of accurate national cancer registration is a prerequisite for this information and forms the basis for many studies. Although education of the population about avoidance of carcinogens and, in some cases, legislation to limit exposure to carcinogens may have an impact on the incidence of specific cancers, such elimination of carcinogens is not always feasible and controlled studies to assess the impact are difficult to maintain.

The rapid advances in molecular biology over the last decade have allowed some understanding of the biological processes underlying carcinogenesis. This knowledge complements our understanding of established disease and may allow the use of drugs earlier to interrupt the process of carcinogenesis. Long-term follow-up in chemoprevention trials allows testing of our theories regarding the aetiology and pathogenesis of cancer. Chemoprevention, if applied to a large section of the population, could have major cost implications but this has to be set against the morbidity of, and lack of effective treatment for, many cancers, together with the high cost of treatment for established disease. Large prevention trials pose many logistic, statistical and ethical problems, most of which can only be answered by carefully designed prospective feasibility and pilot trials.

Breast cancer provides a model of a common tumour for which chemo-prevention may be possible. An initial pilot trial has been encouraging in terms of accrual, compliance and toxicity and has now provided the basis for the establishment of a large multicentre trial to detect whether breast cancer can be prevented or delayed by giving tamoxifen to well women.

FURTHER READING

Byar DP, Piantodosi S (1985) Factorial designs for randomised clinical trials. Cancer Treat Rep 69: 1055

Cancer Statistic Registration, England and Wales (1984) Series MBI, 16. HMSO, London

Cuzick J, Wang DY, Bulbrook RD (1986) The prevention of breast cancer. Lancet i: 83

Greenwald P, Nixon DW, Malone WF, Kelloff GT, Stern HR, Witkin KM (1990) Concepts in cancer chemoprevention research. Cancer 65: 1483

Key TJA, Pike MC (1988) The role of oestrogens and progestogens in the epidemiology and prevention of breast cancer. Eur J Cancer Clin Oncol 24: 29

Love RR (1989) Tamoxifen therapy in primary breast cancer: biology, efficacy and side-effects. J Clin Oncol 7: 803

Millar AB, Bulbrook RD (1980) The epidemiology and etiology of breast cancer. N Engl J Med 303: 1246

Pike MC, Krailo MD, Henderson BE et al (1983) "Hormonal" risk factors, "breast tissue age" and the age-incidence of breast cancer. Nature 303: 767

Powles TJ, Hardy JR, Ashley SE et al (1989) A pilot trial to evaluate toxicity and feasibility of tamoxifen for prevention of breast cancer. Br J Cancer 60: 126

Powles TJ, Tillyer CJ, Jones AL et al (1990) Prevention of breast cancer with tamoxifen: an update of the Royal Marsden Hospital pilot programme. Eur J Cancer 26: 680–689

Sporn MB, Roberts AB (1983) Role of retinoids in differentiation and carcinogenesis. Cancer Res 43: 3034

Tokunaga M, Land CE, Tamamolo T et al (1959) Breast cancer among atomic bomb survivors. In: Boice JD, Fasmeni JF (eds) Radiation carcinogenesis: epidemiology and biological significance. Raven Press, New York

ABOUT THE AUTHORS

Dr Alison L. Jones is a Senior Registrar and Honorary Lecturer on the medical rotation at the Royal Marsden Hospital, London. She has worked closely with Dr T. Powles on his prevention programme.

Dr Trevor J. Powles is a Consultant Medical Oncologist at the Royal Marsden Hospital and Honorary Senior Lecturer at the Institute of Cancer Research, London. He has an interest in all aspects of the medical management of breast cancer and a particular interest in patients with early disease. He has initiated a feasibility and pilot trial on the use of tamoxifen in the chemo-prevention of breast cancer in patients at high risk of developing the disease and the data from this have provided the impetus for a national trial.

24 Issues in the Design of a Tamoxifen Health Trial

RICHARD R. LOVE

In the USA the incidence of breast cancer has increased at rates of 1–2% annually over the last decade during which reliable data have been available. Much of these increases may be due to increased screening with mammography. With these incidence increases, because of aging of the American population, and because of modest treatment success with early-stage disease, the prevalence and visibility of breast cancer have also increased. Despite associated greater concern about breast cancer and considerable study of its etiology, both non-modifiable and especially modifiable causes are not well understood or known. A central role of estrogen in disease development, however, is widely accepted, and thus the general proposition that an "anti-estrogenic" intervention might be successful in suppressing pre-clinical breast cancer enjoys support. Recent data from breast cancer clinical trials employing as adjuvant therapy the longest-used anti-estrogen tamoxifen citrate, combined with rigorous data on other biological effects, have encouraged proposals to evaluate tamoxifen's ability to prevent the appearance of clinical breast cancer [1, 2]. In the USA because of the potential of tamoxifen to favorably affect coronary heart disease, bone disease and overall mortality end-points, in addition to breast cancer incidence, in a proposed clinical "prevention" trial, such an endeavor has been called a tamoxifen health trial (THT). In this article, after a brief review of the biological rationale for such a trial, some detailed consideration of practical, logistic and ethical issues in the design and conduct of this trial will be explored.

THE BIOLOGICAL RATIONALE FOR A TAMOXIFEN HEALTH TRIAL

BREAST CANCER EFFECTS OF TAMOXIFEN

Tamoxifen citrate is a synthetic anti-estrogen with antitumor properties in laboratory animals. Tamoxifen is believed to act primarily by binding to the estrogen receptor in breast cancer cells [3]. This binding appears to prevent estrogen-stimulated cell division and block breast cancer cells

Introducing New Treatments for Cancer: Practical, Ethical and Legal Problems. Edited by C. J. Williams
© 1992 John Wiley & Sons Ltd

at the G1 phase of the cell cycle, possibly modulating stimulatory and inhibitory growth factors. There is excellent evidence from rodent models that long-term tamoxifen can suppress mammary carcinogenesis [4–7].

In treatment of women with primary breast cancer, where tamoxifen is given as adjuvant therapy, when the primary breast tumor exhibits measurable levels of estrogen receptor and/or progesterone receptor protein, prolongation of the disease-free survival is usually seen. In some studies prolongation of overall survival has been seen, and an overview analysis has concluded that tamoxifen does confer survival benefit in post-menopausal node-positive patients. Further, there is a suggestion that when the body burden of tumor cells is smallest, the use of tamoxifen results in approximately a halving of the recurrence rates. The absence of survival benefits from adjuvant tamoxifen in many individual studies may be because only short-term therapy (one to three years) was administered.

The majority of breast cancers in post-menopausal women are estrogen receptor positive at the time of diagnosis. The major tumor-suppressing effect of tamoxifen in rodent cancer model systems compared to its more modest effects in controlling or suppressing established clinical breast cancers in women has suggested a hypothesis about the development of breast malignancies. Breast tumors may begin as clones of estrogen receptor positive cells, which in the course of replication produce estrogen receptor negative daughter cells. If estrogen is required for these cell divisions, then application of tamoxifen earlier in the natural history of the development of these clones, prior to usual clinical detection, might be expected to have a greater impact on tumor appearance than on the suppression of growth of established clones of estrogen receptor positive and negative cells.

The rates of second primary breast cancers in adjuvant tamoxifen treatment trials have supported the prediction that tamoxifen can effectively suppress pre-clinical breast cancer. Overall in four trials the rates of second primary or contralateral breast cancers have been approximately half of those seen in the control or placebo groups [8]. To date the impact of tamoxifen therapy in women with histological evidence of "pre-malignancy" (e.g. atypical epithelial hyperplasia) has not been evaluated because of significant logistical barriers.

The effects of tamoxifen on hormone levels in pre-menopausal women are less completely understood and possibly unfavorable, and in these women the biological effects and detailed symptomatic effects have received only limited investigation. The majority of pre-menopausal women continue to have menses during tamoxifen therapy. Those with ovulatory cycles are clearly at risk for pregnancy. However, tamoxifen should not be administered during pregnancy to avoid the possibility of teratogenesis (although this effect has not been documented). Thus, the current considerations for a prevention trial concern only post-menopausal women.

CARDIOVASCULAR EFFECTS OF TAMOXIFEN

In Western countries, mortality from myocardial infarction in women begins to exceed that from breast cancer in the sixth decade of life and thereafter the mortality rates rise very rapidly. Tamoxifen has significant effects on established risk factors for coronary heart disease (CHD) and stroke.

Total cholesterol and low-density lipoprotein (LDL) cholesterol levels are lowered by tamoxifen treatment. In the Wisconsin Tamoxifen Study, a randomized placebo-controlled, double-blind toxicity trial, total cholesterol was lowered by 26 mg/dl (12%, $p=0.0001$) from 216 mg/dl at baseline to 190 mg/dl at three months [9]. LDL cholesterol was lowered by 20% ($p=0.0001$) from 138 mg/dl at baseline to 110 mg/dl at follow-up. These changes were sustained at these levels through two years of treatment. Minor increases in triglycerides and decreases in HDL cholesterol were seen, each of borderline or no statistical significance depending on the time-point. The total cholesterol and the high-density lipoprotein (HDL)/LDL cholesterol ratios in tamoxifen-treated subjects in this study were statistically improved at all study time-points.

Other studies show similar findings with respect to lowering of LDL and total cholesterol by tamoxifen. No certain picture of tamoxifen's effects of HDL cholesterol has emerged.

In the Wisconsin Tamoxifen Study, with tamoxifen treatment fibrinogen levels were found to decrease from a baseline of 320 mg/dl to 268 mg/dl at six months (-52 mg/dl, $p=0.0003$).

In the Wisconsin Tamoxifen Study, evaluations of systolic and diastolic blood pressure changes over one year showed no differences and no differences in weight, or reported exercise, work activity, smoking habits or fasting glucose levels, developed between the two groups.

The impact these lipid and fibrinogen changes might have on rates of CHD in post-menopausal women is uncertain but likely favorable. Triglyceride levels are not considered to be a major independent risk factor for cardio-vascular disease. Population studies have demonstrated a relationship between fibrinogen levels, myocardial infarction and stroke, with lower levels associated with lower cardiovascular risk. Extrapolations from nine lipid-lowering trials in men with hypercholesterolemia suggest that lowering of total cholesterol by 12% seen with tamoxifen might be associated with decreases of 20% in CHD incidence, and 20% decreases in LDL seen with tamoxifen might be associated with decreases of 30% in CHD incidence [10]. Data in women suggest that a 20% decrease in LDL may result in a 6% decrease in CHD [11].

The directions of changes in total cholesterol, LDL cholesterol, lipoprotein ratios and fibrinogen all *suggest* a favorable impact on CHD risk with tamoxifen treatment. Any stated level of favorable impact, however, can only be a speculation. Further data on tamoxifen's effects on apoliproteins, total and HDL subfractions, blood pressure and body girth changes are needed in healthy women to better predict likely effects on CHD rates.

Further data on the significance of each of these suggested CHD risk factors in older women are also needed. In some large controlled adjuvant studies such as NSABP B14 follow-up of subjects may allow analyses for cardiovascular disease end-points. In a preliminary report from one study, the Scottish trial, among post-menopausal axillary node negative women there have been 18 acute non-cancer deaths in 373 controlled subjects and 5 in 374 long-term tamoxifen recipients.

BONE EFFECTS OF TAMOXIFEN

Bone fractures are a major cause of morbidity in post-menopausal women over age 55. Animal and in vitro laboratory studies indicate that tamoxifen decreases rates of resorption of trabecular bone, with resultant net preservation of bone density. In humans, retrospective studies have suggested no differences in radial or lumbar spine bone density with tamoxifen treatment and prospective studies have suggested increased bone mineral density. In the Wisconsin Tamoxifen Study, a statistically significant preservation of bone density was found in the lumbar spine and a trend to preservation of bone density was found in the radius.

Over time these decreases in trabecular bone loss with tamoxifen would be expected to be reflected in 25% lower fracture rates in a manner similar to the effects from estrogen.

CARCINOGENIC EFFECTS OF TAMOXIFEN

While carcinogenic effects of long-term tamoxifen therapy on the liver and uterus have been suggested, data are both very limited and supportive of extremely low rates at most of these malignancies. In a summary of types of second primary cancers occurring in adjuvant trials, ovarian cancers appeared to be *less* frequent with tamoxifen treatment.

OTHER BIOLOGICAL EFFECTS OF TAMOXIFEN

Other serious biological side-effects of tamoxifen treatment have been suggested, but are of such low frequencies or occur on background rates in normal individuals such as to preclude conclusions about their causative relationships to tamoxifen treatment.

SYMPTOMATIC EFFECTS OF TAMOXIFEN

Major symptomatic effects from tamoxifen treatment are: vasomotor symptoms, gynecological symptoms, depression and nausea. While tamoxifen is very acceptable therapy for women in adjuvant studies where approximately only 4% drop out because of side-effects, the morbidity might result in a much different compliance profile in a study of healthy women.

Vasomotor symptoms of hot flashes (or flushes), flushed face, episodes of sweaty palms and racing heart are increased in frequency and severity in post-menopausal women treated with tamoxifen. After six months of treatment, an additional 17% of tamoxifen-treated subjects over placebo reported moderate or greater hot flashes in the Wisconsin Tamoxifen Study [12]. Treatment for these symptoms is currently limited.

Gynecological symptoms of increased vaginal discharge, vaginal–external genitalia irritation or vaginal bleeding complicate tamoxifen therapy. Approximately 4% of post-menopausal women will complain of moderate or greater such symptoms after six months of treatment. On careful questioning, 35–48% of treated post-menopausal subjects will consistently complain of moderate or greater symptomatic side-effects over the first several months of tamoxifen therapy. Treated women with these symptoms develop heightened anxiety about taking this drug and increased worry about cancer. Long-term compliance with treatment might be expected to be compromised in the presence of these side-effects.

SUMMARY OF BIOLOGICAL RATIONALE FOR A
TAMOXIFEN HEALTH TRIAL

The spectrum of data reviewed above suggest that overall benefits to the health of post-menopausal women might follow long-term treatment with tamoxifen. Specifically a reduced incidence of breast cancer, reduction in coronary heart disease—non-fatal and fatal myocardial infarction and sudden death—and reduction in major fractures can be reasonably hypothesized to accompany long-term tamoxifen treatment. In addition, an overall mortality reduction can also be expected from tamoxifen treatment. It is, however, clear from the rigorous data on symptoms associated with tamoxifen treatment that a significant percentage of tamoxifen recipients will have levels of side-effects which may cause them to stop therapy. Finally, while the biological and clinical data suggest that these hypotheses should be supported in rigorous clinical trials, currently they fall short of adequate to justify acceptance of tamoxifen as an alternative hormone replacement therapy in any non-breast cancer afflicted post-menopausal female population.

CRITICAL ISSUES AND APPROACHES TO A
TAMOXIFEN HEALTH TRIAL

While the critical issues which should be considered in the design and conduct of a tamoxifen health trial are significantly interrelated, here these will be considered in the following sequence: (A) Is tamoxifen a publically acceptable health-promoting intervention? (B) Is now the right time for a tamoxifen trial? (C) Can an adequate trial design be proposed which accommodates the multiple end-points and safety issues of concern? (D) Is such a proposed THT actually feasible? (E) Is such a THT ethically acceptable? and (F) Are the costs in relation to the benefits of a THT acceptable?

(A) IS TAMOXIFEN A REALISTIC INTERVENTION?

The central issues for any new health intervention concern its benefits (does it work?) and its public acceptance. While in the USA there is *some* reluctance to take pills because this is seen as "unnatural", in general we are a pill-consuming society. For the majority of women then the questions center on benefits and risks. For menopausal conditions—symptomatic changes following menopause—at any given time 15–20% of eligible post-menopausal women have been reported to be taking hormone replacement therapy (HRT). This minority of women suggests limited acceptance of HRT: the details are, however, telling. Apparently in recent years women have tended to take HRT for limited times—possibly an average of one year, and possibly 30% of women given prescriptions for HRT never fill them. Short-duration treatment is consistent with the first reason for HRT historically—relief of symptoms. Limited data indicate that concerns about uterine endometrial and breast cancer as side-effects of HRT continue to bother women and probably provide the major explanation for this picture. Given the uncertain situation with respect to breast cancer risk associated with estrogen replacement treatment alone, this is not surprising. Recent studies suggesting modest but nonetheless definite increased risk (estimated relative risk approximately 1.4) of breast cancer with long-term (i.e. greater than six years) estrogen treatment are likely to contribute to continued reluctance of women generally to take estrogen alone for longer periods. This will be even if overall health benefits are presented and emphasized (i.e. that heart disease and bone disease benefits on average significantly outweigh such an increased risk from breast cancer) because Americans tend to be strongly risk aversive; we wish to take no risks at all, and such a decision to take or not to take estrogens alone will likely be framed as one of taking or not taking a risk. With respect to HRT with combination estrogen–progesterone treatment, the paucity of data is likely the major reason women find this less acceptable. In addition some reports have suggested significant increased risk of breast cancer from combination HRT, and the lipid profile associated with progestin treatment is unfavorable. In sum, in the USA HRT to date appears to have had low acceptance because of concerns about toxicity. In general women have focussed on the risks instead of the benefits, even though for estrogen replacement alone these risks are likely far exceeded by benefits.

This picture of concern with toxicity of HRT was reproduced in a survey about participation in a tamoxifen prevention trial. In questioning women who had mammogram screening examinations in Texas, Winn and his colleagues found that the overriding issue about participation was toxicity. It would therefore seem clear that after (if not also before) a THT widespread acceptance of HRT with tamoxifen can only come if there are *not* questions about toxicity, particularly carcinogenicity. It may be instructive to revisit the discussions and debates of 20–25 years ago surrounding the use of oral contraceptive hormones (OCP). Widespread use of OCP has occurred, absent definitive data about cancer risks, but there has certainly been a fraction of women who have never found OCPs to be acceptable "treatment", at least in part in all likelihood because of concerns about toxicity. A THT might be significantly instrumented in facilitating acceptance of tamoxifen as HRT, if safety were demonstrated. These considerations suggest that tamoxifen as HRT, if proven to be health promoting, is a realistic intervention, but in the best of circumstances for a fraction, only possibly a majority of the eligible population. To get to widespread acceptance, however, will likely require a THT or more than one THT, and the same issues will be critical in the complete recruitment and high compliance necessary to a successful THT. These considerations beg the question of when it is appropriate to do a THT.

(B) IS NOW THE RIGHT TIME TO DO A TAMOXIFEN HEALTH TRIAL?

It would seem that the time "window of opportunity" in which to conduct public health trials like a THT is short. On the one hand, it is critical to have adequate data to justify the intervention on the basis of benefits and absence of risks; on the other hand "too much" data leads to adoption of the intervention without rigorous proof of overall health benefits, and compromises the ability of investigators to conduct a trial. With respect to tamoxifen, there appears to be a balance of accepted facts and uncertainties about the suggested benefits of tamoxifen on major disease processes in post-menopausal women. While suppression of pre-clinical breast cancer seems very likely, will the cancers that develop be more lethal or, as has been suggested of breast cancers occurring in the face of estrogen HRT, associated with a better prognosis? While lipid and lipoprotein effects of tamoxifen appear favorable, will these changes actually be reflected in lower rates of CHD in treated post-menopausal women? And, while tamoxifen appears to preserve bone mineral density over the short term, will this preservation continue over longer periods and will it be adequate to result in reductions in bone fracture rates?

Similarly, for the suggested risks of tamoxifen, there appear to be considerable reassuring data about liver and uterine cancers and thrombo-phlebitis, which suggest that these complications are of extremely low or negligible likelihood. In addition, because of the low frequency of these postulated complications, only a large carefully monitored clinical trial is likely to shed any definitive light on their actual occurrence. Thus I would argue that the timing for a THT is right, given particular attention to a prudent and realistic design.

(C) CAN A REALISTIC TRIAL DESIGN BE PROPOSED WHICH ACCOMMODATES THE MULTIPLE END-POINTS AND SAFETY ISSUES OF CONCERN?

The first issue about any clinical trial proposal is: can it be done? As a general strategy, a proposal my colleagues and I have made for a THT addresses this question by suggesting a two–three-year feasibility–vanguard study prior to a full-scale THT [13]. Such an arrangement allows commitment of limited resources to demonstrate that complete and timely subject accrual and adequately high participant compliance can be achieved. In addition, the creation of a cohort of study subjects—a vanguard group—two–three years ahead of the main body of study subjects in duration on study provides a smaller group "at risk" for any unanticipated safety or operational problems.

The major questions then concern the possibility of a design which accommodates safety and appropriate multiple end-point goals. My colleagues and I have proposed a relatively short-term major study—five years duration—with breast cancer incidence, coronary heart disease incidence (non-fatal myocardial infarction, fatal myocardial infarction and sudden death), bone fracture incidence (hip and wrist) and overall mortality as study end-points. Were convincing data obtained on each of these end-points, then widespread use of tamoxifen as HRT could logically be encouraged. Our proposed eligibility criteria allow women at increased risk for breast cancer and osteoporosis, but exclude women with, or at risk for, CHD. Making a variety of conservative assumptions about sample size, my colleague David DeMets has estimated that a full five-year THT trial of 16 000 post-menopausal women would have high power to demonstrate reduction in breast cancer incidence and overall mortality, *and* moderately high power to demonstrate separately reductions in CHD and bone fractures at hip and wrist [14]. Given treatment variations for breast cancer, plus the desirability of reaching conclusions acceptable for public health purposes in a reasonable and achievable period of study, we have focussed on breast cancer incidence instead of mortality. Such a multiple end-point design, however, raises the possibility that one end-point might be reached convincingly significantly in advance of others. For example, a highly statistically significant reduction in overall mortality or CHD incidence might be reached well before a suggested or statistically significant reduction in breast cancer incidence. Should the trial be stopped at that time? There appear to be no simple answers to this question. Clearly the overall goals and purposes of the study need to be considered in the evaluation of results. Ideally, one wants to reach a conclusion about the use of tamoxifen *as HRT for post-menopausal women*. A conclusion about one benefit may be inadequate. In this situation different *benefits* are all of interest. If the trial is continued after benefits have been confirmed in one area, the major consequence is that some women may be deprived of those. This must be seen, however, in light of the overall and hopefully greater benefits to come to many more women because of solid evidence of multiple benefits which may come with continuing the trial. At first consideration, it is not obvious that the potential problem here is so unique. It has recently been reported that in the Physician's Health Trial of aspirin and β-carotene to prevent CHD and cancers, respectively, β-carotene appears to protect against CHD. The decision of the data-monitoring committee for this trial to continue the study given this result and its consquences may provide some ideas as to how such results are handled.

A further issue with respect to realistic design concerns safety. We have identified a number of potential populations which may represent increased risk groups (for side-effects), and have proposed they be ineligible for a THT. Fortunately, these are likely to represent a relatively small fraction of the total population possibly eligible for a THT. Thus we believe safety concerns can be responsibly addressed.

In sum, we believe a realistic study design can be proposed and thus the question of the feasibility of conducting a THT of this design becomes a critical issue.

(D) IS A TAMOXIFEN HEALTH TRIAL ACTUALLY FEASIBLE?

In large prevention trials, success turns on complete rapid recruitment and high compliance. The former issue—recruitment—deserves detailed consideration as there are considerable specific data which bear on the question of success. For compliance, for a THT we believe a feasibility study which assesses this question will be necessary; some aspects of this feasibility study will be considered here.

Population

Several issues are important in the choice of a study population for a THT: the generalizability of the results, the event rate(s) in the populations, the total pool of potential study volunteers, the size of study needed to answer the critical question(s), the feasibility of the entire study, and the total costs of recruitment—considering all resources needed. The ethical concerns about safety for subject volunteers would seem to apply to any population. Two general *post*-menopausal populations appear appropriate for a THT:

(1) Women aged 50–69 at increased risk because of (a) a family history of breast cancer in at least one first-degree relative, (b) two or more surgical breast biopsies, (c) nulliparity or age 30 or greater at first full-term pregnancy. Women in these three groups can easily identify themselves and confirmation of their risk status is not necessary by pathology or radiology review (which is expensive).
(2) "Normal"-risk healthy women aged 55–69.

Unfortunately, the relative risk of breast cancer in the "increased"-risk populations averages two or less. The populations of women with higher relative risks for breast cancer, which are well agreed on, are small and/or complex and costly to identify.

Critical considerations pertaining to these populations are the following.

Generalization

A successful study with one or both populations will be generalizable to large segments of the American population of post-menopausal women.

Event rates

The incidence of breast cancer in these populations is predictable and will depend on the specific mixture of age and risk factors in actual volunteering study subjects. First, specifically, the newest Surveillance, Epidemiology and End Results (SEER) data on incidence of breast cancer combined with projected incidence increases through the coming years can be used to estimate a possible breast cancer incidence figure. Second, published data on the relative risks associated with each of the specific named "increased risk" factors, as well as data on incidence of breast cancer in multiple risk factor subjects from the Breast Cancer Detection Demonstration Project (BCDDP), can be used to estimate breast cancer incidence in increased-risk women.

Finally, the actual risk factor profile of volunteering subjects (age, risk factors) can be combined with the frequently observed "healthy volunteer" effect (which results in an actual event rate of 0.75 compared to predicted in similar studies) to predict a likely breast cancer incidence in a full-scale trial. Whether such an effect might actually be seen in a breast cancer trial is controversial.

Total study population pool

In 1990, the total population of women aged 50–69 in the USA was about 23 million and by 1995 this figure is projected to be 24 million; in 1990 the pool 55–69 was 16 million. Based on published case–control studies of breast cancer risk factors the population prevalence of having a first-degree relative with breast cancer is 7.8%. Thus an estimated 1.8 million women aged 50–69 will have a family history of breast cancer, mostly sisters. Almost 20% of women 60 years of age have undergone surgical (not needle aspiration) breast biopsy. In BDCCP, of women who underwent biopsies one-quarter to one-third had two or more biopsies. Thus 5–7% of all women in a post-menopausal study's age group may have had two or more biopsies at maximum, or 1.15–1.61 million women. Twelve per cent of women 55–64 years were reported in a large American health survey in 1987 to have no full-term pregnancies; an additional 6.3% underwent first full-term pregnancy at 30 or more years. These data suggest that 4.14 million American women fall into this risk category.

Thus the total US pool of 50–69-year-old women at increased risk for breast cancer because of a family history, two or more breast biopsies, or nulliparity or age at first birth $\geqslant 30$ appears at maximum to be 7.3 million $(1.8 + 1.4 + 4.14)$ (obviously some women may be in more than one of these groups and thus the actual figure must be lower).

Feasibility of acquiring adequate numbers
of subjects in these populations

If the actual total pool of increased-risk women is 7.3 million, and the full-scale breast cancer prevention study size required 16 000 *total* subjects (this depends on a number of statistical considerations), then one in every 456 women in the USA would need to be entered on a high-risk only woman study. Geographical dispersion, interest and eligibility restrictions combined with other logistical considerations suggest that these numbers would present a major barrier to complete accrual.

There are no easy, inexpensive logistical approaches to rapidly identifying and accruing a high *fraction* of the total pool of the high-risk women. While working through affected sisters is logical, it is likely to be very inefficient. Lists of high-risk women are dispersed, if they exist at all. Since direct contact with potential subjects is the most efficient way to recruit, the absence of readily available mechanisms to identify such subjects presents a major barrier.

In contrast, for "normal-risk" women (some authors feel that all American women are at "high risk" because the vast majority of breast cancers occur *in the absence of* any identifiable risk factors), identification and successful recruitment of adequate numbers of subjects appears achievable based on population approaches used in other prevention studies. Because incidence increases with age, and the total numbers of normal-risk women are large, a slightly older age group of normal-risk women (starting at 55 instead of 50) is suggested.

Summary of appropriate populations for study

The foregoing discussion suggests that a reasonable general strategy for a THT might be to *target the high-risk populations named for priority recruitment*. The first-phase recruitment experience should optimally be one which is efficient in financial and time costs *and* likely be reproducible over time in the same and other sites.

Compliance

A run-in period should be considered and evaluated in the first phases of a THT. The rationale for this is as follows. High compliance with an intervention over the long periods of time is essential to the success of a prevention trial because, as compliance falls, the sample size necessary to demonstrate a benefit of the intervention with high power rises dramatically. In previous prevention trials a major fraction of individuals who become non-compliant or dropped out of the trial did this in the first few months. In the Physician's Health Trial, one-third of the physicians who initially enrolled dropped out prior to randomization during a run-in period. The power of the trial was increased by having a *smaller* number of very compliant subjects. In colon polyp prevention trials 3–7% of subjects became non-compliant during a placebo run-in period.

In a THT an active-agent, i.e. tamoxifen, run-in period might possibly identify and cause to become non-compliant an even greater percentage of subjects than a placebo run-in period would. This would be due to the added fraction of subjects who would have tamoxifen-induced side-effects. However, such a procedure would likely create problems with different and lower compliance rates in tamoxifen and placebo groups after randomization because different fractions of these groups would then perceive themselves to be taking or not taking tamoxifen. In addition, companion studies of biological effects of tamoxifen on cardiovascular risks and bone could not be conducted with such an active-agent run-in design.

Thus in the feasibility phase of a prevention trial we have proposed that a run-in should be used. Interim analysis of the fraction of subjects who drop out during this run-in and correlates of compliance with the protocol should be conducted so that, should this run-in not be necessary or of limited benefit, it can be dropped early in the trial program.

In sum, careful considerations suggest that a THT is feasible in the USA, but one involving *both* increased risk and "normal-risk" women. While numerically large populations are available, whether adequate compliance can be achieved is uncertain and the conduct of a feasibility study with a test of the usefulness of a run-in study seems appropriate. In these circumstances, the next question concerns the ethics of such a THT.

(E) IS A TAMOXIFEN HEALTH TRIAL ETHICALLY ACCEPTABLE?

Certain ethical questions have been addressed in the foregoing discussions. Two additional considerations seem appropriate here. Pike and colleagues have raised the question of whether the "standard of care" for post-menopausal women is to give estrogen replacement alone and thus whether it is possibly unethical to omit estrogen alone as an option or choice in a THT. An earlier discussion suggested that in fact many women find estrogen HRT alone unacceptable because of concerns about risk of breast cancer—risks which Pike and colleagues accept are real. Thus it is difficult to believe that most women would accept this alternative in a study. An additional question is whether estrogen HRT should be *pro*scribed in a THT. Because of uncertain biological consequences of combined estrogen–tamoxifen HRT and because, taking estrogen by significant numbers of women would likely confound achievement of study objectives, we have elected to proscribe estrogen HRT in our proposal for a THT.

A second general ethical consideration concerns whether in fact a THT, taking all concerns into account, is likely to be successfully completed. It would be unethical to involve women in a trial whose goals are in fact unlikely to be achieved or a trial which is simply non-feasible. This is a major concern and one we believe can only be addressed by having a feasibility study. A THT is a "high-risk" venture, in the sense that at this time it is impossible to know if it can in fact be successfully accomplished. A planning phase, followed by a feasibility phase, are the responsible ways to approach this concern. Lack of support for a full-scale THT after a feasibility study will not mean necessarily that a THT was ill conceived, for hopefully many useful answers to critical questions will be forthcoming from this process and exercise alone.

In sum it appears that a THT is ethically acceptable and thus in the USA the question becomes: is a THT worth the expense and are the resources available to conduct such a trial?

(F) ARE THE COSTS IN RELATION TO THE BENEFITS OF A THT ACCEPTABLE?

Clinical trials testing tamoxifen to prevent breast cancer have been estimated to cost $60–100 million in direct costs, primarily because of their sizes (10 000–20 000 subjects) and durations (five to ten years). Scientists in other research areas may find these possible expenditures great for their perceived return.

Historically, large clinical trials have been found to be cost-effective investments despite their large costs [15]. This is because their impact can be enormous: the widespread application (or non-application in the case of an intervention found useless) involving millions of individuals over long periods of time of a costly intervention (e.g. in the USA tamoxifen currently costs the consumer about $750 a year for a 20-mg daily dose) costs billions and trillions of dollars. The cost effectiveness of a THT is further enhanced because prevention of other chronic processes such as heart and bone disease is also postulated. An example of the consequences of *not* testing an intervention for overall health benefit, with uncertain but costly consequences, is the use of estrogen or other hormone replacement therapy described earlier. While cost-effectiveness analyses considering benefits in heart and bone disease for estrogen alone have been favorable, these have assumed *no* increased risk of breast cancer. Thus the use of estrogen after menopause by American women, now of uncertain *overall* benefit, may represent a very costly public health practice.

Unrelated to the cost directly, the development of clinical trials in breast cancer prevention can be viewed as the setting up of programs in women's health [16]. Such trials will foster a myriad of ancillary studies, both biological and social scientific, from which, if past experience is repeated, much of significance will be learned. As an example, much about the natural history of cervical cancer was learned from screening programs. Even if the primary hypotheses of such trials are not supported (although as indicated above this would be very useful information), the program yields will likely be very great. Women's health in general has received less attention than men's and thus the emphasis in these trials in fact will correct an imbalance in past public health efforts.

CONCLUSIONS

The biological rationale for a THT in post-menopausal women appears well developed. While there are critical issues and questions about the possible success of a THT, several strategies including a feasibility study provide a prudent approach. A THT is a high-risk venture but one justified by the potentially enormous public health benefits in the event of complete success and likely progress in women's health from the exercise itself.

ACKNOWLEDGMENTS

Drs DeMets, C. Furberg, V. C. Jordan, P. A. Newcomb and R. Prentice, in addition to my colleagues of the Tamoxifen Health Trial Group, have contributed ideas and partial reviews of the text presented here.

During the period over which these ideas were developed the author has been supported by grants PDT 302A and B from the American Cancer Society; by grants from ICI Pharma Division of ICI Americas Inc.; and by Public Health Service grants CA-14520 and CA-50243 from the National Cancer Institute, National Institutes of Health, Department of Health and Human Services.

REFERENCES

1. Early Breast Cancer Trialists Collaborative Group (1988) The effects of adjuvant tamoxifen and of cytotoxic therapy on mortality in early breast cancer: an overview of 61 randomized trials among 28 896 women. N Engl J Med 319: 1681–1692
2. Love RR (1990) Prospects for antiestrogen chemoprevention of breast cancer. J Nat Cancer Inst 82: 18–21
3. Jordan VC (1984) Biochemical pharmacology of antiestrogen action. Pharmacol Rev 36: 245–276
4. Jordan VC (1976) Effect of tamoxifen (ICI 46,474) on initiation and growth of DMBA-induced rat mammary carcinomata. Eur J Cancer 12: 419–422
5. Welsch CW, Goodrich-Smith M, Brown CK et al (1981) Effects of an estrogen antagonist (tamoxifen) on the initiation and progression of radiation-induced mammary tumors in female Sprague–Dawley rats. Eur J Cancer 17: 1255–1258
6. Jordan VC, Lababidi MK, Mirecki DM (1990) The antiestrogenic and antitumor properties of prolonged tamoxifen therapy in C3H/OUJ mice. Eur J Cancer 26: 718–721
7. Lemon HM, Pradeep PF, Peterson C et al (1989) Inhibition of radiogenic mammary carcinoma in rats by estriol or tamoxifen. Cancer 63: 1685–1692
8. Fornander T, Cedarmark B, Mattson A et al (1989) Adjuvant tamoxifen in early breast cancer: occurrence of new primary cancers. Lancet i: 117–119
9. Love RR, Newcomb PA, Wiebe DL et al (1990) Lipid and lipoprotein effects of tamoxifen therapy in postmenopausal women with node-negative breast cancer. J Nat Cancer Inst 82: 1327–1332
10. Lipid Research Clinics Program (1984) The Lipid Research Clinics Coronary Prevention Trials results II: the relationship of reduction in incidence of coronary heart disease to cholesterol lowering. JAMA 251: 365–374
11. Bush T, Fried LP, Barrett-Connor E (1988) Cholesterol, lipoprotein, and coronary heart disease in women. Clin Chem 34: 60–70
12. Love RR, Cameron L, Connell B, Leventhal H (1991) Symptoms associated with tamoxifen treatment in postmenopausal women. Arch Int Med (in press)
13. Prentice RL (1990) Editorial: tamoxifen as a potential preventive agent in healthy postmenopausal women. J Nat Cancer Inst 82: 1310–1311
14. DeMets DL, Newcomb PA, Carey P (1991) Design issues for breast cancer chemoprevention trial. Prev Med 20: 101–108
15. Detsky AS (1989) Are clinical trials a cost effective investment? JAMA 262: 1795–1800
16. Furberg C (1991) Organizing multicenter trials: lessons from cardiovascular prevention trials. Prev Med 20: 158–161

ABOUT THE AUTHOR

Richard R. Love is an associate professor in the Department of Human Oncology at the University of Wisconsin, Madison, Wisconsin, USA. While he is trained and practises as a medical oncologist, with particular interest in breast cancer, he has special interest in cancer prevention and screening. For the past several years, he has been investigating the biological effects of tamoxifen and recently has organized the Tamoxifen Health Trial Group to pursue the possibility of a tamoxifen prevention trial in post-menopausal American women.

REPORTING AND CHOOSING NEW TREATMENTS

Notes on Section V

The final section contains eight chapters, each of which discusses aspects of handling data from clinical trials and of using this information in planning future therapy for individual patients or in designing new trials.

Chapter 25 by **Colin Begg** and **Jesse Berlin** was originally published in fuller form in the *Journal of the National Cancer Institute* (1989, 81: 107–115). The authors examine in detail the problem of publication bias—the tendency of researchers only to submit, and journal editors only to accept, trials giving a "positive" result. Because we have generally conducted trials which are too small to detect important but moderate differences (Chapters 4 and 13), decisions on the worth of therapies has often been judged on review of the published literature. The authors' review of such data exemplifies one of the major defects in this process (Chapter 26 discusses others). They make a plea for "major changes in editorial policies and for altering the style and methods of statistical analysis". A major stumbling block is the deeply ingrained need of clinicians to demonstrate statistical significance to "prove" theories. Success in such a venture, as he perceptively observes, gives a powerful push up in the ladder of academic promotion.

One suggestion, already discussed in section I, is assessment of trial methodology and importance by a medical journal *before* the trial starts. If they consider the methodology and question acceptable they may agree to publish the results of the completed trial *whatever* the outcome. This radical suggestion may be unacceptable to journals and it is easy to see the chaos that might ensue if many trials adopted this procedure. Begg and Berlin discuss other strategies including financial support for publication of short negative reports and for major funding agencies to take responsibility for disseminating results. The recent initiative of the National Cancer Institute (NCI) to distribute "clinical alerts" is controversial (Chapters 27–29) and is open to criticism since the studies have not been "peer reviewed" (before starting the trial or following completion).

Lesley Stewart (Chapter 26) examines a more formal way of assessing the overall result of randomized clinical trials. The concept of a systematic overview—meta-analysis—is used synonymously, was developed in the social sciences and has recently been applied successfully to questions in oncology. However, such an undertaking is no simple review of the literature; it is an exhaustive assessment of all *published* and *unpublished* data from *individual* patients in properly randomized trials. Stewart outlines the need for such overviews (inadequate patient numbers in trials) and shows

Introducing New Treatments for Cancer: Practical, Ethical and Legal Problems. Edited by C. J. Williams
© 1992 John Wiley & Sons Ltd

how they should be designed and run. Since the overview secretariat have access to all the data, with the generous co-operation of individual researchers, they have the option to look for inconsistencies in randomization and data collection and can undertake analysis on an "intention to treat" basis.

There is little doubt that the breast cancer overview on adjuvant therapy conducted by the Oxford group has had a major impact on clinical behaviour worldwide. Such an overview, as well as giving the best available answer to a question, may also lead to further questions. The Advanced Ovarian Cancer Trialists Group have formulated questions in early and advanced ovarian carcinoma which are the subject of two new trials. These are designed to be the two largest trials ever conducted in this disease— underlining that international co-operation may be aided by the overview process itself. Although a major undertaking, systematic overviews are cost effective, often providing reliable answers to contentious questions and suggesting appropriate new lines of research.

The next three chapters introduce and discuss the relative merits of the decision of the NCI in the USA to circulate "clinical announcements" or "clinical alerts". The first of these concerned the announcement which strongly supported the use of adjuvant chemotherapy in pre-menopausal women with breast cancer which did *not* involve the axillary lymph nodes. Because of this I asked **William McGuire** and his colleagues in San Antonio to review their perspective on the clinical advantages and disadvantages of such a treatment policy (Chapter 27). It is clear from their assessment of the situation that there are radically different opinions on the merits of adjuvant chemotherapy in this group. Treatments of all such women would be "over-treatment" in 70% or so since they were not destined to relapse. Of the remainder there is evidence of delay in recurrence and based on this it is assumed that survival will also improve (though this remains to be demonstrated). McGuire and his co-workers along with other researchers in breast cancer are especially interested in developing methods of detecting the minority of patients in this group who are destined to relapse. They argue that treatment of these women would be logical and ethically more acceptable than blanket treatment of all women in this group—most of whom will be at unnecessary risk of acute and long-term toxicity. They state that "over enthusiastic claims of treatment success must not be allowed to substitute for sound clinical judgement based on peer-reviewed scientific study". It must be said that their views are not shared by all breast cancer researchers— others would support the routine use of adjuvant chemotherapy in all pre-menopausal node-negative breast cancer. However, this is not the real subject of this debate—the crux is, if there is disagreement amongst researchers how should such data be handled and whether a "clinical announcement policy" is appropriate.

Michael Friedman (Chapter 28) writes on behalf of the NCI putting forward their rationale for this policy. Briefly, the policy of clinical announcement or alert by-passes the normal peer review process, thus speeding up the dissemination of information; the implications of this approach, however, go far beyond this. Friedman takes us through the perceived responsibility of the NCI to ensure appropriate dissemination of information from its clinical trials and the methods they use to achieve this. They envisage a clinical announcement as a brief report sent to clinicians which summarized important new studies describing new information. Their stated aim is to "reduce the interval between identifying an effective therapy and wide-spread adoption of that therapy". In principle they advocate a clinical announcement when a new treatment is identified that measurably improves survival or quality of life in cancer patients (with reasonable certainty) and when such treatment is generally available.

Friedman acknowledges that such announcements from such a national agency may cause concern and he stresses that they should not be taken to be an authoritative directive dictating therapy. Rather they should be regarded as educational in intent. The process of initiating and deciding on an eventual announcement is described and this is followed by discussion of the announcement process with reference to the announcements on breast and colon cancer. Friedman accepts that the present process is not yet optimal but states that the policy will be justified if there is a reduction in cancer deaths.

George Omura (Chapter 29) feels along with others that the policy of clinical announcements is well intentioned but ill advised. He reviews the process of presentation of scientific information with checks and balances provided by "peer review" and he acknowledges that it is currently cumbersome and often slow but argues that there are dangers in short-circuiting the process. He discusses the early dissemination of unpublished interim data from breast cancer and colon cancer studies by the NCI and the outcry this provoked amongst physicians and the considerable media coverage that followed.

Omura reviews the detailed debate that has taken place in the literature on these two topics. This very much seems to examine the validity of the conclusions of the "alerts" rather than the process itself. By showing that many workers do not accept these conclusions he undermines the whole procedure. He also examines the attitude of cancer researchers to the whole process—the defence by officials of the NCI and criticisms by others. This debate is not finished; the *Journal of the National Cancer Institute* (1991, 83 (4)) carried a report of a meeting of 25 medical editors, scientists and journalists to help the National Institute of Health to hammer out guidelines for clinical announcements—a tacit acceptance that all was not right. Since the article by Lindon Schwab concludes that "NCI guidelines are a step in the right direction" the controversy is unlikely to have been put to rest. However, the programme is firmly in place and a further clinical announcement on colon cancer has recently been published.

The main areas of debate remain: (a) there is no peer review and process of questioning; (b) some studies are NCI sponsored; are they and the investigators in a position to give an independant review? (c) despite their disclaimer, publication of an announcement by the NCI puts the individual physician under pressure—especially in the USA, where the threat of litigation is greater; (d) simultaneous announcement to the press increases this pressure since patients reading or seeing uncritical coverage of the "alert" will demand treatment; (e) because the communication is brief and lacking in detail the individual clinician is not in a position to make informed decisions; (f) alerts to date have been premature in that the encouraging results have primarily concerned disease-free survival and not survival; (g) informed decisions can only be made after publication of a peer-reviewed paper followed, most importantly, by editorials and letters dissecting and questioning the trial—this cross-examination is missing from an alert since it only contains positive opinion and does not have a section presenting the contrary view. From the fuss over the first breast-cancer alert it is clear that such a critique could have been included—or would this be too objective, defeating the object, which is a rapid change in clinical habits?

Consensus conferences have been introduced in the past decade or so in an attempt to define "best care" for patients. **Tony Smith** (Chapter 30) tackles the problem of consensus on cancer treatment. He highlights the major variation in approach to a common tumour such as breast cancer and examines the reasons for this trend, which is disquieting to patients and the general public. He rapidly identifies gross inadequacies in current clinical research: over-enthusiasm in uncontrolled phase II trials, often promoted by charities and research organizations; inadequate phase III trials which are far too small; and lobbying by doctors, research organizations and pharmaceutical companies. This results in a literature which is almost impossible to assess objectively. Smith suggests that it may not be in the interests of these parties to carry out large, effective studies in case they fail to support the hypothesis they promote. Quoting a number of distinguished academics and editors, he throws doubt on the usefulness of consensus conferences—even experts cannot produce the judgment of Soloman if the appropriate trials have not been done. As Skranbanek puts it, "consensus conferences are like convocations of bishops seeking the truth"; unlike bishops we do have concrete ways of testing "facts". Smith concludes that lack of direction is due to a failure to produce convincing evidence from clinical trials and underlines the fact that internationally only 1% of cancer patients are recruited into phase III clinical trials.

The laissez-faire attitude may, according to Smith, be challenged by the introduction of medical audit, though whether clinicians will audit the overall outcome of their treatment strategies is open to question. Many seem more ready to audit aspects of care rather than prospectively assess their overall results, a much larger task. One way of overcoming this may be to persuade clinicians of the advantages of including patients in large-scale studies of the sort discussed in Section II. As Smith says, maybe auditors should be asking "why weren't the patients enrolled into a trial?" We should be avoiding the approach of "what would you do if it were your wife?" (Hayes, *Journal of Clinical Oncology*, 1991, 9: 1–2) posed in an editorial discussing a paper reviewing the variation in practice and failure of clinicians to respond to results of clinical trials (Belanger et al., *Journal of Clinical Oncology*, 1991, 9. 7–16). If we do demonstrate that a new, and possibly toxic, treatment improves outcome, how should we decide when to use this treatment? Adjuvant chemotherapy for breast cancer is a good example of the problem. For every 100 women given adjuvant chemotherapy for stage II breast cancer, 50 or so will not benefit for they would not have relapsed anyway, 40 or so gain no benefit because they relapse despite the therapy, which leaves about 10 patients deriving benefit. However, the other 90% or more of patients have undergone all the side-effects of chemotherapy for little or no gain. How should we decide on when and in whom to offer or to use such treatments? One way of gaining help is to ask patients who have had such treatment, and this is the approach used by **Alan Coates** and **John Simes** in Chapter 31.

Clinicians spend much of their life making decisions but, as the authors of this chapter point out, few have had *any* formal teaching of decision theory. At present decisions are arbitrary and often fail to consider the wishes of the recipient. The authors use breast cancer as an example and base their survival data on the overview (Chapter 27) of the Early Breast Cancer Trials Group conducted in Oxford. As mentioned above, this suggests a 10% improvement in survival at five years of treated patients with stage II disease. Interestingly, they estimate that survival benefit may only be 1–2% in good-risk stage I patients—see discussion of clinical alert on this subject (Chapters 27–29).

Coates and Simes have approached the problem of decision making in this context by going directly to patients; they distrust the concept of a surrogate system (see Chapter 32). Their study of women receiving adjuvant chemotherapy asked patients to estimate what gain, in terms of extra survival time or of improved proportion of long-term survival, would make the experience of adjuvant chemotherapy worthwhile. Attitudes towards taking risk were also studied.

The major outcome of the study was that most *patients* felt that modest improvements in outcome justified the chemotherapy. These differences are often less than required by clinicians when they decide for patients if they will offer the treatment. No study is perfect and this one has its flaws. Only patients completing at least three cycles of chemotherapy were included (so that they could properly assess the impact of treatment); thus patients not referred, refusing treatment or dropping out early were excluded. In addition, assessment of attitudes was taken after therapy at a time when patients were personally motivated, because they had taken the gamble, to have a positive attitude that they had benefited. Since only few benefit it would be interesting to assess attitudes in all patients at a later time—including those who are failing despite therapy (there were too few in this study to reliably answer this question).

Particularly interesting is the finding that family situation affects attitudes to the usefulness of such therapy. This is fairly obvious if we think about it but cannot be taken into account by any system that fails to consult the patient. It also underlines that the results of this study cannot be translated to the next patient who walks through the door. This study does, however, give weight to the decision that it is right and reasonable to talk to that patient about the pros and cons of therapy and to reach a joint decision as to what plan is best for them. Such decisions, if they are to be valid, must be based on solid information; a recent paper (Fetting et al., *Journal of Clinical Oncology*, 1990, 8: 1476–1482) suggests that patients over-estimate benefit because of vague doctor–patient communication. This, as Coates and Simes point out, is an extremely complex decision.

William Mackillop and his co-workers (Chapter 32) take a different route, preferring to examine the validity of treatments (and of clinical trials) by using the clinician as an expert surrogate. Their major concern is the ethics of individual clinical trials and not of treatment of the individual patients, and for this reason I believe the approach is valid, despite Coates and Simes' dislike of surrogates for clinical decision making—the decisions discussed in this chapter are at this stage probably largely the responsibility of the clinician since until the trial(s) is completed there are no facts to present to the patient. Complex clinical concepts may be difficult for patients to weigh up even when there are data but this may be overwhelming if decisions are ringed by uncertainty and opinion.

At present some of the decisions on the ethics of trials are left to research ethics committees (Chapter 7 and Notes on Section I), though these often lack the expert input to make complex clinical judgments. Since it is inappropriate to leave the individual clinician to decide whether a trial is ethical on complex clinical grounds, MacKillop and his colleagues have used the expert surrogate system to assess attitudes to a number of clinical trials, especially in lung and urological cancer.

Presumably, they argue, if a trial is ethical then most experts would, viewing themselves as a patient, be willing to be entered into that trial. Clearly this has not always been the case, since in the study of lung cancer experts the majority of clinicians would have refused the study and in one case 89% found a trial unacceptable for themselves. When presented with these results 40–60% of doctors surveyed said that trials with a large clinician-disapproved rating should never have gone ahead. Later studies suggested that a consent rate of two-thirds was required by most doctors (and non-experts) for the study to be seen as ethically acceptable.

The situation is made somewhat more complex by the suggestion that a high refusal rate by experts may be acceptable if this is made up of a high frequency of refusal for *both* arms. In this situation, described as *clinical equipoise* by Friedman, the trial may still be ethical. Only one study fitted this bill; the rest of the trials remained "unethical" because clinicians largely agreed why they would refuse to be included into the study (poor efficacy and high toxicity). Recently Korn and Baumrind have taken the concept of clinical equipoise further by suggesting that potential trial patients are examined and investigated by a team of doctors. Where they have different opinions on the optimal trial treatment the physician who will care for the patient will be the one who favoured the treatment to which the patient was subsequently randomized. Although an attractive idea it seems far too cumbersome to work in practice.

Based on these studies Mackillop suggests that impartial expert surrogates be used to assess the ethical nature of cancer trials, thus avoiding the problems of committee decisions.

They then go on to assess whether this approach can be used to make decisions on management controversies—a consensus conference in another guise? Their studies underline major variations in practice between clinicians, specialities and between countries. These come as no surprise to those in the field but are rather disturbing. My own prejudice is that like consensus conferences such a practice can only underscore differences—without the data on which to make decisions, we are only defining what particular groups think. The finding of widely different practices would be useful in suggesting important large-scale clinical trials, provided we can overcome clinical prejudices. This is of course the situation of clinical equipoise where, for instance, radiotherapists may passionately hold the view that radiotherapy after surgery is the best treatment and surgeons feel that it holds no benefit—the perfect situation for a large-scale *simple* trial asking a straightforward question.

The paper by Belanger and co-workers mentioned above reports a worrying though not entirely unexpected trend—the failure of so-called experts (medical oncologists in this case) to respond to the results of large trials and of an overview. So far these have *all* failed to show any survival benefit for adjuvant chemotherapy in post-menopausal women with stage II breast cancer. Despite this, 80% of US oncologists recommended such treatment. Whilst this might be influenced by the financial rewards of such treatment, physicians were at least consistent in that 86% said they would select such treatment for themselves when asked to act as a surrogate. The majority would enter patients into a trial comparing two chemotherapy regimes in such patients (without a no-treatment control) even though such treatment had not been validated.

This survey is extremely worrying in that: (a) it throws doubt on the validity of expert surrogates (especially when such surrogates have such varied opinions around the world); and (b) that their opinions fly in the face of large-scale trials and systematic overviews. It is urgent that we try to assess why so many clinicians choose to ignore negative data, preferring to go on believing in a treatment.

25 Publication Bias and Dissemination of Clinical Research*

COLIN B. BEGG and JESSE A. BERLIN

At some point in the course of a clinical trial, the investigator begins to consider the manner in which the study results will be disseminated. This may happen early in the trial as initial results begin to become available. Indeed, the more striking the results are, the more ambitious the publication plans are likely to be.

Reporting of the results may occur in various ways. The investigator often communicates the general findings by word of mouth to interested colleagues and may present an abstract at one or more conventions. If the circumstances demand, there may even be a press release to encourage transmittal of the findings to the general public. Eventually, an article may be written for publication in a medical journal. Another variable in this process is the decision regarding the journal to which the article should be submitted. The more striking the results are the greater is the impetus to target a prestigious general medical journal rather than a specialty journal. It is not uncommon for this entire process to occur while the trial is in progress. Early publication provides the opportunity for subsequent follow-up publications to further advertise the conclusions of the study or, on rare occasions, to contradict them.

Clearly, the vehicles used for disseminating the results and the timing of their use are extremely variable. The *manner* in which the results are presented is also very unstructured. Prior to preparation of an abstract or manuscript, the following sequence of events usually takes place. First, the data are reduced to an interpretable summary. Then there is interpretive analysis of the data, which often involves testing of statistical significance and reorganization of the data, usually in an interactive manner. The investigator may have some prior beliefs or hypotheses, and the analysis may be directed toward "proving" the hypotheses. Eventually, an inference will be drawn, possibly supported by statistical confirmation (e.g. $p < 0.05$).

*Originally published in the *Journal of the National Cancer Institute*, 1989, 81: 107–115 (73 refs). Supported by Public Health Service Grant CA-35291 and CA-38493 from the National Cancer Institute, National Institutes of Health, Department of Health and Human Services

Introducing New Treatments for Cancer: Practical, Ethical and Legal Problems. Edited by C. J. Williams
Published 1992 by John Wiley & Sons Ltd

There are a variety of other opportunities for subjective input in the process of analysis, such as the decision to exclude certain categories of patients (e.g. ineligible or without measurable disease), to perform separate analyses in selected subgroups of patients, or to adjust for selected covariates with statistical modeling. In fact, the fragmentation of the analysis into a variety of seemingly distinct issues may lead to a number of separate publications, a device that is partly responsible for the remarkable volume and expansion of the literature. This phenomenon is encouraged in the competition for academic promotion and lamented for its role in degrading the quality of published medical research.

When study results are reported, they are often presented in an advocacy style. Statistical significance, if it is achieved, may be used as "proof" of a theory, such as the assertion that treatment A produces longer patient survival than treatment B. It is widely believed by authors of articles that the advocacy style is necessary to attain publication. If no theory is proved or disproved, what reason is there for an editor to use valuable journal space for the article?

The process of information dissemination as outlined here contrasts markedly with conventional wisdom and current practice regarding the design and conduct of cancer clinical trials. In particular, trials sponsored by the National Cancer Institute (NCI) undergo a thorough review and approval process prior to implementation. In addition, details of the protocol and the specific objectives of the study are registered in the NCI-sponsored International Cancer Research Data Bank (ICRDB). There are requirements for conformity to conventional standards of good study design, such as the use of randomization for comparative trials, statistical projection of an adequate sample size, and definition of the patient population. Moreover, these methodologic standards for clinical trials are broadly accepted by the research community as being beneficial in that they encourage a scientific approach to clinical research.

In summary, clinical cancer research, especially the design and conduct of the trials, is increasingly performed in conformity with reasoned scientific principles. The methods of statistical analysis have also changed as a result of the many new specialized techniques, particularly those for survival analysis, even though statistical analysis in practice still has a very strong subjective component. In contrast, the system of reporting results of trials is extremely haphazard and unscientific. Many factors influence the reporting process, including the "significance" of the results, subjective data interpretations, and the preferences and relative enthusiasm of investigators and journal editors. Results are frequently presented in an advocacy style, which is not in conformity with the tradition of scientific objectivity.

The thesis of this review is that the present system is unsatisfactory. A major consequence of the problems in the system is publication bias, the systematic error that is entirely a product of selective publication [1].

PUBLICATION BIAS AND ITS CONSEQUENCES

Publication bias has two distinct though often related components, a subjective component and an objective component. The subjective component comprises some of the phenomena already mentioned; for example, the exaggerated claims that are stimulated by the advocacy style of presentation common in research papers. This bias, in other words, involves the "biased" opinion of the investigator and is often reflected in the tone of the presentation, the literature cited, and the interpretation of the evidence, rather than in the objective data. The phenomenon is hard to measure, but it has actually been studied by Chalmers [2], who cross-tabulated the opinions presented and the specialty of the author in various types of studies, including studies of prophylactic radiotherapy for breast cancer. Chalmers demonstrated significant association.

The objective component of publication bias is a more subtle and serious problem, since it is reflected in the "objective" data. The problem occurs because the decision to publish is often influenced by the results of the study. Specifically, it is widely believed and is demonstrated empirically in the section Empiric Studies of Cancer that the chance of publication is greater if the results of a study are statistically significant than if the results are not significant. Consequently, the literature contains a preponderance of "significant" trials relative to those that are unpublished. Many of these published trials may have false-positive results, since statistical variation ensures that the results in trials of ineffective agents are significant with at least 5% probability. (In reality, the chance of false-positive results is much higher because of the use of selective statistical analyses, subgroup analyses, sequential analyses, and other common methods that interfere with the validity of the mathematics.) Publication bias affects even straightforward data summaries such as estimates of median survival and response rates. Consequently, abstraction of summary data from published reports is hazardous. This fact has especially serious consequences for meta-analysis of published data, in which data from several studies are aggregated, and for decision analysis, since these methods are often heavily dependent on summaries of published data.

The primary causes of objective publication bias are editorial and author preferences, in addition to selective analytic maneuvers and other subjective influences. There is a perception that many journal editors give preference to reports of study results demonstrating statistical significance, and this has even been stated explicitly as editorial policy. As a result, authors are more inclined to submit articles with striking or significant findings and less likely to spend time on studies that are "uninteresting."

Investigators have attempted to examine these issues and to distinguish the relative importance of author and editorial preferences. A recent study of randomized clinical trials involving a survey of authors demonstrated that a substantial proportion of studies remain unpublished [3]. Moreover, 55% of the published trials demonstrated a trend favoring a new therapy, compared with 14% of the unpublished trials. After studying the reasons for failure to publish, the investigators concluded that author preferences were the dominant reason and that these were usually based on negative results and/or general lack of interest in pursuing the project to completion. The investigators inferred from these results that author preferences are a more important cause of publication bias than editorial preferences.

It seems likely that the decisions to submit and accept manuscripts are based on many complex factors, including the size or expense of the trial and the "quality" of the work. Sacks et al. [4] examined outcomes of published studies on the efficacy of six important types of therapy, including 5-fluorouracil for colon cancer and BCG for melanoma; they classified the studies as randomized or based on historic controls. The trends for the therapy trials were strikingly similar: most of the non-randomized trials demonstrated the effectiveness of the new treatment and most of the randomized trials showed no effect. At least some of this trend may be due to publication bias; since randomized trials generally involve a greater commitment of time, authors may be more inclined to follow through to publication. Conversely, historic comparisons can be assembled from a database with relative ease and are therefore easily discarded if the results are uninteresting.

Selective publication seems even more likely in relation to studies conducted in less controlled settings, like phase II trials, especially since these studies usually have relatively small sample sizes. Although many phase II studies are registered with NCI and designed with precise end-points, they are often characterized by arbitrary start and stop dates, which create the potential for selective reporting of positive results. Moreover, it may be more difficult to publish a study with negative results in this setting even if the author takes the trouble to prepare a manuscript. A well-known example is Moertel's report of 21 studies of 5-fluorouracil in advanced colon cancer [5] which demonstrated response rates ranging from 8% to 85%. It is notable that response rates in the large studies ranged from 12% to 31%, while the studies reporting very high response rates were generally small.

Calendar time can also have an impact, since early studies tend to be "exploratory", while later ones are "confirmatory" (designed to replicate a previous study). Uninteresting exploratory studies are more likely to be discarded prior to publication.

In addition to these technical factors, financial incentives may have an influence. In a review of clinical trials published in prestigious medical journals, Davidson [6] classified the trials into those that were "pharmaceutically supported" and those that were funded by other means; 89% of the pharmaceutically supported studies had results favoring the new therapy, compared with 61% of the other studies.

What are the consequences of publication bias? The most immediate consequence is that objective data reported in the literature cannot necessarily be accepted at face value. This finding has important implications for those who abstract published data, especially for formal quantitative analyses. The use of meta-analysis of published data [7] is particularly susceptible to bias, especially if the studies tend to be biased in the same direction, namely, toward a positive association. If the aggregated sample size is large, the results may appear to be extremely precise and convincing even though the observed association is entirely due to bias. There are other related hazards in assembling published data for meta-analysis; for example, the retrieval of studies using MEDLINE or other computerized searches may be very incomplete.

Data in the literature are also used extensively in decision analyses and cost-effectiveness analyses in which the decision options facing a physician are examined quantitatively by comparing costs and potential benefits. Virtually every decision analysis uses objective data abstracted from the literature, so the impact of publication bias is potentially extremely serious.

Publication bias is not merely a phenomenon that is apparent when data from the literature are aggregated; it applies to reports of single studies in all fields of science. A major consequence is that temporary prominence may be given to studies that are eventually found, via subsequent replicative investigations, to have false-positive results. This can have an impact on the practice of medicine by investigators for whom the credibility of the literature is high. To the extent that this is true, erroneous results and claims may strongly influence medical practice, although the little evidence that exists on the diffusion of results of individual trials into medical practice appears to show that individual studies have little immediate impact.

EMPIRIC STUDIES OF CANCER

This section focuses on studies of cancer clinical trials. The goal is to ascertain the magnitude of the bias so we can realistically appraise the seriousness of the problem.

One study involves 246 consecutively published comparative cancer clinical trials [8]. The trials were identified by a MEDLINE search of all trials published during 1986. The trials cover a wide variety of therapies and cancers and would be expected to show great diversity in the effects observed. All but three of the trials were published once during 1986; the remaining three were published twice. The analysis focuses primarily on sample size as the key factor for identifying bias, since there are compelling theoretical reasons why the bias should be large for small studies and should become progressively smaller as the sample size increases. In contrast, a major premise of the study is that the true differences in treatment results in the clinical trials should generally be unrelated to sample size; that is, the ranges of treatment results should be similar in large, medium-size, and small studies. Consequently, if the *observed* mean effects are related to sample size, the differences can be explained by publication bias.

The results of the study for the three major end points are presented in Table 1. For each end-point, there is an extremely strong association between the sample size and the observed average treatment effect. For overall survival, the average small study ($\leqslant 50$ deaths) demonstrated an average of 54% improvement in the results of the superior treatment over those of the inferior treatment, compared with an average of 13% for large studies (> 100 deaths). The trend is even more striking for disease-free survival. When the data are stratified on the basis of whether the study was randomized, there is evidence that the bias is present in both the randomized and non-randomized studies, which confirms the conventional wisdom that randomized trials are better protected against bias.

A variety of other study characteristics were examined. The results suggest that the differences in treatment effects among single-center trials are greater than those among multicenter trials, although the differences are consistently large only for survival. This finding may be due to increased pressure in the co-operative groups for publication regardless of the results of the trial. The studies were also classified and compared with regard to the circulation of the journal of publication, but no trends were apparent.

A completely different design for identifying bias was used by Simes [9] in his examination of comparative trials of therapy with single alkylating agents versus combination chemotherapy in advanced ovarian cancer. He

Table 1. Treatment results[a]

End-point	Sample size[b]	All studies[c] (%)	Randomized studies[c] (%)	Non-randomized studies[c] (%)
Overall survival	$\leqslant 50$	54	19	86
	51–100	35	28	55
	> 100	13	0	35
Disease-free survival	$\leqslant 50$	79	55	116
	51–100	36	30	48
	> 100	0	0	15
Response rate	$\leqslant 50$	17	12	33
	51–100	11	11	15
	> 100	0	0	0

[a]From Berlin et al., *Journal of the American Statistical Association*, 1989, 84: 381–392.
[b]For overall survival, values = no. of deaths. For disease-free survival, values = no. of patients with relapse. For response rate, values = total no. of patients.
[c]For overall survival and disease-free survival, values = average (geometric mean) percentage increase in survival with relapse in patients receiving superior versus inferior treatment. For response rate, values = mean difference in response rates between treatments compared.

Table 2. Meta-analysis for treatment of advanced ovarian cancer: significance of treatment results[a]

Status of trial	Results	
	Significant	Not significant
Published/not registered	3	9
Published and registered	1	7
Registered/not published	0	6

[a]From Simes, *Statistics in Medicine*, 1986, 6: 11–30.

identified the trials from two sources: MEDLINE searches of published articles and the NCI registry of cancer trials. Then he conducted follow-up on the unpublished registered trials by mail. The novelty of this approach is that the registry provides a sampling of studies that is uninfluenced by publication bias (objective), since the trials are registered at the design stage before any results are obtained. In principle, this provides a general sampling frame for meta-analysis that circumvents publication bias.

Simes [9] analyzed 26 studies, some of which were published, some published and registered, and some only registered (Table 2). We might expect that the unregistered published studies were most likely to be biased, and indeed, three of the 12 studies in this group had significant results, compared with one of the eight published registered trials and none of the six unpublished registered trials. When an unbiased meta-analysis restricted to the registered studies was performed, there was little observed difference among treatment results. In contrast, a meta-analysis based only on published studies demonstrated a statistically significant superiority for combination chemotherapy (Table 3). The number of studies in this meta-analysis is too small to yield conclusive results, but the findings support our presuppositions regarding the expected effects of publication bias.

Another study (M. Dubrow and C. B. Begg, unpublished data) involved phase II trials of treatments for melanoma. The design was similar to that of the Simes study [9] even though the trials were not comparative. The same sources were used: MEDLINE searches of published articles and the

Table 3. Meta-analyses for treatment of advanced ovarian cancer: p-values and median survival ratio[a]

	Published studies	Registered studies
No. of studies	16	13
Pooled p-value	0.02	0.24
Pooled median survival ratio	1.16	1.06
95% confidence interval	1.06–1.27	0.97–1.15

[a]From Simes, *Statistics in Medicine*, 1986, 6: 11–30. Summary data were insufficient for analysis in four studies.

NCI registry of cancer trials. Published and registered trials were matched on the basis of the drugs used in the study, the institution or co-operative group that conducted the study, and the sequence of dates of registration and publication. A total of 141 registered trials and 241 published trials were identified.

The average response rates are classified by sample size and registration status in Table 4. Surprisingly, these data do not demonstrate any association between outcome and sample size, although almost all such studies are relatively small (i.e. <50 patients). The response rates in the non-registered studies are clearly higher in all categories. However, the most striking result of this study is the observation that only 46 (33%) of the 141 registered trials were published. Admittedly, a few of the registered unpublished trials may have been "in the pipeline" at the time the study was done. This can be modeled by analyzing the times from registration to publication and treating the unpublished studies as "censored". Such an analysis reveals that almost all studies of this type, if published, are published one to eight years after registration. After adjustment of the analysis to accommodate the chances that the recently registered studies will be published eventually, the revised estimate of the long-term chance of publication is 40% ± 10%.

In summary, these empiric studies highlight several aspects of publication bias. The results of the first study of comparative trials (Table 1) demonstrate a strong association between outcome and sample size. The presence of such associations has often been used in the context of meta-analysis to infer publication bias. The results of the study of ovarian cancer (Tables 2 and 3) suggest that there is a bias in favor of publishing more studies with positive results and that this trend is greatest for non-registered studies. The results of the third study, which involved phase II trials in melanoma, confirm that the trend to publish more studies with positive results is greater for non-registered studies and demonstrate that the overall chance for publication of phase II studies is low. It does not confirm the association between outcome and sample size, although almost all phase II studies have relatively small sample sizes.

Table 4. Response rates in published phase II melanoma trials[a]

Sample size	Average response rate (No. of studies)	
	Registered studies	Non-registered studies
<20	9% (13)	22% (46)
20–39	13% (21)	17% (93)
≥40	13% (12)	19% (37)

[a]M. Dubrow and C. B. Begg, unpublished data.

STRATEGIES FOR REDUCTION OF BIAS

In recent years, commentators have suggested a number of different proposals that have direct or indirect bearing on the prevention or reduction of publication bias. These proposals can be grouped into four broad categories. The first proposal concerns methods of performing retrospective corrections for publication bias in the context of meta-analysis. The remaining proposals deal with research policy as it is targeted at journal editors, funding agencies such as NCI, and authors of research reports.

We first consider retrospective methodologic correction techniques for meta-analysis. One strategy commonly used in psychology studies is to speculate on the number of unpublished studies. This method can be used to limit the degree to which publication bias may have inflated any apparent associations and to calculate an adjusted p-value. However, the number of unpublished studies is hard to estimate. One can try to track down unpublished studies by writing to interested investigators, although this can be a painstaking process. Alternatively, if a registry of trials is available, it can be used as the source of studies. With this method, one can determine which unpublished studies require follow-up. Some commentators believe that when unpublished data are included, there is a risk of lowering the quality and credibility of a meta-analysis, since data from unpublished studies, which have not passed peer review, may be less reliable.

Other methods have been based on the premise that the analysis involves only published studies. A popular, informal technique is the funnel graph, a plot of treatment efficacy versus sample size. Any apparent association between the two factors is indicative of bias; in the absence of bias, the plot should have the shape of a pyramid. If this graph shows no evidence of bias, the investigator can be more certain that it is appropriate to proceed with the meta-analysis of published studies.

Finally, more formal methods use "weight functions" to model the probability of publication as a function of the p-value. Investigators have studied this method theoretically using the extreme sampling assumption that all statistically significant studies are published, and they have used generalizations of this model to accommodate more realistic, smoother weight functions.

All of these methods are based on fairly strong assumptions, and the current consensus seems to be that although these methods may be valuable tools, long-term policy measures aimed at reducing publication bias are required.

It has been suggested by several authors that editorial policy regarding the statistical methodology of clinical trials should be changed. Newcombe [10] has recommended that the decision of editors to accept or reject a study should be made prospectively, prior to the initiation of the study, on review of the protocol. This follows an earlier suggestion by Kochar [11] that manuscripts should be reviewed on the basis of the methods used in the study rather than the results, perhaps by blinding the reviewer to the results. This suggestion would have no impact on the author's choice of whether to try to publish a study. However, if it were recognized that there is an accepted place for trials with negative results in the literature, the problem might be alleviated. It has also been suggested that journals should be provided with financial incentives to make space for short reports of negative results and that studies with negative results should be recorded by title only. Some commentators have drawn attention to the need to revamp the peer-review process, and others have highlighted the poor standards of statistical analysis in medical reports. The bias due to sequential analysis and publication of ongoing trials (Chapter 15) has been recognized in the suggestion that if an interim analysis is published, the author should be required to provide published confirmation of the results on completion of the study. Some journals, including the *Journal of the National Cancer Institute*, provide methodologic guidelines for authors. A conference of medical editors was held in 1989 to provide a forum for discussion of general issues regarding the role of journals, including peer review.

A more radical idea is for the major funding agencies, in particular NCI, to take an active role in the dissemination of the results from the studies they fund. NCI is already extensively involved in the prospective registration of cancer trials through its sponsorship of the ICRDB. As well as being useful as an ideal source for meta-analysis, the registry is also extremely valuable in promoting collaboration and in helping physicians to identify available clinical trials. However, this activity reflects the preoccupation at the National Institutes of Health with peer review at the planning stage of research, in contrast to other agencies, which give more attention to the conduct and completion of research studies. The present system governing the publication of results is largely uncontrolled. Cancer trials, if published at all, are published in a remarkably broad range of specialized and general medical journals. This system could be radically streamlined if NCI were to provide new and more effective vehicles for information dissemination; for example, a standardized data summarization format could be developed and linked to the computerized registry. Investigators of NCI-sponsored studies would be required, within a reasonable time after completion of the study, to report the data in the standard format so that the results would be available on-line to subscribers. These reports could even be published routinely by NCI. Moreover, the system need not preclude the option for investigators to publish their results in journals in the conventional way. For the system to be effective, the standardization of the reporting is important, and some broad agreement would be necessary on the format of the data summaries. In addition, investigators would have to recognize that they do not have proprietary control over the data. This is not an insurmountable task, given our collective experience with cancer trials in the past few decades. Indeed, there have been various calls in recent years for better standardization of the reporting of clinical trials, especially in the form of the abstracts [12]. The cancer research community and NCI in particular have the opportunity to provide leadership in this task, in view of the resources available (computerized registration of studies) and the long-term experience with clinical trials.

This plan, if implemented, could have substantial impact on the need for our fourth strategy, dealing with the role of the investigator in dissemination of research results. At present, the opinions and incentives of the author have a large impact on the manner in which results are both interpreted and reported. If NCI provides a format for data standardization in the registry, the objective data can be reported dispassionately, without the subjective inferences that are believed by many to play a major role in the creation of publication bias.

This point of view may be surprising to readers, in view of the central role that statistical inferences play in the current system of research reporting. It is important to reflect on the historic development of statistical theory and its role in shaping this system.

The theoretical foundations for classical statistical approaches, the significance test in particular, were developed in the early part of this century by scientists who faced a very different scientific world than we face today. There were relatively few research institutions, and investigators worked under the generally realistic assumption that their study was unique. It is not surprising that they developed an analytic tool, the significance test, designed to make *definitive* inferences from an individual study without reference to any other information. Also, since relatively few investigators were conducting research, they probably had little doubt that their results would be published and found no need for the flamboyant claims that characterize many contemporary submissions.

Now the scientific world is entirely different. Issues in cancer research, for example, are characterized by the breadth of the scope of the research rather than the uniqueness of individual studies. Therefore, the interpretation of the results of one's own study involves the integration of information from a variety of other sources. Moreover, this interpretation should also be made with the recognition that subsequent research is inevitable and that the individual study is merely one contribution to the accumulating evidence on the topic at hand. Thus, the foundation of the significance test, based on a definitive interpretation of an individual study, with its attendant encouragement to the advocacy style of analysis and interpretation, is much less appropriate for contemporary scientific inference.

There is nothing new about this point of view. There has been a growing disquiet among statisticians regarding the deleterious effects of significance testing, although the technique still has many supporters. One epidemiology journal has even strongly advised against the use of significance testing.

However, if a system were available for the routine publication of objective summary data, as outlined here, the impact of significance testing on the supply of research information would be curtailed, and we would all have the opportunity to make our own inferences about the available, objective information.

DISCUSSION

The existence of publication bias has been recognized for many years, though only recently have attempts been made to study it quantitatively. In medicine, this phenomenon is usually reflected in the preponderance of studies with (false) positive results in the literature. It is believed to be caused by a variety of factors, including editorial and author preferences, with author preferences prompted to some extent by the perception that a positive or significant finding will increase the chances of the article being accepted and will draw attention to the finding. Another proposed cause is the advocacy style of statistical analysis and reporting, with the study by itself expected to provide a definitive conclusion. The few empiric studies of the problem suggest that publication bias is associated with (small) sample size, whether or not the study is registered, and design features such as (absence of) randomization. The results of a study of registered phase II cancer protocols indicate that many of these studies are never published; current research using records of institutional review boards should shed further light on the issue of what proportion of studies conducted are never published. Finally, beyond the objective data, the tone and style of research reporting are important causes of bias and other misconceptions.

A variety of proposals have been suggested for dealing with these problems. They include the creation and expansion of registries of clinical trials and other scientific investigations, although the field of oncology is already relatively well served in this regard. It has been suggested that editorial policy should be changed to encourage peer review of manuscripts on the basis of methods rather than results or even peer review at the design stage with a subsequent guarantee of publication for prospective studies. A more radical suggestion is that the major funding agencies (e.g. NCI) should take greater responsibility for ensuring the dissemination of the funded research. The need for NCI to take a more active role in this area is evidenced by the recent initiative to distribute the Clinical Alert about findings regarding the treatment of node-negative breast cancer (Chapter 28). A more comprehensive approach would involve the creation of vehicles for the efficient reporting of studies. An on-line system of standard reports linked to the registry of trials would be invaluable. In fact, the raw data collected should be in the public domain, with patient names undisclosed. One can envisage a library of computer files containing a standardized minimal data set; however, the complexity of this task cannot be overlooked, in view of the range of data items collected in clinical studies.

Finally, investigators should be encouraged to make better use of accepted measures of summarized data rather than relying on significance testing when the study is clearly not definitive. We must recognize that concurrent studies are often similar and that each investigator is a contributor to the global research effort rather than the author of a unique and conclusive report, and this should be reflected in the statistical methods used.

There are a number of qualifications to this discussion. First, the arguments have been based on the premise that publication bias has a seriously distorting effect on medical research. There are those who believe that the problem is exaggerated. Their argument is: (a) that studies with negative results, especially exploratory studies, are less important than studies with positive results; (b) that the sophisticated observer is able to suitably discount exaggerated claims; (c) that confirmatory studies and anecdotal evidence will eventually contradict false-positive results; and (d) that the present system may be an efficient vehicle for developing a consensus. It is difficult to disprove such assertions. It is evident, however, that the present system of disseminating research is haphazard and uncontrolled, and we are largely ignorant about its effects on the diffusion of medical information and about the consequences of any change.

The empiric studies that were used to quantify publication bias and identify its correlates have been criticized on the grounds that they may also be biased. It is certainly true that the studies are all both retrospective and exploratory. However, the likely existence of publication bias is evident to any investigator who is actively involved in research. The empiric studies simply reflect the magnitude of the problem, and it seems to be large. The results suggest that sample size is a strong risk factor for bias. Should small studies, therefore, be discouraged? Some investigators believe that the greatest efforts should be concentrated on large studies of selected issues. Small exploratory trials, however, play a valuable role in the formulation of new ideas and the discarding of ineffective hypotheses prior to the start of large trials; therefore, they seem essential to the scientific process. Small trials need not be discouraged. We must simply interpret the results with appropriate caution, and we must find ways to ensure that the small trials and negative results are recorded.

A major theme of this review has been the role of statistical significance testing and the advocacy style of analysis in the creation of publication bias. It is important, however, to distinguish bias in the reporting of objective data from the natural enthusiasm of the investigator for the research. Enthusiasm and advocacy are integral features of human commitment, and their presence in the discussion section of a publication has a positive influence in stimulating the reader's interest and stirring controversy. Scientific speculation is also an essential ingredient. Problems relating to publication bias occur when the style of analysis and its consequences interfere with the reporting of the objective data, and it is by the structured reporting of prospective studies that we can best circumvent this problem.

It is important to distinguish between phase III comparative studies, which are relatively large and often conducted in a co-operative group setting, and the more exploratory phase I and II studies, which are much smaller and usually not randomized. From our empiric investigations, it is clear that publication bias is a much more serious problem in phase I and II studies. However, in these exploratory studies, commitment and enthusiasm play an important role in stimulating investigators to develop new theories and try new ideas, often in very small pilot trials. Small, flexible studies are entirely appropriate in this setting, and the advocacy style of reporting is almost inevitable. We emphasize that our recommendations regarding the structured reporting of studies are especially important for this type of study and are designed to ensure that the *data* are objectively reported, even though the theories and hypotheses are speculative.

The journals play a central role in the process of research dissemination. However, if the on-line standardized reporting of trials were to become a reality, it seems inevitable that the primary role of the journals would change. Currently, their primary role is reporting original research; in their secondary functions they serve as a medium for education and for reviews of the literature and as a forum for debates on controversial issues. If reporting of research studies outside the journal system were more standardized, the major role of the journals would tilt toward their present secondary functions. These functions used to be the primary role of the journals in the early days of medical journalism, before the relatively recent enormous expansion of the medical research effort.

In summary, the scientific world has become increasingly complex in recent years. The scope of cancer research is vast, and investigators must now struggle, using modern library science methods, to keep abreast of the relevant literature, most of which is still published in independent journals. A major consequence of the system is publication bias. It seems likely that information technology will continue to evolve rapidly. We need to harness this evolution to encourage the efficient dissemination of scientific information. The NCI is in a unique position to provide leadership in directing these changes by structuring the system to facilitate dissemination of the results of studies in the cancer clinical trials program.

ACKNOWLEDGMENTS

This work was supported by Public Health Service grants CA-35291 and CA-38493 from the National Cancer Institute, National Institutes of Health, Department of Health and Human Services.

REFERENCES

1. Begg CB, Berlin JA (1988) Publication bias: a problem in interpreting medical data. J R Stat Soc A 151: 419–463
2. Chalmers TC (1982) Informed consent, clinical research and the practice of medicine. Trans Am Clin Climatol Assoc 94: 204–212
3. Dickersin K, Chan S, Chalmers TC et al (1987) Publication bias and clinical trials. Controlled Clin Trials 8: 343–353
4. Sacks HS, Chalmers TC, Smith H (1983) Sensitivity and specificity of clinical trials: randomized versus historical controls. Arch Intern Med 143: 753–755
5. Moertel CG (1984) Improving the efficiency of clinical trials: a medical perspective. Stat Med 3: 455–466
6. Davidson RA (1986) Source of funding and outcome of clinical trials. J Gen Intern Med 1: 155–158
7. L'Abbe KA, Detsky AS, O'Rourke K (1987) Meta-analysis in clinical research. Ann Intern Med 107: 24–233
8. Berlin JA, Begg CB, Louis TA (1989) An assessment of publication bias using a sample of published clinical trials. J Am Stat Assoc 84: 381–392
9. Simes RJ (1986) Confronting publication bias: a cohort design for meta-analysis. Stat Med 6: 11–30
10. Newcombe RG (1987) Towards a reduction in publication bias. Br Med J 295: 656–659
11. Kochar MS (1986) The peer review of manuscripts: in need for improvement. J Chronic Dis 39: 147–149
12. Huth EJ (1987) Structured abstracts for papers reporting clinical trials. Ann Intern Med 106: 626–627

ABOUT THE AUTHORS

Colin B. Begg has a variety of research interests in biostatistical theory and applications, primarily in the area of medical oncology. His methodo-logical research encompasses clinical trials, epidemiological studies, evaluations of diagnostic technologies and medical imaging trials. More recently he has been studying meta-analysis techniques and publication bias.

After receiving his PhD from the University of Glasgow, Dr Begg spent a year at the State University of New York at Buffalo before taking an appointment at the Harvard School of Public Health, where he remained from 1977 until 1989. He is currently Chairman of the Department of Epidemiology and Biostatistics at Memorial Sloan-Kettering Cancer Center, and Professor of Biostatistics at Cornell Medical School.

Jesse A. Berlin received his undergraduate training in biology at Yale College. He went on to earn a Master of Science degree in natural resources at the University of Michigan, where he collaborated on research in health promotion. He completed a Doctor of Science degree in biostatistics at the Harvard School of Public Health under the direction of Dr Begg.

Dr Berlin's research interests have been in the area of meta-analysis—the combination of analytical results from different studies. In particular, he has devoted much effort to exploring the application of meta-analytical methods to epidemiological results. He is currently involved in epidemiological research at the University of Pennsylvania, in the Clinical Epidemiology Unit.

The work presented here stems from Dr Berlin's doctoral research performed under the guidance of Dr Begg.

26 The Role of Overviews

LESLEY STEWART

Overviews or meta-analyses originated in the social sciences, but the methods involved are equally applicable to any quantitative discipline. The use of this technique to combine formally the results from similar clinical trials began to appear in the medical literature in the mid-1970s and has gained prominence in cancer research during the late 1980s. As with any other new research tool, the acceptance of overviews has not been without difficulty; there is contention over certain issues and there remain some sceptics who dispute the use of the technique at all. Generally, however, overviews are perceived as a useful analytical addition to clinical research. This chapter aims beyond this, and in addition to describing overview methodology proposes that the overview process can lead to unprecedented levels of international collaboration out of which can grow something potentially even more valuable than the analysis itself.

THE NEED FOR OVERVIEWS

In oncology it is seldom the case that a novel form of therapy shows such marked improvement over standard treatment that a single clinical trial furnishes conclusive evidence of its increased efficacy. Recently it has become generally accepted that despite the desire to find miracle cures and "magic bullets", moderate survival improvements are generally the best that can be hoped of new treatments. It has also been realized that these moderate benefits can be both clinically worthwhile and extremely important in terms of their public health consequences.

The problem is that with such moderate effects it is difficult to establish whether observed differences between treatments are real or due to the play of chance. This difficulty arises because the reliability of trial results depends on the degree of scatter or distribution of events around the mean effect for each treatment. Greater numbers of events in each arm of a trial lead to better-defined distributions and narrower confidence intervals, so that there is increased reliability in detecting differences between treatments. In other words detection of moderate treatment effects requires large clinical trials. Figure 1 illustrates this principle: assuming a baseline survival rate of 50% at two years for a standard treatment, then a typical two-arm trial with 400–500 patients is capable only of detecting treatment effects in

Introducing New Treatments for Cancer: Practical, Ethical and Legal Problems. Edited by C. J. Williams
© 1992 John Wiley & Sons Ltd

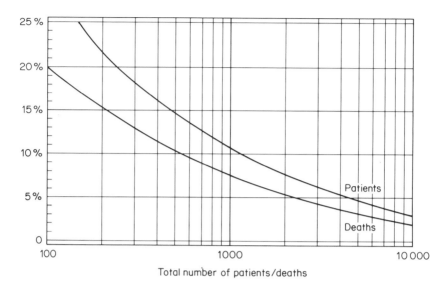

Total number of patients/deaths

Figure 1. Percentage improvement in survival detectable with various sample sizes (adapted from Freedman [1])

excess of 15% (i.e. an increase from 50% to 65% or more). To detect reliably a 10% difference requires twice this number, while a 5% difference would require thousands of patients. Until the late 1980s it was virtually unheard of for cancer clinical trials to plan to recruit anything like these numbers and many trials involved fewer than 100 patients. Consequently there are numerous areas of oncology where many such small or medium-sized clinical trials have addressed the same or similar therapeutic questions, but owing to the lack of patient numbers the results from these trials have been inconclusive. Consequently the therapeutic issues have remained unresolved. The inference often drawn from such a collection of equivocal and sometimes conflicting results is that there is no difference between the treatments in question. In fact, owing to the potentially large effect of random fluctuation in small clinical trials, the distribution of the results is often consistent with the possibility of a moderate treatment benefit.

In such situations the desire to amalgamate existing information is intuitive and making informal comparisons across studies is an almost inevitable hazard of reading the medical literature. Traditionally this informal approach to pooling data has been propagated by the ubiquitous review article, commonly written by an eminent physician and thereby presenting an apparently authoritative view of the treatments in question. Yet despite the reviewer's best efforts and intentions this means of reaching consensus can be seriously flawed.

Usually only published results are considered and the reviewer is often at the disadvantage of having to review his or her own data as well as that of others. Most importantly there is often simply too much confusing and conflicting information to make sensible deductions from a mere qualitative reading of the published texts. An overview or meta-analysis is based on the same underlying philosophy of amalgamating information, but differs importantly in that it offers a *formal quantitative method of combining the results* from similar clinical trials. Thus in the absence of definitive large-scale randomized studies, and given the unreliability of the review process, an overview often offers the best means of clarifying a confusing clinical situation. In fact, the scope of overviews is wider than this in that they serve as a link between past and future research. The summary and synthesis of existing information that they provide serves the dual purpose of providing the best estimates of relative efficacy for existing treatments and of identifying future areas of study.

Both the terms "overview" and "meta-analysis" (the two can be used synonymously although the former tends to be preferred in the UK and the latter in continental Europe and North America) have been used to describe techniques that range from calculations based on figures taken from a few fully published papers to those founded on carefully collected individual patient data from all known randomized clinical trials. Clearly the latter, which tend to be known as systematic overviews, are the more reliable, and it is on these that this chapter concentrates.

The fundamental assumption of any overview of studies addressing similar questions is that although the size of treatment effect may vary from trial to trial these are likely to be in the same direction, although in a small number of cases this direction may be reversed by chance alone. Thus, although the direction of treatment benefit may be obscured in an individual trial, when all the evidence is considered the nature of the treatment effect will be reflected in the overall pattern of individual trial results and some form of summation of these results will provide an estimate of the average treatment effect.

It is extremely important to understand this assumption since the most common objection to the methodology of overviews is based on the misconception that studies which have different eligibility criteria and which come from different patient populations are being crudely combined. In fact, the only direct comparisons that are made are between the arms of each randomized study in turn and it is only the *results* of these individual within-trial comparisons which are combined. Although it would be wrong to assume that the effect of a treatment administered slightly differently to patient populations who may vary in a number of important characteristics would be to produce exactly the same reduction in the risk of death, it is reasonable to assume that the net effect will be in the same direction.

DESIGN OF SYSTEMATIC OVERVIEWS

A good rationale is perhaps even more critical in an overview than in an individual trial, given the potentially influential status that large numbers of patients can provide. The design of an overview is based on avoiding both random and systematic errors in order that they are not so substantial as to obscure moderate treatment effects. Although random errors cannot, by their very nature, ever be eliminated they can be minimized by including large numbers of patients. Systematic errors or bias can occur through bad design or flawed analysis but can be minimized by adhering to the following general principles.

INCLUDE ONLY PROPERLY RANDOMIZED CLINICAL TRIALS

The implicit potential bias in non-randomized studies, which is well documented, is the reason that overviews should be restricted to include only randomized controlled clinical trials. However, not all studies described as randomized clinical trials can be assumed to be free from bias since some randomization methods may be insecure. For example, alternative allocation, randomization by birthdate and even the sealed envelope method do not ensure that treatment allocation is blind.

If a clinician may, whether unwittingly or not, determine the treatment to be allocated to the next patient and on the basis of this information decide whether or not to enter that patient into the trial, then bias can result. Each individual case where there is any potential problem with the randomization procedure must be considered very carefully indeed before being included in or excluded from the overview. Individual patient records are invaluable in this respect since they permit certain checks on the integrity of randomization such as testing for imbalances in prognostic factors.

INCLUDE ALL RELEVANT PUBLISHED AND UNPUBLISHED TRIALS

As there is considerable evidence that both journal editors and investigators themselves are more likely to publish trials with "positive" results (see Chapter 25), all relevant randomized studies should be included in an overview in order to avoid this potential publication bias. This principle is not universally accepted and those disputing its validity would claim that the quality of unpublished data which has not been subject to "peer review" is unreliable. This criticism can be largely circumvented by obtaining the trial protocol and individual patient data so that the overviewer can check both the data and trial design for flaws or inconsistencies, thus in a sense performing the "peer review" himself. Conversely it should be noted that publication of an apparently sound manuscript does not guarantee the quality of the actual data. Data and protocols have to be examined equally thoroughly for both published and unpublished studies.

ANALYSE ON "INTENTION TO TREAT"

All patients entered in a trial should be analysed according to the treatment that they were allocated at randomization irrespective of whether or not they actually received that treatment.

Many trial reports exclude high proportions of patients, often for spurious reasons, and this can give rise to a huge potential for bias. For example, consider a hypothetical study in which a control arm of no adjuvant treatment is compared to one in which post-surgical chemotherapy is administered.

A number of patients may die postoperatively but before receiving chemotherapy. If these patients are excluded from the survival analysis (reports doing this are far from uncommon) then clearly the results will be biased in favour of the chemotherapy; essentially the very poor prognosis patients have been removed from the treatment but not the control arm. Obtaining individual data for each and every patient randomized is obviously necessary if such a trial is to be re-analysed according to the intention-to-treat principle.

COMMON OBJECTIONS TO OVERVIEWS

Even if the above principles are followed there are some commonly cited objections to the methodology and usage of overviews that can be raised: one widely expressed concern regarding overview design is that trials vary in quality and that combining results from "good" and "bad" studies in some sense dilutes the results of the "good" trials. As a consequence it has been suggested that trials should be assessed and in some way weighted to take account of this. However, a good systematic overview circumvents this need in a number of ways:

(1) If the question that the overview poses is well formulated, then any trial with a poor overall rationale will not meet the overview eligibility criteria.
(2) Exclusion of improperly randomized trials will tend to remove "poor-quality" studies since the randomization procedure is probably the most common and most important source of flawed trial design.
(3) Collection of individual patient data allows the original data to be checked. This does not rely on data from the published article; it is often the written article and not the trial itself that is of poor quality.
(4) Use of "hard" end-points such as survival leave little room for any subjective interpretation which can result in bias and poor-quality data.

Additionally, if trials were to be weighted for quality by the overviewers, then this could in itself be a potential source of bias on their part. It is also important not to alienate investigators who may be less keen to collaborate in the knowledge that their publications are to be assessed for quality and scored publicly.

A similar concern is that when the results of trials with different eligibility criteria are pooled, responsive and non-responsive patient populations are being combined, so that the net effect will be to see no difference between treatments. However, it is generally true that although different patient populations may show responses that differ quantitatively they are unlikely to be qualitatively different. Further, it can be argued that a cross-section of patient types from a number of different trials is more likely to reflect the real world of heterogeneous patient types and therefore to reflect more accurately the type of treatment effects that are achievable outside clinical trials. This does not of course mean that the characteristics of patient populations can be ignored or that there will never be identifiable subgroups that respond differently to treatment. Clearly each overview needs to be considered on an individual basis and this problem will be reflected in the nature of the questions that the overview addresses.

Other more general criticisms concern the impact that overviews can have on prospective randomized trials. One fear is that important ongoing studies can be disrupted by the results of a meta-analysis. This can of course be perfectly legitimate in certain circumstances, for example, if an overview reliably shows a significant and worthwhile benefit for one type of treatment over another then it would be unethical to continue a trial that compared these two treatments. The concern remains that if incorrect conclusions are drawn from an overview, then valuable trials can be stopped or fail to recruit. This particular problem is not restricted to the misinterpretation of overviews—the same can be true of individual trials. However, the large number of patients involved in an overview can lend much weight to the conclusions drawn, even if they are based on misinterpretation. This particular problem emphasizes the importance of good reporting practice; the onus must be on the overviewers to present the results in a manner that will minimize misinterpretation or misrepresentation.

Another fear is that overviews encourage small individual studies rather than participation in large collaborative trials. It is difficult to imagine a situation where trialists deliberately set up small trials a priori with insufficient patient numbers to answer the questions posed with the justification that they may at some point in the future be incorporated into an overview. In contrast the prospect of performing a number of co-ordinated parallel trials holds a certain appeal. In such situations individual institutions or groups may have minor differences in protocols as dictated by local conditions and perhaps perform their own randomization, but eventually the data from all the trials will be pooled in an overview. The advantage of such prospective overviews is that there are cases where it is simply not feasible to recruit thousands of patients from around the world into a single study, and here it is surely advantageous to co-ordinate activity in such a way that will yield meaningful results. In point of fact the evidence from cardiovascular research suggests that overviews actually promote the setting up of large randomized trials through the collaboration and goodwill that they can generate [2].

PRACTICAL ASPECTS OF PERFORMING A SYSTEMATIC OVERVIEW

A great deal of effort is involved in performing a systematic overview and it is certainly not a task to be undertaken lightly or on a part-time basis. For example, it is estimated that the Advanced Ovarian Cancer Overview, initiated by the British Medical Research Council, required a minimum of two person-years (excluding the time of those preparing the raw data) from initiation to presentation of the results of the initial survival analyses at the first collaborators' meeting. Figure 2 illustrates the series of steps which are involved in performing such an overview and which are described in more detail below.

INITIAL DESIGN PHASE

Since good design is of the utmost importance in an overview, it is important to draft a protocol at an early stage and this should certainly be done before embarking upon data collection.

This functions both to set out clearly the aims of the overview and to identify any potential problems. It can also be used to demonstrate the scientific rationale and serious intent of the overview to trialists, persuading them that if they supply their data for analysis it will be used wisely. With the same aim of initiating co-operation it is extremely important to remember at all times the vast effort that has gone into each individual trial and that the data from these belongs to the original investigators. It is necessary to establish from the outset the extent of involvement of trialists and the publication procedure. The large international systematic overviews in oncology [3–5] have been based on the formation of a collaborative group of trial investigators, with publications and presentations being made in the name of the group, and it seems likely that this contributed significantly to their success.

It is of course crucial to pose the correct question(s) in terms of what is important therapeutically, what data are available and what constitutes an exciting project, since the overview must have a wide appeal if it is to

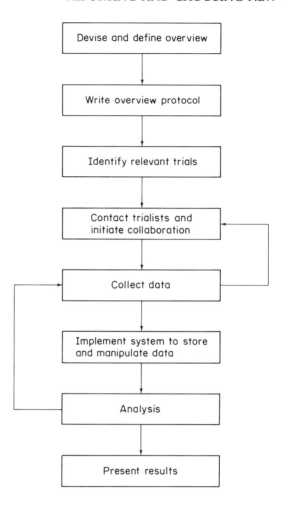

Figure 2. Stages involved in performing a systematic overview

generate enough enthusiasm from trialists to carry it through to completion. Overviews should be performed in situations where there is genuine confusion over trial results and where sufficient data are available to be analysed in a sensible manner. The questions that the overview poses should be formulated in a way that will yield meaningful results. Here there may be a trade-off in defining precisely the form of comparison(s) to be made. For example, if a comparison of chemotherapies is restricted to include trials using only exactly the same drugs administered in identical conditions, then each comparison will necessarily include fewer patients than groupings of functionally equivalent drugs.

IDENTIFYING ALL RELEVANT TRIALS

This is a major undertaking, in itself requiring considerable time and effort to reach an exhaustive listing of relevant trials, especially in the case of unpublished studies. A good starting point is to perform a bibliographic search using on-line databases such as CANCERLIT and MEDLINE.

These searches should be supplemented by cross-checking the reference lists of existing trials, review articles and textbooks, since computer-aided searching techniques can be imperfect and database entries incomplete. CLINPROT, which is part of the National Cancer Institute's PDQ (Physicians Database Query) system, is extremely useful in identifying ongoing studies especially in the USA, and the UK Cancer Coordinating Committee Trials Register provides a similar means of identifying British trials. Meeting abstracts are an invaluable source of information on trials which have never been reported fully, even if searching through all the entries in a particular field is somewhat laborious.

Identification of unpublished studies is undoubtedly the most difficult task and one which depends largely on word of mouth. One means of discovering these studies is to send questionnaires to known trialists and experts in the field, asking them to supplement a provisional list of trials with any further trials (published or unpublished) that they or colleagues may have performed. Another route is to approach pharmaceutical companies with a particular research interest in the field and ask them to list trials that they have either performed or sponsored.

Inevitably the outcome of this searching process is to produce an initial list of plausible trials many times the length of the final one. Although a good many trials can be disregarded after an initial reading of the abstract, inevitably numerous published articles and protocols have to be read in order to determine exactly which trials meet the overview eligibility criteria.

This monumental task of providing a listing of all revelant trials is one which may eventually be much simplified if, as has been proposed by many people [6], an international cancer registry is established and all cancer clinical trials are prospectively logged with the registry. Since trials would be registered from the outset there should be no selectivity in the reporting process and the register would therefore form an unbiased, though not necessarily exhaustive, sample of trials upon which overviews could be based.

CONTACTING TRIALISTS AND INITIATING COLLABORATION

Even the apparently straightforward task of making contact with trialists can be both difficult and extremely time consuming, given that addresses taken from publications can be out of date and tracing authors can be problematic. It is obviously difficult to obtain data from a large number of people who naturally may be protective or possessive of their studies. The success of any overview will owe much to devoting a large amount of time and energy to explaining the need for and rationale of the overview to the original investigators. This involves communication by letter, fax, telephone and where necessary by site visits. Naturally the best selling point for a project is that it is a good one, but trialists also need to be assured of the serious intent of the overviewers. This task has undoubtedly been made easier by the success of the Breast Cancer Overview [1, 2], since the very feasibility of systematic overviews has been demonstrated. Collecting individual patient data can require much work on the part of the trialist, who may even have to go back to original patient notes in the case of old studies, although with more and more trials being maintained on computer this may be less of a problem in the future.

Even with minimal data collection it is important not to underestimate the amount of time required to perform the simple administrative tasks involved in keeping track of a large number of studies and vast number of patients, and to keep in close contact with many investigators worldwide. One encouraging point is that data collection is inevitably a "bandwagon" process; the more people that have already agreed to collaborate and provide data, the easier it is to persuade others to do the same.

COLLECTING AND COLLATING INDIVIDUAL PATIENT DATA

A very important, although not highly visible, aspect of an overview is in the design, implementation and maintenance of a system on which to store and manipulate individual patient data from each participating trial. Although no hard and fast rules can be made about what type of computational approach is most appropriate (it will depend largely on the expertise available to the overviewers and will vary from one overview to another), it is recommended that considerable thought be given to this matter at an early stage. Clearly when dealing with data from thousands of individual patients an efficient and reliable means of storage and retrieval is required. The resulting system should facilitate easy keyboard entry and be able to transfer information from other systems via electronic and magnetic media with minimal programming. It should also be flexible enough to incorporate modifications that may be necessary as new types of information need to be stored or different means of data manipulation carried out.

This side of an overview is all too easily overlooked and is seldom mentioned in the literature; it is, however, of vital importance to the success of the project and is certainly an aspect of an overview which should not be underestimated.

STATISTICAL ANALYSIS

The statistical techniques most frequently employed in meta-analyses are based on the Mantel–Haenszel method of combining data over a series of 2×2 contingency tables. Note that although discussion here refers only to survival, the methods described may also be applied to surrogate end-points such as recurrence. Basically this involves comparing the observed and expected numbers of deaths on treatment and control within each individual trial. There are a number of ways of doing this, the simplest of which utilizes the proportion of patients dead and alive at one or more time points. For each individual trial the overall death rate within the study is used to calculate the expected number of deaths that would occur if there was no difference in survival between the two arms of the trial. A worked example of this is shown in Table 1. The difference between the actual observed (O) and this expected (E) number of deaths is then calculated for the treatment arm, giving the $O-E$ value. A negative $O-E$ value indicates that the treatment group has fared better than the control group, whilst a positive $O-E$ value indicates the opposite.

These individual $O-E$ values can then be summed for the treatment group. If the treatment has no effect then each individual $O-E$ value could be either positive or negative and differ only randomly from zero. Likewise the overall $O-E$ value from all the studies will differ only randomly from zero if the treatment is not beneficial. If, however, the treatment does have a beneficial effect then there will be a trend for each individual $O-E$ value to be negative, and the overall summated value to be clearly so.

Table 1 shows how these $O-E$ values can be used to calculate odds ratios (OR) for each trial. This OR, which is approximately equal to the hazards ratio, represents the ratio of the odds of death among the treatment group patients to the corresponding odds of death among the control patients. An OR value of 1.0 represents equal risks or no difference between treatments, while a value of 0.5 indicates a doubling in survival chances for patients in the treatment arm. A pooled OR can be calculated by summing the individual $O-E$ and variance values in such a way that the pooled OR represents a weighted average of the individual mortality ratios where the individual trials which contain the most information (usually the largest trials) influence the estimate most.

Figure 3 illustrates the standard means of graphical representation of this type of information. The mortality ratio for each study is plotted as an occluded square, whose size is directly proportional to the amount of information in any one trial. Horizontal lines extend outwards from this to display the confidence intervals. A vertical line is drawn through unity to indicate the point where there is no difference between treatments. Trials indicating an advantage for the treatment will lie to the left of this line and those showing advantage to the control will lie to the right. Trials indicating

Table 1. Hypothetical example of the statistical methods used in overviews

Suppose there are four trials comparing surgery plus adjuvant chemotherapy versus surgery alone and that the number of deaths on each arm of these trials are those given below:

	Treatment	Control	p-value
Trial A	22/40	28/42	0.27
Trial B	24/40	30/40	0.16
Trial C	14/20	12/20	0.52
Trial D	44/100	56/100	0.09

Thus for trial A there are 40 patients on the treatment arm, of whom 22 have died. None of these trials show a statistically significant difference between the number of deaths on the treatment and control arm. Thus a qualitative examination of these trials, as would happen with a review article, offers no good evidence that adjuvant chemotherapy improves survival. A quantitative pooled analysis can be performed as follows: for trial A the expected number of deaths (E), $O-E$ value ($O-E$), variance (Var) and odds ratio (OR) can be calculated as shown below.

	Treatment	Control	Total
Dead	22	28	50 (D)
Alive	18	14	32
Total	40 (n_t)	42	82 (N)

Expected number of deaths on treatment $O-E$ *value*

$E \quad = (D/N)n_t$ $O-E = 22 - 24.4$

$\quad = (50/82)40$ $\quad\quad = -2.4$

$\quad = 24.4$

Odds ratio

$OR \quad = \exp (O-E/\text{Var})$ $*\text{Var} = [E(1-n_t/N)(N-D)]/(N-1)$

$\quad\quad \exp (-2.4/4.9*)$ $\quad\quad = [24.4(1-40/82)(82-50)]/81$

$\quad\quad = 0.61$ $\quad\quad = 4.9$

Values can be calculated in the same way for trials B, C and D to produce the following table.

	$O-E$	Variance	Odds ratio
Trial A	-2.4	4.9	0.61
Trial B	-3.5	4.4	0.51
Trial C	1.0	2.3	1.54
Trial D	-6.0	12.6	0.62

Overall odds ratio for all trials

$OR \quad = \exp [\Sigma(O-E)/\Sigma \text{ Var}]$

$\quad\quad = \exp (-10.4/24.2)$

$\quad\quad = 0.65$ (95% c.i.'s$=0.44$, 0.97)*   *Confidence intervals$=$
$\quad\quad\quad\quad\quad\quad\quad\quad\quad\quad\quad\quad\quad\quad\quad\quad\quad\quad \exp [(\Sigma O - E/\Sigma \text{Var}) \pm (1.96/(\sqrt{\Sigma} \text{ Var}))]$

Conclusions

Although none of the individual trials in this hypothetical example showed a significant difference between treatments, the overview analysis shows a significant survival advantage for patients treated with adjuvant chemotherapy with a 35% reduction in the odds of death for these patients.

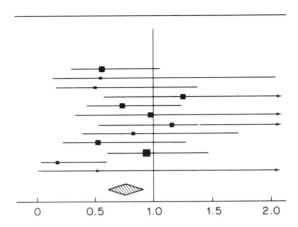

Figure 3. Mortality ratios plotted for a hypothetical example

a significant result will lie wholly to one side of the line, i.e. the confidence interval will not straddle it. The overall pooled OR is shown as a hatched lozenge whose extremities denote the overall confidence interval.

A good visual impression is gained from this type of plot, in that any trends are immediately apparent and an idea of the increase in precision of the combined estimate is gained by the short length of its confidence intervals relative to the confidence intervals of the ORs for individual studies.

When survival information is available on a year-by-year basis as is available from tabular or individual patient data, a number of calculations can be performed to provide $O-E$ values at, for example, 1, 2, 3, 4 and 5+ years. Summing these figures for each trial over time gives a log-rank type statistic for a year of death analysis and calculation of the overall OR now represents the annual odds of death.

In many cases it may be more appropriate to calculate the actual hazard ratios (HRs) rather than using ORs. Here the log-rank expected values are calculated, taking into account the time to each event in the treatment and control group, and the variance is the log-rank variance. The easiest means of doing this is via a standard statistical package such as BMDP. Once the $O-E$ and Var values have been calculated the calculations proceed as before with the overall HR value equivalent to $\exp[\Sigma(O-E)/\Sigma\text{Var}]$ but using the log-rank $O-E$ and Var. This method requires that the duration of survival is available for each individual patient but has the important advantage of providing a more sensitive analysis.

THE COLLABORATIVE GROUP MEETING

There are a number of reasons why it is important to the success of any major overview to hold a meeting of all collaborators. The trialists themselves deserve to have the opportunity to hear first hand the overview results, to air their opinions and publicly accept or reject the findings of the overview—it is after all their data. Since a major problem in clinical research is the dissemination of information and the transfer of results from research into practice, if the overview results are debated and endorsed by an international group of experts it will have a far greater chance of making an impact on clinical practice. Finally, and extremely importantly, the immense potential in assembling such a group of specialists for generating and promoting future collaboration must not be overlooked. This is an area that needs to be exploited fully since such a meeting is an ideal opportunity for assessing the state of the art in existing treatments and providing a platform for deciding what areas of treatment need clarifying or what new studies are needed in the future. Indeed it provides an excellent chance of initiating or promoting the large-scale clinical trials that overviews are sometimes seen to be in competition with.

EXAMPLES OF SYSTEMATIC OVERVIEWS

THE BREAST CANCER OVERVIEW

It is probably true to say that overviews have gained credibility in the medical world largely owing to the efforts of the Oxford group, whose stringent approach in the use of the technique culminated in the Breast Cancer Overview [3]. This, the first systematic overview of its kind, examined the question of whether or not adjuvant tamoxifen and cytotoxic chemo-therapy reduced mortality in breast cancer. The overview was conducted on behalf of the Early Breast Cancer Trialists Collaborative Group and at first publication had collected data from 61 randomized clinical trials involving a staggering 28 896 women worldwide.

The study illustrates very well the principles of good overview design: there were clear-cut questions that needed to be posed, since confusion existed over whether or not adjuvant systemic treatment of operable breast cancer was desirable. Although it was agreed that such treatment extended disease-free survival, worries that this was counterbalanced by poor activity in patients who relapsed meant that there was no consensus on whether this effect was translated into survival advantages. Every effort was made to obtain information on all relevant published and unpublished trials which were identified from bibliographic sources on computer databases and published texts, meeting abstracts, cancer registries and from discussion with the trialists themselves. Proper randomization technique was a prerequisite for trial inclusion and the analysis was, at least initially, restricted to the hard end-point of survival. Individual patient data were obtained from all but four collaborative groups and extensive checks were made on each of these data sets for any irregularities or sources of bias.

The role of tamoxifen was evaluated by combining the results from all randomized clinical trials in which the treatment arms within any one trial differed only by the addition of tamoxifen.

There was great variability in the apparent treatment effect between the 28 studies which fitted this description, the wide confidence intervals of each of these reflecting the unreliability of separate individual estimates. The combination of the results from these trials showed a reduction in the annual odds of death ratio by 16%, which is equivalent to an absolute increase of 5% in the survival rate of five years for the tamoxifen arm. This is a highly significant result ($p=0.00001$), which cannot be attributed to chance.

When the same comparison was made according to age group, dividing patients into women younger than 50 years and women of 50 and over it became apparent that this effect was only clear in older women. A significant effect was not demonstrated in the younger age group, although smaller numbers of patients in this group produced wider confidence intervals, and hence even the meta-analysis of the 3652 women in this group is not as accurate as might be wished.

For the 31 trials that compared adjuvant chemotherapy with no chemotherapy there was an overall improvement in five-year survival rates of 4% in the treated patients. In this case the clearest effect was in younger women (under 50 years) whose improvement in survival was from 66% to 73%. For older women there was no clear evidence for a reduction in mortality.

Although it is now virtually impossible to hold a discussion about either overviews or the treatment of early breast cancer without mentioning the Breast Cancer Overview, that is not to say that it was immediately universally accepted; indeed much controversy followed in its wake. Much of this was in direct consequence of its publicity before publication, since the first meeting of collaborators was attached to the National Institute of Health Consensus Development Conference on the Adjuvant Chemotherapy for Breast Cancer, and the overview undoubtedly influenced the conclusions of the conference before the results had even been debated fully by the trialists themselves.

It was also an unfortunate, although perhaps predictable, consequence of the overview that indirect comparisons between chemotherapy and tamoxifen treatment were made by some readers even though the overview publication (published three years after the conference) warned against doing just that. Consequently the notion that tamoxifen was the treatment of choice for older women and chemotherapy the treatment of choice for younger women came about even although no randomized clinical trial had actually addressed this question.

At the time fears were expressed that the overview would lead to early closure and disruption of ongoing studies, and indeed there was some evidence that the number of patients being entered into trials comparing chemotherapy in older women dropped after the conference. It was also feared that the overview would encourage individual small studies rather than large collaborative ones. However, in the same way that overviews in cardiovascular disease have stimulated large-scale clinical trials such as ISIS-1 and ISIS-2 [6], a number of large trials examining the optimum duration of tamoxifen have now begun.

As well as the obvious public health consequences of the Breast Cancer Overview (it is estimated that 1000 women's lives may be saved each year in the UK alone in consequence of its findings) this project has been a landmark in the history of overviews, setting a future standard and providing a model for other similar studies. A number of lessons can also be learned from it, for example the importance of prompt publication and the importance of emphasizing the collaborative aspects of the overview, specifically its role as a potential springboard for new prospective projects in future overviews.

THE ADVANCED OVARIAN CANCER OVERVIEW

This international systematic overview was initiated by the British Medical Research Council (MRC) Gynaecological Cancer Working Party and carried out on behalf of the Advanced Ovarian Cancer Trialists Group (AOCTG) by the MRC Cancer Trials Office in Cambridge [4].

This is another good example of an area in oncology where an overview was clearly indicated: ovarian cancer is a common disease, being the fifth most common cancer of women in the world [7] and the most common cause of death attributable to gynaecological malignancy in Europe and North America. Survival rates are low, around 5–10% at five years for FIGO stages III and IV. Thus even a small improvement in survival could have important public health consequences. Following surgery, chemotherapy is accepted as standard treatment for advanced disease, but there is no general consensus about the most appropriate forms of chemotherapy, and standard treatments vary between Britain, Continental Europe and North America. Although individual randomized clinical trials have confirmed significantly higher response rates for combination and for cisplatin-based chemotherapy, they have not adequately demonstrated a corresponding improvement in survival.

The Advanced Ovarian Cancer Overview was therefore initiated to attempt to resolve important pre-existing clinical questions regarding the use of chemotherapy in the treatment of this disease. These questions, which had not been resolved by the numerous inconclusive trials reported in the literature, concerned the relative merits of single-agent and combination chemotherapy and the role of platinum in treatment.

The overview gathered information from 45 clinical trials and 8139 women from around the world, much of this data being previously unpublished. Even with such large numbers of patients no firm conclusions regarding optimal chemotherapy could be reached. However, there was an indication of a survival advantage for women treated with a platinum-based combination of drugs over those treated with non-platinum-based drugs, or with platinum alone. The results also showed there to be no difference between cisplatin and carboplatin in terms of relatively short-term survival (up to four years) although further follow-up on this particular comparison is required.

When these results were presented at the first collaborative group meeting, it emerged that an appropriate trial in advanced disease would be to compare high-dose carboplatin with the CAP regimen (cyclophosphamide, doxorubicin and cisplatin).

International collaboration within the group was possible and such a trial, icon-2 (International Collaborative Ovarian Neoplasm study-2), has been launched together with a similar trial comparing immediate platinum-based treatment versus no immediate treatment in early-stage disease. Each of these trials plans to recruit 2000 patients and as such will be the largest clinical trials ever initiated in advanced ovarian cancer.

Thus new trials, to be run under the auspices of the AOCTG, have been initiated as a direct consequence of this overview and as such provide direct evidence against the criticism that overviews detract from large prospective clinical trials.

THE ROLE OF OVERVIEWS IN CANCER RESEARCH

It is clearly the case that the best possible means of addressing a therapeutic question is by performing a large randomized clinical trial. In the past the importance of trial size has not been recognized fully and for this and other reasons many small and inconclusive randomized trials have been carried out. Overviews can be used to formally combine the results of such studies which have considered similar questions to achieve greater statistical stability and to establish more reliably if there is a real difference between treatments. Further, they can do so in a relatively short period of time compared to initiating new prospective studies. Given that in many cases it is possible that there is already sufficient information available from previous randomized studies to resolve therapeutic issues and given the relative speed of the overview process, it could be considered unethical not to carry out a formal review of existing information. In any event, it is clearly sensible to consider all the available evidence in depth before embarking upon a new large prospective study.

The point is often lost that it is inevitable that reviews will continue to be carried out, both as preparation for new trials and to summarize the results of research for the practising clinician. It is surely better that these take the form of proper quantitative overviews than qualitative review articles.

Overviews do not attempt to replace large clinical trials but they do attempt to formalize the review process and put it on a quantitative footing.

If from now onwards all clinical trials were run on a scale capable of detecting the minimum degree of difference between treatments that is judged clinically worthwhile, then clearly there would be no need to perform overviews in the future. However, in reality it is unlikely that this will always be possible and for a variety of practical, political and economic reasons many small to medium-scale trials will continue to be performed. As long as this practice continues there will be a need for overviews in one form or another. In this case the concept of the prospective overview has to be considered seriously. Although it can be argued that when this degree of planning and co-operation are in force the same effort might be better employed in organizing large-scale multicentre trials, there are cases where this is just not possible. In such situations the idea of a prospective overview should be welcomed.

Just as there can be "bad" clinical trials, so there can be "bad" overviews; it is therefore essential that principles of good design and conduct should be adhered to and that the methodology used should be reported fully in publications so that the reader can interpret the results in the correct context. For example, it is important to distinguish between systematic and non-systematic overviews. While small, quickly performed meta-analyses can be useful in some circumstances they are potentially biased since not all randomized patients and not all studies are included in the analysis; the reader should therefore be alerted to interpret them with care.

As already pointed out, a great deal of effort has to be employed in a systematic overview both on the part of the trialists and the overviewers.

The degree of collaboration needed for the success of such a project can only be advantageous; not only do the overviewers and trialists work together but the trialists themselves can co-operate. Holding a meeting of investigators seems vital to the success of overviews and it is to be hoped that this will become a standard feature of overviews in the future. At these meetings an international group of experts meet and focus on one particular problem, exchanging ideas and debating the results of the overview. In addition the meeting provides an excellent forum for initiating future collaboration. Indeed it is a perfect opportunity to design or even launch the large trials that overviews are often seen to be in competition with. In this way an overview can play an important part in identifying particular areas of confusion, reliably assessing the existing treatments, and in identifying and initiating new areas of research.

In conclusion, large international systematic overviews are both time consuming and demanding; they are, however, relatively inexpensive high-profile projects which provide a rapid turnover of information. Thus the future of overviews in cancer research seems assured.

REFERENCES

1. Freedman LS (1989) Size of clinical trials: what are the current needs? Br J Cancer 59: 396–400
2. ISIS-2 Collaborative Group (1988) Randomised trial of intravenous streptokinase, oral asprin, both or neither among 17,187 cases of acute myocardial infarction. Lancet ii: 349–360
3. Early Breast Cancer Trialists' Collaborative Group (1988) Effects of adjuvant tamoxifen and cytotoxic therapy on mortality in early breast cancer. N Engl J Med 329: 1681
4. Advanced Ovarian Cancer Trialists Group (1991) Chemotherapy in advanced ovarian cancer: an overview of randomised clinical trials. Br Med J 303: 884–892
5. Ovarian cancer meta-analysis project (1991) Cyclophosphamide plus cisplatin versus cyclophosphamide, doxorubicin and cisplatin chemotherapy of ovarian carcinoma: a meta-analysis. J Clin Oncol 9: 1668–1674
6. Simes RJ (1986) Publication bias: the case for an international registry of clinical trials. Clin Oncol 4: 1529
7. Parkin DM, Laark E, Muir CS (1988) Estimates of the worldwide frequency of sixteen major cancers in 1980. Int J Cancer 41: 184–197

ADDITIONAL SUGGESTED READING

Statistics in Medicine (1987) Vol 6 (3). Proceedings of the Workshop on Methodological issues in Overviews of Randomised Clinical Trials May 1986. Wiley, Chichester.

ABOUT THE AUTHOR

Lesley Stewart has been employed by the British Medical Research Council as Overview Co-ordinator since 1988. She is based at the MRC Cancer Trials Office in Cambridge, where she is responsible for running the overviews initiated by the MRC Cancer Therapy Committee. Her background is mainly in the biological sciences and she has strong interests in the fields of computing and statistics. She completed an honours degree in Zoology at Glasgow University before taking an MSc in computing and statistics at York University. This was followed by gaining a PhD in ecology at the University of East Anglia. She is currently involved in both the theoretical and practical aspects of overviews. In addition to the Advanced Ovarian Cancer Overview she is at present involved in overviews of superficial bladder cancer, advanced bladder cancer and lung cancer.

27 Treatment Decisions in Axillary Node-Negative Breast Cancer Patients

WILLIAM L. McGUIRE, ATUL K. TANDON, D. CRAIG ALLRED,
GARY G. CHAMNESS and GARY M. CLARK

There is now evidence in prospective randomized clinical trials that adjuvant endocrine therapy and adjuvant chemotherapy can be of benefit in certain axillary node-negative (ANN) breast cancer patients. This has led to recommendations that most if not all ANN breast cancer patients should be considered for some form of adjuvant therapy [1]. The alternative point of view is that since the majority ($\sim$70%) of ANN patients enjoy long-term survival following surgery and/or radiotherapy, it is inappropriate to recommend adjuvant therapy for all of these patients [2]. Probably all would agree that if we had good methods to distinguish those ANN patients who are "cured" from those destined to recur, only the latter should be treated. It is our purpose to briefly review the evidence supporting the use of prognostic factors and finally to provide a framework from which prognostic factor information can be used directly to make treatment decisions.

TUMOR SIZE

The relationship between the size of the primary tumor and recurrence and survival has received considerable attention. In the earliest large series, Fisher et al. found that increasing tumor size was indeed related to the likelihood of recurrence [3]. This was particularly evident within subsets of axillary nodal involvement.

Rosen and colleagues studied 474 ANN breast cancer patients with a median follow-up of 18.2 years [4]. Probability of recurrence by 20 years was only 14% of patients with tumors 1 cm or less, but 31% in those with tumors 1.1–2 cm.

The largest series examining the role of tumor size in ANN breast cancer patients is from the Surveillance, Epidemiology and End Results (SEER) Program of the National Cancer Institute. This program has collected cancer survival data on nearly 10% of the general population of the USA. Between 1977 and 1982 a total of 13 464 ANN breast cancer patients were investigated

Introducing New Treatments for Cancer: Practical, Ethical and Legal Problems. Edited by C. J. Williams
© 1992 John Wiley & Sons Ltd

for the relationship between tumor size and five-year survival [5]. The results of this study are illustrated in Table 1.

The data show that ANN breast cancer patients with tumors less than 2 cm in size enjoy excellent survival rates. Since approximately 42% of ANN patients have tumors less than 2 cm, tumor size alone or in combination with other factors will be extremely important in deciding upon adjuvant therapy in ANN patients.

NUCLEAR GRADE

Several histological grading systems have been described and shown to have prognostic value in the evaluation of breast carcinoma. The two most frequently used are those of Scarff–Bloom–Richardson (SBR) and Fisher. Both take into account the architectural arrangement of cells, the degree of nuclear differentiation and the mitotic rate, although each system utilizes distinct and differently weighted histological criteria.

The role of these grading systems has recently been evaluated in ANN patients. Fisher et al. studied nuclear grade in 879 ANN patients treated by surgery without systemic adjuvant therapy [6]. Because of the small number of patients classified as nuclear grade 1, they collapsed nuclear grades 1 and 2 into a category called "good" and nuclear grade 3 into a category called "poor". The data show a statistically significant difference in both recurrence and survival between patients with nuclear grade good and poor tumors. One objection to this approach of combining nuclear grade 1 and 2 into one category is that the excellent prognosis usually seen in the nuclear grade 1 patients is diluted out by this procedure.

Regardless of the nuclear grading system used, nuclear grade or its equivalent can identify a small subject of ANN patients at very low risk of

Table 1. Five-year adjusted survival in relation to tumor size in axillary node-negative breast cancer patients

Size (cm)	No. of Patients	Five-year survival
<0.5	269	99.2
0.5–0.9	791	98.3
1.0–1.9	4 668	92.3
2.0–2.9	4 010	90.6
3.0–3.9	2 072	86.2
4.0–4.9	845	84.6
≥5.0	809	82.2
Total	13 464	

Adapted from reference [5].

recurrence and death from breast cancer. A final note must be made regarding the issue of interobserver reproducibility. This has been discussed extensively and, while it may be a problem for some pathologists, it should be remedied with additional training.

ESTROGEN RECEPTOR

Since the initial observations of Knight et al. in 1977 the measurement of estrogen receptor (ER) has become standard practice in the evaluation of patients with primary breast cancer. Many investigators have reported a significant advantage in disease-free survival for ER-positive ANN patients, whereas others fail to show a benefit. The lack of consistent findings is usually attributed to a lack of quality control of assay methodology, patient selection, small numbers of patients studied, etc.

Many of these factors would not pertain to the larger series reported by the NSABP [6] or collected in San Antonio. A summary of these data is illustrated in Table 2. In this combined series of 2853 ANN patients, the five-year disease-free survival difference between ER-positive and ER-negative tumors is highly significant, but the magnitude of the difference is only 8–9%. This has led some investigators, including ourselves, to conclude that ER *by itself* is not a sufficiently strong factor on which to base a treatment decision [7]. As we will see, however, combining ER with tumor size and oncogene expression can be very useful.

PROLIFERATIVE RATE AND PLOIDY

Proliferative rate as determined by the percentage of cells in the DNA synthetic phase of the cell cycle (percentage S-phase) does not require fresh tissue or prompt assay; it can be performed later on frozen tissue or on formalin-fixed paraffin-embedded material. Percentage S-phase was found to be higher in aneuploid and ER-negative breast tumors, and in tumors

Table 2. Relationship of estrogen receptor with five-year disease-free and overall survival in axillary node-negative breast cancer

	No. of patients		Disease-free survival (%)			Overall survival (%)		
	ER+	ER−	ER+	ER−	p-value	ER+	ER−	p-value
Fisher et al. [6]	525	300	74	66	<0.001	92	82	<0.001
San Antonio series	1422	606	76	67	<0.001	84	75	<0.001

with poor histological grade. Perhaps more important, recent reports demonstrate that increased percentage S-phase predicts for early recurrence or poor survival in ANN and also in axillary node-positive (ANP) breast cancer patients. That this is not a universal finding may be best explained by the variability resulting from various methods currently used to calculate percentage S-phase, particularly in aneuploid tumors with overlapping cell populations. Work in progress in San Antonio and elsewhere with newer S-phase modeling programs is leading to more accurate determinations and more striking clinical correlations. Some suggest that DNA flow cytometry may even be useful in the future in predicting response to chemotherapy.

Ploidy can be determined by DNA flow cytometry or static cytophotometry. The majority of breast tumors are aneuploid, having an abnormal DNA content. Most workers agree that aneuploidy is associated with ER negativity and poor histological grade. Some report an association with tumor size or nodal status. Most important are the reports of aneuploidy predicting for shortened disease-free survival or overall survival.

Both ploidy and S-phase were measured in 395 specimens of node-negative breast cancer by Clark et al. [8]. Thirty-two per cent of the 345 specimens that could be evaluated were diploid and 68% were aneuploid. The probability of recurrence within five years was 12% in patients with diploid tumors and 26% in those with aneuploid tumors ($p=0.02$). The probability of recurrence in patients with diploid tumors and low S-phase was 10% at five years, as compared to 29% in those with diploid tumors and high S-phase ($p=0.007$). Similar differences in overall survival were found. In this series of patients, patients with aneuploid tumors could not be separated on the basis of S-phase into groups with differing probabilities of relapse and survival. However, early results from a co-operative group clinical trial in ANN patients using improved S-phase modeling techniques do show that S-phase can discriminate between high and low probability of relapse within the aneuploid ANN population.

HER-2 ONCOGENE

In 1987 Slamon et al. published a pilot study of 86 ANP breast cancer patients correlating HER-2 oncogene amplification with recurrence and shortened survival [9]. Subsequent attempts to confirm a relationship between HER-2 amplification or elevated expression and outcome have not always been successful.

With regard to ANN patients, though most reports on HER-2 have been negative [10], the data from Paik et al. are noteworthy [11]. In a retrospective study of 292 ANN patients, they found an association of HER-2 overexpression with decreased survival among women with tumors of good nuclear grade. In this subgroup, HER-2 overexpression was associated with an approximately fivefold increase in mortality rate ($p = 0.00001$). A similar finding is as yet unpublished from Allred and colleagues in San Antonio, who retrospectively evaluated a group of 325 ANN patients assigned to the observation arm of a clinical co-operative group trial. These patients had tumors <3 cm and were ER positive. HER-2 overexpression in purely invasive tumors within this otherwise good risk group predicted early recurrence.

It would therefore seem that despite the controversies regarding the role of HER-2 amplification or expression in predicting clinical outcome, there may be a role for HER-2 expression studies in selected subsets of ANN patients. For those ANN patients with purely invasive ductal carcinoma (without any ductal carcinoma in situ component) who fall into the usual good risk categories (tumor <2 cm, ER positive, or nuclear grade 1) with an associated five-year disease-free survival probability of 85% or better, HER-2 overexpression may well identify the few patients within the group destined for early recurrence.

CATHEPSIN D

Cathepsin D, whose proenzyme secreted form was originally identified in breast cancer cells as 52K, has been extensively studied, especially in France. These workers found cathepsin D to be estrogen dependent in breast cancer cells in vitro, and to be abnormally processed as well. It is proposed that cathepsin D might facilitate cancer cell migration and invasion by digesting basement membrane, extracellular matrix and connective tissues, though it would be necessary for the cells to develop a sufficiently acidic micro-environment to allow autoactivation of the proenzyme. The mechanism of the reported mitogenic action of secreted cathepsin D is unknown.

Along more clinical lines, 396 Danish breast cancer patients were studied retrospectively for the overexpression of cathepsin D. Patients with high cathepsin D had a shorter disease-free survival and a trend for shorter overall survival. Multivariate analysis revealed a prognostic impact of cathepsin D which was independent of ER, tumor size and lymph node status. A study from France also correlated cathepsin D expression with the clinical outcome of 122 breast cancer patients. Even in this relatively small series, cathepsin D was a good predictor of metastatic disease, especially in node-negative patients, in whom the relative risk of recurrence was seven to ten times that of the cohort with low cathepsin D.

In San Antonio, we examined the level of cathepsin D in 199 ANN patients and found an association with aneuploidy, but none with estrogen or progesterone receptors, tumor size or age of the patient [12]. For disease-free survival, cathepsin D status was predictive of outcome particularly among those with aneuploid tumors; the actuarial five-year recurrence

Table 3. Cathepsin D in axillary node-negative breast
cancer ($n = 199$)

	Actuarial 5-year recurrence
Diploid	22%
Aneuploid	
Low cathepsin D	29%
High cathepsin D	60%

Adapted from ref. [12].

rates of aneuploid tumors were 60% among women with high levels of
cathepsin D, and 29% among those with low levels, as compared with
22% for all diploid tumors (see Table 3). We conclude from these three
independent series from three different countries that cathepsin D is an
independent predictor for recurrence and death in node-negative breast
cancer.

TREATMENT DECISIONS IN ANN PATIENTS

Having reviewed the relative merits of the prognostic factors in ANN
patients, how can we use them in making rational treatment decisions? The
steps in this process are illustrated in Figure 1. The first step in the process

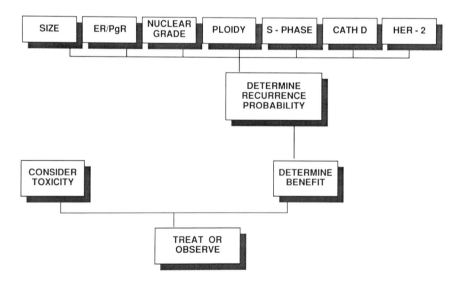

Figure 1. A scheme to use prognostic factors to arrive at a treatment decision in
axillary node-negative breast cancer

is to determine a recurrence probability for the patient based upon the results of the prognostic factor studies. In most cases tumor size and ER/PgR (progesterone receptor) will be known, though ER/PgR in small tumors may have to be evaluated by immunohistochemistry. Nuclear grade may also be available from the hospital pathologist, particularly if he or she has had special training in breast histopathological grading. Ploidy and S-phase are now routinely available from reference laboratories covering all of the USA. HER-2 expression studies and cathepsin D measurements are not yet as widely available as flow cytometry, but soon will be offered by most reference laboratories.

The second step in the process is to calculate the anticipated benefit of adjuvant chemotherapy or endocrine therapy for the particular patient with a defined risk of recurrence. This can be done by using data from the published adjuvant trials in ANN patients and calculating a general proportional reduction in the risk of relapse and then applying it to the particular patient. For example, a patient with tumor size <1 cm and otherwise good factors will have a five-year risk probability of <5%, which equates to an anticipated benefit of <2% from adjuvant tamoxifen or <3% from CMFP (cyclophosphamide/methotrexate/5-fluorouracil/prednisone) chemotherapy. Conversely, a patient with an aneuploid, high cathepsin D tumor has a risk probability of 60% and anticipated benefit of 15% for adjuvant tamoxifen and 30% for adjuvant CMFP.

The third and final step is to weigh the anticipated benefit against the risks and costs of treatment. It should be emphasized at this point that the benefit we are calculating is only a delay in eventual recurrence, which may or may not translate into a survival advantage and is most probably not a cure. Regarding risks and side-effects, concerns with tamoxifen include the occurrence of thrombophlebitis in one of 100 women with a rare death from pulmonary embolism, the striking increase in endometrial carcinoma in more than one of 100 women and, most worrisome, the unknown effects of long-term tamoxifen administration on the liver, cardiovascular and skeletal systems. The financial burden of more than $5000 in the USA for a complete five-year course of the drug alone is another factor. For adjuvant chemotherapy, approximately 30% of patients will develop severe neutropenia which will lead to a treatment-related death in as many as one in 250. As more intensive regimens are introduced in efforts to increase benefits, more treatment-related deaths will occur. What are the longer-term risks of adjuvant chemotherapy in ANN patients? We really don't know, but we might expect some small increase in second malignancies depending on the regimens used, or an increase in cardiovascular disease or osteoporosis in pre-menopausal women who have premature ovarian failure from chemotherapy.

At this point we can begin to weigh benefit versus risk. Consider the patient with a <1 cm tumor and otherwise good factors, with a 95% five-year disease-free survival and a 98% five-year overall survival. The absolute benefit of tamoxifen therapy would be <2%, and of CMFP chemotherapy <3% if the same proportional reduction in recurrence observed in the overall population (26% and 52% respectively) was achieved in these particular subsets. Thus approximately one or two patients of every 100 treated would benefit in terms of delayed recurrence and, hopefully, longer survival. The known side-effects of tamoxifen therapy would be 1% thrombophlebitis with a rare pulmonary embolism and death, and 1.1% endometrial carcinoma. It is important to note that this high incidence of endometrial carcinoma was seen in women taking twice the usual dose of tamoxifen and has not yet been reported in other trials, and also that the low-grade endometrial carcinoma seen following tamoxifen therapy should be highly curable. Considering adjuvant chemotherapy for this patient would mean weighing a 2–3% chance of benefit against a 30% chance of severe neutropenia and even a one in 250 chance of a treatment-related death.

Following the above three steps will identify at least 50% of ANN breast cancer patients who are at a sufficiently low risk for recurrence ($\leqslant 10\%$) that the probability of a treatment benefit will be minimal and observation only could be recommended. This would include ANN patients with ER-positive tumors <2 cm, or nuclear grade 1, or low S-phase tumors, provided there is no overexpression of either cathepsin D or HER-2 oncogene. In the last analysis, the final decision regarding adjuvant therapy of ANN breast cancer rests with the particular patient. It is the responsibility of the practicing oncologist to help the patient evaluate her prognostic factors, arrive at an understanding of her particular risk of recurrence, and within this context weigh the potential benefits and risks of adjuvant therapy. Overenthusiastic claims of treatment success must not be allowed to substitute for sound clinical judgment based on peer-reviewed scientific study.

ACKNOWLEDGMENT

This work was supported by NIH grants CA11378 and CA30195. William L. McGuire MD is a Clinical Research Professor of the American Cancer Society.

REFERENCES

1. DeVita VT (1989) Breast cancer therapy: exercising all our options. N Engl J Med 320: 527–529
2. McGuire WL (1989) Adjuvant therapy of node-negative breast cancer. N Engl J Med 320: 525–527
3. Fisher B, Slack NH, Bross IDJ et al (1969) Cancer of the breast: size of neoplasm and prognosis. Cancer 24: 1071–1080

4. Rosen PP, Groshen S, Saigo PE, Kinne DW, Hellman S (1989) A long-term follow-up study of survival in stage I ($T_1N_0M_0$) and stage II ($T_1N_1M_0$) breast carcinoma. J Clin Oncol 7: 355–366
5. Carter CL, Allen C, Henson DE (1989) Relation of tumor size, lymph node status, and survival in 24,740 breast cancer cases. Cancer 63: 181–187
6. Fisher B, Redmond C, Fisher ER, Caplan R et al (1988) Relative worth of estrogen or progesterone receptor and pathologic characteristics of differentiation as indicators of prognosis in node negative breast cancer patients: findings from National Surgical Adjuvant Breast and Bowel Project Protocol B-06. J Clin Oncol 6: 1076–1087
7. McGuire WL (1988) Estrogen receptor versus nuclear grade as prognostic factors in axillary node negative breast cancer. J Clin Oncol 6: 1071–1072
8. Clark GM, Dressler LG, Owens MA, Pounds G, Oldaker T, McGuire WL (1989) Prediction of relapse or survival in patients with node-negative breast cancer by DNA flow cytometry. N Engl J Med 320: 627–633
9. Slamon DJ, Clark GM, Wong SG, Levin WJ, Ullrich A, McGuire WL (1987) Human breast cancer: correlation of relapse and survival with amplification of the HER-2/*neu* oncogene. Science 235: 177–182
10. Tandon AK, Clark GM, Chamness GC, Ullrich A, McGuire WL (1989) HER-2/*neu* oncogene protein and prognosis in breast cancer. J Clin Oncol 7: 1120–1128
11. Paik S, Hazan R, Fisher ER et al (1990) Pathologic findings from the National Surgical Adjuvant Breast and Bowel Project: prognostic significance of erbB-2 protein overexpression in primary breast cancer. J Clin Oncol 8: 103–112
12. Tandon AK, Clark GM, Chamness GC, Chirgwin JM, McGuire WL (1990) Cathepsin D and prognosis in breast cancer. N Engl J Med 322: 297–302

ABOUT THE AUTHORS

William L. McGuire MD is a Professor of Medicine and has been Chief of the Division of Medical Oncology since 1975. He received his medical training at Western Reserve University and University Hospitals in Cleveland, Ohio, and a fellowship at the National Cancer Institute. He has received the Gibson D. Lewis Cancer Research Award from the State of Texas, and an American Cancer Society Clinical Research Professorship. His research interests include investigations of the biology of human breast cancer with emphasis in the fields of gene regulation, hormone receptor molecular structure, drug resistance, and new markers for predicting the recurrence and overall survival in breast cancer patients.

Atul K. Tandon PhD is a Research Assistant Professor of Medicine. He received his doctorate in immuno-endocrinology of reproduction from the All-India Institute of Medical Sciences, New Delhi, India, and fellowships at Hyogo Medical College, Nishinomiya, Japan, and at the University of Texas Health Science Center at San Antonio, Texas. His research interests include biochemical factors associated with drug resistance and clinical behavior of human cancers.

D. Craig Allred MD is an Associate Professor of Pathology. He received his medical training at the University of Utah and the University of Connecticut, and a fellowship at the University of Connecticut Health Center. His research interests include immunohistochemical evaluations of prognostic factors in human breast and lung cancers.

Gary C. Chamness PhD is a Research Associate Professor of Medicine. He received his doctorate in biochemistry from the University of California at Berkeley, and a fellowship at the University of Texas Health Science Center at San Antonio, Texas. His research interests include the development of new estrogen and progestin analogues for precise cytochemical localization of their receptors in human breast cancers, and evaluation of factors for predicting clinical outcome of breast cancer.

Gary M. Clark PhD is a Professor of Medicine. He received his doctorate in biostatistics from the University of Washington. His research interests include the design of clinical trials and pre-clinical investigations, and the evaluation of factors for predicting clinical outcome of breast cancer.

28 The Clinical Announcement Policy of the National Cancer Institute

MICHAEL A. FRIEDMAN

The National Cancer Institute (NCI) of the USA is charged with the responsibility for eliminating human malignant disease. This enormous responsibility is carried out by supporting basic laboratory investigation, clinical trials, and general education, technology transfer and implementation. Whether the goal is cancer prevention, therapy or rehabilitation, a set of similar considerations hold. In order to achieve the desired goals, information must be generally available. Once new knowledge is reliably identified, what are the most appropriate means for information dissemination? Historically, the peer review publication mechanism (such as a journal article) has been the most widely accepted method of displaying data and recommendations. However, the review and publication of any particular piece of work may be far from orderly, predictable or even timely. Delays of one year or more may occur depending on a journal's publication priorities, the length of the queue of accepted articles and publication policy preference. While such delays may be regrettable with respect to an arcane pre-clinical study, they are completely unacceptable if patient benefit is compromised.

INTRODUCTION*

The NCI and the extramural investigators it supports share an ethical obligation to disseminate the results of federally supported clinical investigation. The NCI, as the disburser of federal funds, and the clinical investigators, as the recipients of public moneys and trust, both recognize the duty to disseminate new information of substantial, practical clinical impact as rapidly, responsibly and effectively as possible. Additionally, the NCI is directly accountable by law to the public in matters relating to

---

*Portions of this chapter are identical to Guidelines presented to the National Cancer Advisory Board meeting on 14 May 1990 and are used with the permission of the Subcommittee Chairman.

Introducing New Treatments for Cancer: Practical, Ethical and Legal Problems. Edited by C. J. Williams
Published 1992 by John Wiley & Sons Ltd

information dissemination. Possessing both the authority and the responsibility, the NCI has the obligation to ensure appropriate dissemination of information derived from its extramural clinical trials. In order to provide equality in access to information, it becomes necessary to make certain clinical trials data generally available. If only some certain selected physicians have access to these data then best care will be provided only to a limited subset of all potential patients. Certainly in a free society it should be choice, not chance, which dictates therapeutic options. One method employed by the NCI to disseminate information is the Clinical Announcement (CA).

The CA is a brief communication that is directed primarily at practicing physicians and summarizes the results of crucial clinical studies. It includes a background description of the disease setting, the study design(s), minimal details of therapy, and data on efficacy and toxicity. It cautions that there are limitations of interpretability of the data and encourages further consideration. The CA is intended to bring new information to the attention of clinicians, in order to reduce the interval between identifying an effective therapy and widespread adoption of that therapy.

To date there have been two public announcements made by the NCI. The first was a Breast Cancer Clinical Alert issued in May 1988. This described a series of clinical trials of adjuvant systemic therapy for completely resected breast cancer patients whose axillary lymph nodes were uninvolved with tumor (so-called "node negative"). A clear benefit in disease (recurrence)-free survival was demonstrated for both the estrogen receptor positive and estrogen receptor negative cohorts with tamoxifen and cytotoxic chemotherapy, respectively. These studies were formally published in the *New England Journal of Medicine* in February 1989 [1–3]. The second announcement was a Colon Cancer Clinical Update issued in October 1989 which described the overall survival advantage conferred on those receiving adjuvant 5-fluorouracil (5-FU) + levamisole after undergoing a complete resection of a stage III colon adenocarcinoma (Dukes C). The Breast Cancer Alert was initially sent to about 13 000 and the Colon Cancer Update to almost 34 000 physicians and surgeons.

In principle, a CA should be considered when the clinical trials process identifies a new treatment or prevention procedure that measurably improves survival or the quality of life of a defined group of cancer patients with reasonable certainty, and when that intervention is available to the general public.

Unfortunately, the issuance of a statement from a prestigious and powerful national agency like the NCI can be a source of concern to some individuals. The CA is not to be construed as an authoritative directive dictating a therapy for all patients. It is an educational document, presenting facts and informed opinions on options to be considered by the practicing physician. It is not a means of delegating (assigning) health care resources nor is it a proposal for a comprehensive standard of care. It is not a "Federal Mandate" for a uniform "Practice Plan".

The primary motivation for issuing a CA is to promote delivery of effective therapies to cancer patients, a goal shared by all parties. The question is not whether a CA will ever be issued; rather, it is how best to utilize this powerful tool.

CAs are based on general confidence in a system and a mechanism. Implicit is a confidence in the validity of the data generated and the analyses employed, the respect of the NCI for the prerogatives and concerns of the investigators, and the legitimate responsibilities of all parties to disseminate information to the patients.

GUIDELINES FOR DEVELOPMENT AND ISSUANCE OF A CLINICAL ANNOUNCEMENT

The proposal to issue a CA may be initiated by either the investigators or the NCI, but both must agree to proceed. Collegial co-operation is fundamental to this entire process. To date the experience has been with phase III therapeutic trials carried out by the investigators supported through NCI's Clinical Trials Co-operative Groups. These groups have an exemplary record of appropriate quality control and assurance mechanisms.

In both the cases noted above, the announcements were based upon the body of evidence available about the disease and its therapy. Recognizing the dangers of publication bias, the decision to issue an announcement should ideally be based on a thorough, quantitative review of all relevant clinical trials, not merely focused on one positive (and possibly anomalous) study.

The size of the treatment benefit should be estimated by considering the relevant clinical data and the magnitude of that benefit should be deemed worthy, compared to cost and quality of life considerations. A significant improvement in overall survival is the ideal stimulus for issuing a CA. However, in selected situations a carefully documented meaningful increase in improvement in quality of life, complete response rate, disease-free survival or other surrogates could merit a CA. Likewise, the description of some important new toxicity might also qualify.

TYPICAL CHARACTERISTICS OF CLINICAL TRIALS DATA SUITABLE FOR CLINICAL ANNOUNCEMENT

The following represent general guidelines acceptable for motivating and directing public announcements. Usually the proposed intervention is evaluated in a randomized study with a "control group" representing a widely accepted standard treatment. Ideally, the trial would confirm a positive randomized study (one that, preferably, is published). The trial must have sufficient sample size and include representative patients so that the results may be expected to be valid and generalizable. Under extraordinary circumstances a single, dramatic unrandomized trial could also be considered as a candidate for an announcement.

The data analysis must be conducted in accordance with the protocol designated statistical design. The target sample size must be achieved and follow-up must conform with the statistical design. A sequential analysis plan to be used and the critical p-value for declaring significance at an interim analysis must be clearly specified before the trial is even initiated. The overall results for survival or disease-free survival should be statistically significant when all data are analyzed—with no exclusion of eligible randomized patients and an acceptably low lost-to-follow-up rate (ideally $\leqslant 5\%$). Subset analyses would not be considered unless separate accrual and monitoring were used for each subset. The data should also be sufficiently mature relative to the disease's natural history (predicted event rate).

The trial should be evaluated and reviewed by a formal Data Monitoring Committee whose composition and function are designated at the trial initiation. This committee should contain a Cancer Therapy Evaluation Program, NCI representative and at least one clinician and statistician who are not directly involved with this particular trial. This committee makes the initial recommendation concerning public announcement, publication, etc.

ONCE A CANDIDATE STUDY IS IDENTIFIED

A full report of the data should be available to physicians concurrent with the distribution of the CA. This may be in the form of a conventional printed publication or through an unconventional system. It may be electronically available via computer link (from a scientific journal or via the Physicians Data Query network). If previously unpublished data are the basis for a CA, a publication must be accessible in a peer-reviewed format in a reasonably timely fashion. The NCI stands ready to assist the study Principal Investigators in securing rapid journal consideration and (once accepted) dissemination of information. Journals with rapid, flexible review policies or with full text available eletronically at the time of acceptance (e.g. *Annals of Internal Medicine*) are especially attractive. This speediness does not imply a less rigorous review; it merely connotes efficiency and flexibility.

The responsibility for reviewing the available evidence regarding the candidate intervention should be delegated to a subcommittee of the NCI's Division of Cancer Treatment Board of Scientific Counselors and National Cancer Advisory Board, made up of skilled investigators and statisticians selected by the Director, NCI and Study Principal Investigator. This small committee should advise the NCI on whether a CA should be issued and could help draft the CA.

The data, tone and format of the CA would be mutually established by the NCI and investigators with the review and concurrence of the Principal Investigator and statistician of the clinical trial that is the subject of the CA. The summary data and the CA draft could then be reviewed by segments of responsible bodies such as the NCI Executive Committee, Chairman of the National Cancer Advisory Board, Chairman of the Board of Scientific Counselors for Division of Cancer Treatment, and the Physicians Data Query Editorial Board.

Relevant extramural organizations would also be offered an opportunity to review and comment on the draft CA. Such organizations could include the American Society for Clinical Oncology, American College of Surgeons, American Society for Therapeutic and Radiation of Oncology, American Cancer Society, etc. This review would concentrate on the tone and content of the announcement and would identify the appropriate audience. This review would not necessarily imply a formal approval of the CA by such organizations.

Once finally approved by the Director of the NCI, the CA would be mailed to all the appropriate physicians prior to a public (lay) media announcement. The public announcement would be co-ordinated by the NCI Press Office and those of organizations participating in the announcement, a press conference would be held if appropriate, and would be a joint effort of the Principal Investigator(s) and the NCI.

THE CLINICAL ANNOUNCEMENT PROCESS

The principal utility of the CA has historically been in the communication of new therapeutic results. There are other potential roles for the CA including the description of untoward treatment-related side-effects. In all cases, it is meant to serve the public's interest.

These guidelines describe the usual process for issuing an announcement and considerable peer advice and participation is anticipated. However, given the mission of the NCI in Cancer and AIDS, in rare instances it may be necessary that one or more steps of this process will be waived by the Director of the NCI if there is an unexpected and urgent need for information dissemination.

How should public announcements be judged? In what sense is one successful? Both the quality of the data and the effectiveness of the announcement need to be considered. With respect to the former, the crucial issues are consistency (fidelity) and validity (accuracy). To use the Colon Cancer Update as an example, the toxicity and efficacy data were consistent throughout the entire process from October 1989 to February 1990. Both the journal publications that were the bases for the announcement bore data essentially the same as the announcement and hence would be counted as a success [4, 5]. The judgment of biological or clinical validity is somewhat more complicated. However, these data were carefully reviewed by two journals, and the Oncologic Drug Advisory Committee of the Food and Drug Administration without challenge. Most critically, these data were examined by a Consensus Development Conference convened by the National Institutes of Health in April 1990. This panel recommended that levamisole and 5-fluorouracil be considered the best available treatment and the standard of care for stage III colon cancer patients. Evaluation by virtually every segment of the clinical and research communities resulted in the endorsement of the NCI Clinical Update issued in October 1989.

In order to assess the effectiveness of the public announcement process the general pattern of practice must be assessed. Such a comprehensive analysis is not currently possible. Partial data are available from an American College of Surgeons survey which revealed that 74% of 2816 responding physicians changed their practice to include a consideration of levamisole + 5-fluorouracil after the announcement (data from the American College of Surgeons). Additionally the NCI, as part of its group C drug effort, supplied levamisole for nearly one-third of all new stage III colon cancer patients in the USA. It would be reasonable to assume that with greater familiarity with the primary study data and the commercial availability of levamisole even greater numbers of patients will have access to this therapy.

For the stage I breast cancer Clinical Alert the cycle of public and private review is almost as complete. A Consensus Development Conference was held on 18–21 June 1990, and the value of adjuvant systemic therapy for selected node-negative patients was affirmed.

At any rate, the ultimate test of the effectiveness of the NCI public announcement is the demonstrated reduction in cancer deaths. Recognizing that it may take many years to document an increase in the cure rate, a full and complete judgment must be suspended.

It would be foolhardy to assume that the announcement process is optimized. Improvements can and will be instituted when the next opportunity arises. Certainly there are difficult issues generated by the NCI effort to rapidly disseminate information. But how fortunate we are to be discovering information of such importance to the progress of care for cancer patients.

REFERENCES

1. Fisher B, Redmond C, Wickerham L et al (1989) Systemic therapy in patients with node-negative breast cancer: a commentary based on two National Surgical Adjuvant Breast and Bowel Project (NSABP) clinical trials. Ann Intern Med 111: 703–712

2. Mansour EG, Gray R, Shatila AH et al (1989) Efficacy of adjuvant chemotherapy in high-risk node-negative breast cancer: an intergroup study. N Engl J Med 320: 485–490
3. Fisher B, Costantino J, Redmond C et al (1989) A randomized clinical trial evaluating tamoxifen in the treatment of patients with node-negative breast cancer who have estrogen-receptor-positive tumors. N Engl J Med 320: 479–484
4. Moertel CG, Fleming TR, Macdonald JS et al (1990) Levamisole and fluorouracil for surgical adjuvant therapy of colon carcinoma. N Engl J Med 322: 352–358
5. Laurie JA, Moertel CG, Fleming TR et al (1989) Surgical adjuvant therapy of large bowel carcinoma: an evaluation of levamisole and the combination of levamisole and fluorouracil. The North Central Cancer Treatment Group and the Mayo Clinic. J Clin Oncol 7: 1447–1456

ABOUT THE AUTHOR

Dr Michael Friedman is Associate Director of the Cancer Therapy Evaluation Program, Division of Cancer Treatment, National Cancer Institute. This program is responsible for the clinical development of new cytotoxics and biologicals, the NCI-sponsored therapeutic clinical trials program, and a substantial grant portfolio related to identifying better therapies for cancer patients. Currently, he is also the interim Associate Director for the Radiation Research Program. He co-ordinates the bilateral therapy programs with several countries (including Japan and the USSR). He is involved in a variety of oncology-related activities through committee and professional memberships (American College of Physicians, American College of Surgeons, Accreditation Council for Graduate Medical Education, American Society for Clinical Oncology, International Union Against Cancer, and European Organization for Research and Treatment of Cancer) and serves on a number of editorial boards (*Journal of the National Cancer Institute, Cancer, American Journal of Oncology*). A graduate of Tulane University (BA) and the University of Texas Southwestern Medical School (MD), Dr Friedman completed his post-doctoral training at Stanford University and the National Cancer Institute. He previously served as Chief of the Clinical Investigations Branch at the Division of Cancer Treatment and as the Director of the Cancer Research Institute at the University of California at San Francisco.

29 Clinical Cancer Alerts: Less than Wise

GEORGE A. OMURA

The recent advent of the National Cancer Institute "Clinical Alerts" and "Updates" is well intentioned but ill advised. Given the virtual certainty that more will be forthcoming, it seems appropriate to review some of the problems associated with those reports regarding the adjuvant chemotherapy of node-negative breast and node-positive colon cancers.

An underlying problem in interpreting new cancer treatments is the phenomenon of "minimal residual disease". When treatment produces a complete remission (disappearance of palpable, visible or otherwise measurable disease), the patient may at that point be cured or may be harboring microscopic amounts of residual cancer somewhere in the body (micrometastases) which cannot be detected by currently available means. In a population of patients who are at risk for recurrence (by growth of the micrometastases into macrometastases), the only way currently to accurately assess the value of a new treatment program is to conduct a large-scale clinical trial in which adequate numbers of patients are randomly assigned either to no further treatment or to the new therapy; prolonged follow-up of these patients is necessary before one can begin to judge the value of the new treatment. With some types of cancer, the recurrence will routinely appear within months, but in breast cancer, for example, recurrence may not be apparent for many years. In the absence of a scientific breakthrough that reliably identifies minimal residual disease, the identification of new curative treatments for cancer requires properly designed multicenter trials and lengthy follow-up.

Traditionally, progress in medical science has been reported at medical meetings with a formal presentation. This is typically followed by a question and answer session, which may be more interesting than the presentation itself from the standpoint of placing the new findings in some perspective. Then a full written report is submitted to a medical journal for publication. The review process varies from journal to journal, but many prestigious journals employ a peer review process in which one or more authorities on the subject provide written critiques, including questions, to the editor and authors. As a result, some papers are revised many times before publication; some are rejected. The process may take months. In time the results are confirmed or refuted and the report placed in proper perspective.

Introducing New Treatments for Cancer: Practical, Ethical and Legal Problems. Edited by C. J. Williams
© 1992 John Wiley & Sons Ltd

The peer review and publication process takes too long in this electronic age. In particular, some journal reviewers procrastinate excessively, well beyond their deadlines. To what extent more thoughtful reviews come from procrastinators is unclear. Certainly the process could be accelerated. But instantaneous reviews cannot and probably should not be expected from a knowledgeable critic. At any rate, all the relevant data should be available for review when decisions about medical practice are made, even if the individual attending physician doesn't actually review them.

Instances of partial release of new information before formal publication have led the *New England Journal of Medicine*, for example, to refuse to publish reports that have been excessively publicized ahead of time. At the same time, there has been intense and increasing interest on the part of the public in reports of medical progress. This seems especially true with respect to cancer, since it is so common, since it is an emotionally charged subject and since considerable expenditure of public funds has been devoted in the past two decades to cancer research.

In this setting, a summary of unpublished interim results of adjuvant therapy trials in node-negative breast cancer was sent to 13 000 oncologists in 1988; in 1989 another summary report was distributed on the use of adjuvant fluorouracil plus levamisole in node-positive colon cancer prior to publication. The details of these reports and their shortcomings are of interest.

Women with breast cancer involving the axillary lymph nodes frequently have a recurrence after surgery alone, while the majority of node-negative patients are cured with local measures. That is not, however, a large majority, so the possible value of adjuvant systemic therapy has been investigated in several randomized multicenter trials. The National Surgical Adjuvant Breast and Bowel Project (NSABP) initiated protocol B13 [1] in 679 node-negative, estrogen receptor negative cases in 1981, comparing no further treatment to sequential methotrexate 100 mg/m² followed by fluorouracil 600 mg/m² intravenously on days 1 and 8 every four weeks with leucovorin 10 mg/m² by mouth every 6 hours for six doses starting 24 hours after each dose of methotrexate. Therapy was to begin 14–35 days after mastectomy and continue for one year (12 courses). Protocol B14 [2] was begun at the same time in node-negative estrogen receptor positive cases randomizing a placebo versus tamoxifen 10 mg twice a day for five years; 2644 patients were accrued to that study (*New England Journal of Medicine*, 320: 479). An intergroup study [3] was begun in June 1981 comparing observation to prednisone 40 mg/m² and cyclophosphamide 100 mg/m² by mouth on days 1–14 and methotrexate 40 mg/m² on days 1 and 8 plus fluorouracil 600 mg/m² intravenously on days 1 and 8 for six four-week cycles in node-negative women with estrogen receptor negative tumors or in estrogen receptor positive tumors at least 3 cm in diameter; 536 patients were accrued to that study.

The interim results of these adjuvant trials showing a statistically significant improvement in disease-free survival (but no difference in overall survival) were reviewed by the sponsoring agency, the NCI, in the spring of 1988:

> Both the National Cancer Institute and its advisors felt a responsibility to provide this information to the women of the country through the press and to physicians who needed advance notice, by direct mail. The PDQ (Physician Data Query) list of 13 000 physicians who care for patients with cancer was used in mailing the Alert. The PDQ Board also recommended that any new protocols for studying the treatment of node-negative breast cancer should include a treatment arm as their control. [4]

The ensuing Clinical Alert stated in a three-page summary that "although the median follow-up is only three to four years, adjuvant systemic therapy has resulted in statistically significant improvement in disease-free survival in all three studies". The document went on to say that "outside of a trial setting, the hormonal and chemotherapy treatments described represent credible therapeutic options worthy of careful attention".

This communication evoked considerable press coverage (although a press conference was not employed) and numerous comments from physicians. The *Washington Post* (20 May 1988) reported:

> New studies suggest that breast cancer patients whose underarm lymph nodes show no evidence of cancer should nevertheless undergo post-surgical treatment to prevent recurrence of cancer. A description of the findings in the studies was sent to 13 000 oncologists last week by the National Cancer Institute in an unusual "Clinical Alert" which bypasses formal publication of the results in a medical journal or even their presentation at a medical conference.

The front page of the *New York Times* (21 May 1988) had a story with the headline "Cancer Drug Therapy Urged For All After Breast Surgery". Under a paragraph entitled "Exclusion of Small Group" the story by Gina Kolata went on to say:

> The only group of women excluded from this advice are those who, like Nancy Reagan, had such very small tumors that they were restricted to the milk gland, where breast cancer starts. These cancers had not even spread within the breast and so they could not have spread throughout the body, necessitating chemotherapy or hormone therapy according to Dr DeVita (Dr Vincent DeVita Jr, Director of the National Cancer Institute). Breast cancer specialists noted that the new research provided no guidance for women who have had surgery for early breast cancer in the past but who did not have additional treatment. Dr DeVita said that he would advise women with early breast cancer who had surgery six months ago or less and who did not have additional drug therapy to consider drug treatment now. But he added, it's a judgment call.
> The studies used three treatments, including two chemotherapy regimens and a hormonal therapy. In all three studies the women who had additional

therapy were less likely to suffer a recurrence of the cancer within three or four years of its removal. Dr DeVita said that such results have always translated into an overall survival advantage as the patients are studied for longer periods. Women and their doctors still will have to decide which drug regimen to use.

In a supplemental article (21 May 1988) the *New York Times* reported on the circumstances of the Clinical Alert:

Dr Vincent T. DeVita Jr, Director of the National Cancer Institute, explained that when he heard the new data presented at a Cancer Institute Advisory Board Meeting May 9, he felt he had to notify doctors immediately. He asked the researchers for permission to send their results in a letter to the cancer specialists.

He also took the unusual step of calling Dr Arnold Relman, Editor of the *New England Journal of Medicine*, to ask if the publication would still publish the results if he announced them as he had. The Journal does not publish papers if the results have already been reported widely, but Dr Relman, according to Dr DeVita, said this would be no problem because the results were so important.

Eleanor Nealon of the Institute's Press Office said the entire episode was unusual. She said it would have been difficult to set up a news conference because the main researchers had gone to a week-long meeting in New Orleans and the Institute did not want to wait until they were back to announce the results.

Parenthetically it might be noted that the meeting referred to was the annual sessions of the American Society of Clinical Oncology and the American Association for Cancer Research.

In response to the Clinical Alert, Balch and Singletary commented [5]: "Unfortunately the incomplete dissemination of information about these trials and the exaggerated interpretation of the results by the lay press and others have led to considerable confusion about specifically which node-negative breast cancer patients should receive post-operative chemotherapy or hormonal therapy as 'standard treatment.'" They went on to say:

Three issues must be addressed before adjuvant chemotherapy or hormonal therapy can be utilized as standard practice for the entire cohort of patients: 1. Are the patients entered into these clinical studies representative of the entire universe of node-negative breast cancer patients? If not, is there an identifiable subset of "high risk" node-negative breast cancer patients for whom this treatment is justified? 2. Does the statistically significant difference in disease-free survival at four years actually translate into an equally significant difference in overall survival between the treatment arm and the control arm? 3. Does the benefit of systemic chemotherapy or hormonal therapy outweigh the risks, complications and costs of treatment?

Finally, they noted, "these three clinical trials are well-designed and important studies that will contribute to the scientific literature. It is the interpretation of their results and their application to the standards of treatment that we question. In our opinion the current information from these three clinical trials does not clearly justify adjuvant therapy for the entire universe of patients with node-negative breast cancer."

Lee [10] remarked:

> there remain some important questions about the merits of this new approach to the dissemination of scientific information. At the least it means a sharing, if not a usurpation, of the main functions of the major peer-reviewed medical journals. Whereas published articles are subject to peer review, statements made by public officials are the sole responsibility of such officials. Whether this practice is acceptable to the scientific community remains to be seen.

Merz [6] quoted DeVita as saying that using the Clinical Alert to disseminate data "was in a sense an experiment that may change how journals treat data, and we're anxious to get feedback".

Spratt and Greenberg [7], following up on a 1988 commentary in the same journal by Dr Spratt, expressed concern about failure to consider cost–benefit ratios and failure to exclude late toxicities.

Prosnitz [8] worried about the medical–legal implications if a physician fails to employ systemic adjuvant therapy for a woman with node-negative breast cancer and relapse subsequently takes place. He went on to note, "it would have been much more appropriate to expedite the publication of the pertinent study results in peer review journals, convene a consensus development committee, and have that group issue a recommendation".

Cady [9] noted that the distribution list of the Clinical Alert "ignored the fact that almost all patients with node-negative breast cancer had been handled exclusively by surgeons . . . (moreover) the Clinical Alert, even in its revised form did not distinguish between non-invasive and invasive breast cancers!" To make it entirely clear that he disapproved, Dr Cady went on to say, "the use of unpublished data in the Clinical Alert was a disservice to science, the medical profession and particularly the public. The fact that this Clinical Alert caused enormous anxiety, confusion, and uncertainty in patients, the public and the profession merely exemplifies the penalties for such a disorderly process."

When the reports in question, B13, B14, the Intergroup Study as well as Ludwig Trial 5 [11] of the Ludwig Breast Cancer Study Group (which reported a disease-free survival benefit for a single course of CMF) were finally published in the 23 February 1989 issue of the *New England Journal of Medicine*, there was additional comment. Editorials by William L. McGuire and DeVita accompanied the papers. McGuire [12] expressed concern that relatively few patients actually benefited since most were already cured by local measures, that the possibility of late toxicity was not excluded, that the economic cost is considerable and that proper use of other prognostic factors could sort out patients at a very low risk of recurrence without adjuvant therapy.

DeVita, no longer the Director of NCI, still had a very optimistic view of the results [13], noting an "impressive reduction in the risk of recurrence", "minimal toxicity" and that "the markers of prognosis beyond those used in the studies are either still too controversial or not widely available for general use".

The 17 August 1989 issue of the *New England Journal of Medicine* contained seven presumably representative letters accumulated over the five months after publication of the studies, concerning several points which helped to put the reports in perspective—points which could not be debated a year earlier when the Clinical Alert was issued, for lack of adequate details, but which remained timely much later. Concerns were expressed about treating all node-negative patients, about the relatively brief follow-up, and about short-term and long-term toxicity. A very interesting point was made by Buckman et al. [14] that in NSABP B13 methotrexate plus fluorouracil "did not produce a statistically significant difference in the incidence of distant metastatic disease. The only significant difference between adjuvant methotrexate and fluorouracil and surgery alone was with respect to local or regional recurrence."

Tannock [15] viewed even the published data as premature, expressing concern that early differences in relapse-free survival did not necessarily predict differences in overall survival ten years later.

Pritchard, writing in the *Annals of Internal Medicine* [16], noted that:

> delay in relapse while clearly desirable and likely representing a biologic effect that can be exploited in future trials, may not be a sufficient outcome measure to justify the use of adjuvant systemic therapy, outside of clinical trials, at least until clear gains in overall quality of life can be shown. Furthermore, we need to know much more about the long-term effects of both tamoxifen and chemotherapy in this setting before recommending either as routine therapy for women with node-negative breast cancer.

One of the NCI officials [17] acknowledged the controversy but summarized what he perceived to be the principal objections as "A. Many physicians who should have received the Clinical Alert did not; B. The contents of the Clinical Alert were incomplete; C. NCI has no business telling physicians how to practice medicine; and D. A direct mailing that bypassed the normal processes of peer review is an inappropriate vehicle for disseminating medical and scientific information."

Everyone reviewing this matter will have his or her own interpretation, but it would seem that a key issue is the prematurity of the conclusion that patients with node-negative breast cancer should receive adjuvant therapy. If that recommendation were unassailable, most of the complaints could be dismissed as carping, but the matter is actually quite complex. On the one hand, an early impact on disease-free survival does not necessarily translate into improved survival, and there is no certainty that the cure rate will be improved. On the other hand, progress is ongoing in sorting out the minority of node-negative patients who might stand to benefit from adjuvant therapy, from the large majority who are already cured by mastectomy or equivalent local measures. Several points can be made.

Rosner and Lane [18] reported that patients with lesions 1 cm or less had an excellent survival, especially if the primary was well or moderately well differentiated. Fisher et al. acknowledged that the NSABP trials provided no information on most such cases because they were too small for receptor determination by the cytosol method, a requirement for entry in those trials [19].

The Ludwig Group [20] reported on 921 cases classified as node negative by routine examination; serial sectioning revealed micrometastases in 83; the latter had a significantly poorer survival than those whose nodes remained negative on serial sectioning.

Several groups have employed DNA flow cytometry to assess prognosis in node-negative cases. Clark et al. [21] observed that aneuploidy was unfavorable, with disease-free survival at five years of 74% compared to 88% for those with diploid tumors. In diploid cases a high S-phase fraction was unfavorable, with $70\% \pm 13\%$ surviving disease-free at five years versus $90\% \pm 3\%$ when the S-phase fraction was low. Significant differences in overall survival were also noted. Sigurdsson et al. [22], Joensuu et al. [23] and Lewis [24] have made similar observations.

Recent studies of cathepsin D, an estrogen-induced lysosomal protease, indicate that high levels of this protein, which may facilitate invasion and metastasis, represent an adverse prognostic factor in node-negative disease [25, 26]. A contradictory report [27] was based on a small number of cases, but reflects the need for further study of cathepsin D.

McGuire et al. have summarized the current information on prognostic factors in node-negative breast cancer [28]. They reviewed tumor size, nuclear grade, estrogen receptor status, ploidy, S-phase fraction, cathepsin D level and HER-2/NEU oncogene expression as factors which could provide an estimate of the risk of recurrence in an individual patient with node-negative breast cancer. An approximation of the risk–benefit ratio from adjuvant therapy in that patient could then be arrived at. At this juncture such an approach is not highly refined, but it does clearly make the points that we are not dealing with a homogeneous risk group, that many patients will be over-treated with a blanket approach, and that ongoing research is likely to refine the known prognostic factors and identify new ones.

Many of the interested parties were assembled in June 1990 at an NIH "Consensus Development Conference on the Treatment of Early Stage Breast Cancer". In addition to addressing questions about "breast conservation" treatment, the participants observed that the majority of such patients are cured with local treatment, that the rate of relapse is decreased by chemotherapy and by tamoxifen but that the pros and cons of adjuvant treatment should be discussed with each patient, and that patients with small tumors ($\leqslant 1$ cm) don't require adjuvant therapy. The Consensus Meeting was not ready to agree on the clinical value of prognostic factors other than tumor size. Pending the publication of the conference summary, there has been no formal reaction, but newspaper accounts of the meeting included comments such as "panel of experts offers little guidance to women" (*Washington Post*, 26 June 1990) and "a meeting of experts convened in Washington last week to tackle the issue was a disappointment" (*Boston Globe*, 25 June 1990). The latter article went on to quote a member of the audience as saying that "the decision of the NIH panel not to endorse systemic therapy for these women after the NCI essentially did two years ago, is really a step backward".

Although the Consensus Conference did not endorse McGuire's view of prognostication, it did not necessarily represent a step backward; rather, it seemed to underscore the prematurity of the breast cancer Clinical Alert.

As noted above, the NCI staff acknowledged some of the problems with the details of the breast cancer Alert [17] shortly after it was issued; nevertheless, they were undeterred with respect to the wisdom of the basic approach. Thus, in mid-1989 when positive results were observed from an NCI-sponsored adjuvant trial in node-positive (Dukes C) colon cancer, another report was distributed. This communication, identified as "National Cancer Institute Update", was mailed on 2 October 1989 to 35 000 physicians, surgeons and major institutions treating cancer patients. The Update "describes the efficacy and the availability of adjuvant levamisole and 5-fluorouracil (5-FU) through a group C protocol, for patients with completely resected Dukes C colon cancer. This treatment substantially reduces the risk of dying of recurrent colon cancer." Parenthetically, group C refers to investigational drugs which the National Cancer Institute makes available for treatment of patients with very specific indications. In the case of levamisole, it has in fact been available as an anti-helminthic agent in other countries but not in the USA.

The basis for the conclusion that this regimen was indicated was in essence two multicenter trials: one published by the North Central Cancer Treatment Group [29] (NCCTG) at the time of the Update, and one unpublished intergroup study, which was said to be "confirmatory". A third study was also referred to but was discounted because of the small number of patients studied [30]. The Update was viewed by some as an improvement over the Clinical Alert because some of the information was "published" (some subscribers received the relevant issue of the *Journal of Clinical Oncology* on 10 October 1989), because survival benefit rather than merely improvement in disease-free survival was reported, and because the distribution list was broader. The reaction to the Update seemed more subdued, perhaps because the report was thought to be more credible or because the medical community was getting used to the NCI process.

A close look at the colon Update suggests that at least in some measure it is misleading. First, it talks about increasing the "cure rate" when there is unfortunately no basis for that interpretation of what has been observed and reported. Second, the NCCTG trial is referred to on page 1 of the Update as showing a survival benefit (for patients with completely resected Dukes C colon cancer), but on page 2 it is acknowledged that that finding was in subset analysis, while an overall survival benefit was not shown ($p=0.09$). Finally, the "confirmatory" intergroup study (unpublished at the time of the Update) was in fact the first study that gave a seemingly clear answer, but those data were not provided in the Update.

One very brief paragraph is provided in the Update about the results of the intergroup trial. Since the NCCTG trial was not definitive, to what extent is the intergroup trial confirmatory? Did it merely provide more suggestive data? Is that what was confirmed? We can't really tell from what is given in the Update. Presentation of all the data would have been much better, although, as mentioned earlier, that might have created difficulties with subsequent publication in certain journals.

The intergroup paper [31] was published in the *New England Journal of Medicine* on 8 February 1990. As noted above, the NCCTG paper appeared in the *Journal of Clinical Oncology* in October 1989 [29] and the Update was mailed on 2 October 1989. Was the four-month interval between the Update and the intergroup publication important? One really can't say. How many patients were begun on adjuvant treatment during that interval and how have they fared since then? It would be interesting to know how much levamisole was distributed by the NCI from October 1989 until June 1990 when Janssen Pharmaceutica was allowed by the Food and Drug Administration to market the drug.

The intergroup report indicated that 1296 patients with resected colon cancer that either was locally invasive (stage B_2) or had regional nodal involvement (stage C) were randomly assigned to observation or to treatment for one year with levamisole combined with fluorouracil (5-FU). Levamisole was given by mouth 50 mg every 8 hours for three days, repeated every two weeks for one year. 5-FU was given by rapid injection $450\,mg/m^2$ daily $\times 5$, no earlier than 21 days after surgery. Twenty-eight days after the start of 5-FU, weekly treatment with 5-FU was begun with $450\,mg/m^2$ i.v. and continued for 48 weeks unless toxicity occurred. Patients with stage C disease could also be randomly assigned to treatment with levamisole alone. The median follow-up time was three years (range, 2–5½).

Among the patients with stage C disease, therapy with levamisole plus 5-Fu reduced the risk of cancer recurrence by 41% ($p<0.0001$). The overall death rate was reduced by 33% ($p=0.006$). Treatment with levamisole alone had no detectable effect. The results in the patients with stage B_2 disease were equivocal and too preliminary to allow firm conclusions. Toxic effects of levamisole alone were infrequent, usually consisting of mild nausea with occasional dermatitis or leukopenia, and those of levamisole plus 5-FU were essentially the same as those of fluorouracil alone, i.e. nausea, vomiting, stomatitis, diarrhea, dermatitis and leukopenia.

The intergroup paper was generally convincing, but with some reservations: interim analysis was used, the stage B study was inconclusive but reported with the stage C results, later treatment was actually better than early-onset treatment (21–35 days versus 7–20 days for initiation of therapy) with respect to recurrence, and the median follow-up was only three years. Finally, the beneficial effect of the combination remained unexplained.

There remains a clear need for a follow-up report of the intergroup study; late recurrences and late effects of treatment are of concern. A recent Consensus Conference [32] acknowledged that longer follow-up is indicated.

How does 5-FU plus levamisole work? Although there are various speculations, it is generally agreed that levamisole alone is not a reproducibly useful anticancer agent, whether as an immunomodulator or otherwise; it was not consistently better than observation in the NCCTG trial. The mechanism of action of the combination is unclear, as discussed in the only two relevant letters to the editor published by the *New England Journal of Medicine* (323: 197–198) in the months following publication of the intergroup report. What about 5-FU without levamisole? The earlier information about that subject was either ignored or misquoted, but is of interest to review in light of the "new" results.

Since the development of 5-FU in the late 1950s, several multicenter trials of adjuvant 5-FU in colon cancer have been carried out. These were similar in that they involved relatively small numbers of patients and their results were generally negative even though the treated patients fared slightly better than the controls. Some investigators interpreted such results as supporting the use of adjuvant therapy [33]. At that point the NSABP initiated a large trial, CO1 (1166 patients with Dukes B and C colon cancer) using 5-FU plus methyl CCNU plus vincristine versus bacille Calmette–Guérin (BCG) versus no further treatment [34]. The combination chemotherapy regimen had been briefly popular in treating metastatic colon cancer. The use of BCG by scarification was then in vogue as a form of non-specific immunotherapy. The chemotherapy group showed an improvement in disease-free survival ($p=0.02$) and overall survival ($p=0.05$) compared to observation. The outcome was confused somewhat since the BCG arm also showed a survival benefit compared to control. The latter finding was explained as the result of a diminution in deaths that were non-cancer related.

In addition to the quirk regarding BCG, there were other concerns about the CO1 study. Similar studies by the Gastrointestinal Tumor Study Group [35], the Southwest Oncology Group [36], the VA Surgical Oncology Group [37] and the Cross Cancer Center [38] were negative. Two-thirds of the patients in the NASBP trial were "pre-randomized" [39]; that technique, although of considerable interest, has not been widely accepted (Chapter 14). Methyl CCNU is leukemogenic. The study included Dukes B cases, which have not as yet shown a benefit in the intergroup study. The level of significance of the NSABP trial was "borderline" at $p=0.05$. Finally, an Eastern Co-operative Oncology Group Study had shown no advantage of adding methyl CCNU to 5-FU [40].

In the meantime, Buyse et al. [41] carried out an exhaustive meta-analysis of colorectal adjuvant therapy, which appears to have been misquoted on more than one occasion since then. Both colon and rectal studies were included and radiotherapy as well as chemotherapy trials were analyzed. They concluded "some overall survival benefit from adjuvant therapy (up to 1986) cannot be excluded but it is likely small". With regard to the seven studies in which 5-FU was administered (possibly in addition to other drugs) for a period of at least one year, there was a statistically significant survival difference ($p=0.03$). Clinically the effect was very modest, with the improvement in five-year survival only 3.4%, but an effect was seen nevertheless. In fact, the benefits of chemotherapy in other types of cancer sometimes prove to be much smaller than what we have assumed in the past, and it is possible that the long-term benefit of 5-FU plus levamisole in colon cancer will prove to be more modest than the interim results of the intergroup study suggest. It is unfortunate that the recent trials did not include an arm of 5-FU alone; conceivably that would have done as well as the combination.

Thus, either the information on adjuvant therapy of colon cancer is new and is based on two individually ineffective treatments which miraculously work when combined, or the information is old, merely a confirmation of what had been observed in earlier 5-FU trials, which were not appreciated because of the modest long-term benefits. In that case, why all the fuss now?

Levamisole is generally well tolerated, but there are some practical problems with this agent which raise concerns about compliance, both in the trials already completed and in future medical practice. First is the fact that not all patients take oral medicines as prescribed, regardless of the importance of the treatment and even if there are no side-effects. Second, the wholesale cost of a full course of levamisole (excluding other costs, such as that of the 5-FU) in the USA is in excess of $1000; this may be covered by some but not all insurance programs. Finally, it has been reported to produce "antabuse"-like (disulfiram) side-effects in association with alcohol, which may discourage some patients from taking it faithfully.

Although not as likely as with node-negative breast cancer, a substantial fraction of Dukes C patients are cured with surgery and would not benefit from any adjuvant treatment. In the NCCTG study, a multivariate analysis indicated that stage, location, grade and performance score were significant for recurrence (B_2 lesions and rectal lesions were included in that study). The same factors (except performance score) were significant for survival.

In the intergroup study (rectal cancers were excluded), depth of invasion, number of involved nodes and grade were significant for recurrence. The same factors plus location of the primary and obstruction were significant for survival.

Other parameters such as DNA ploidy [42, 43] and chromosome abnormalities [44] are currently being evaluated. Although prognostication about colon cancer is not as developed as in breast cancer, progress will undoubtedly occur in the next few years and will require modification of the blanket recommendation now in place. Better treatment regimens may also emerge for those at high risk.

In an article entitled "Medical Data: Who Should Hear it First?" by Gina Kolata in the *New York Times* (22 May 1990), Dr Charles Moertel, the senior author of the intergroup study of 5-Fu plus levamisole, was quoted as saying:

> I seriously question if there is any time when the well-developed scientific method of insuring truth should be bypassed . . . I can assure you that many of the delays attributed to peer review are in fact necessary delays. Investigators have sent in manuscripts that are inadequate or where the data are misrepresented or inappropriately analyzed. Those who think they can bypass the process of peer review are perhaps those most in need of this process.

The same article suggested that the traditional approach is to keep data "secret" until publication, when in fact virtually all important studies are presented at medical meetings, sometimes well in advance of publication, and may be "covered" by the press, so it is difficult to say that the data are really ever secret. For example, the NCCTG trial interim results were presented in May 1986 [45] complete with press release.

Having lots of pre-publication publicity is no assurance that a study will be favorably received by reviewers. Henderson [46] asked:

> But can peer review operate in the emotional environment that surrounded the publication of the node-negative trials, after the prior judgment of the clinical alert on these trials and the front-page publication of this judgment in the *New York Times* and most other newspapers in the country? If the *New England Journal of Medicine* (*NEJM*) had refused to publish the articles, there would likely have been a public outcry that important information was being withheld from physicians who had a need to know. Even though these reports would almost certainly have been published elsewhere, rejection by the *NEJM* would have resulted in a delay of at least 4 to 6 months. These reports now have the prestigious imprimatur of *NEJM* and its readers will reasonably assume that the papers have passed the rigorous peer-review process for which that journal is justifiably respected throughout the world. Is it possible that on this occasion the editors decided that the public good was better served by relaxing its usual rigorous standards? If so, we must ask if the end really justified these unusual means.

The wisdom of issuing the Clinical Alerts is a subject of continuing debate. Peggy Eastman reported in the April 1990 issue of *Oncology Times* on a special meeting of the National Cancer Advisory Board of the National Cancer Institute held on 31 January 1990. According to this article, NCI Director Samuel Broder MD and other NCI officials strongly defended the institute's right to issue Clinical Alerts. The interests of patients and the public at large "are supreme and over-ride all other interests, such as those of investigators, the organization or institution sponsoring a clinical trial, the scientific peer community, NCI and private sector pharmaceutical companies", Dr Broder said.

Taking the opposite viewpoint was Saul A. Rosenberg MD of Stanford University. Dr Rosenberg said there is "no justification" for bypassing peer review and releasing research results before publication in a respected, reviewed journal. He warned, "the dogmas of today are disproved tomorrow. I do not accept the premise that NCI has the mission or the responsibility to protect the public from cancer. It's much more complicated than that."

Another consideration, presumably not touched on at that meeting, is the reality that NCI is a publicly funded institution which must compete for funds with innumerable science and non-science activities of the federal government. One hopes that the need for publicity and to be in favor with Congress are not considerations when Clinical Alerts are issued.

Medical progress has an ebb and flow; that is unlikely to change. If a truly important, unequivocal medical advance were to occur, it would deserve to be reported broadly and expeditiously, on the nightly TV news and next morning's newspaper. The developments discussed above regarding breast and colon cancer are not so straightforward, and need to be put into perspective before they can be applied to individual patients.

In summary, one can view the colon adjuvant story in at least three ways:

(1) This was in fact important new information which needed to be disseminated imediately.
(2) This was nothing new: the basic information, that 5-FU-based adjuvant treatment was beneficial, was already available from Fisher, Higgins or Buyse, and the fuss had to do with the magnitude of the benefit expected.
(3) The results were subject to change, subject to varying interpretation, achieved by an undefined drug interaction, and best put into perspective in the usual way, with review and debate in the medical community, rather than in the media.

At this juncture the first view is least convincing.

The node-negative breast adjuvant story seems premature both because a survival benefit has not yet been demonstrated and because it emerged in the midst of multiple leads for better defining different risk categories within that group of patients.

As already noted, the phenomenon of Clinical Alerts and Updates is probably here to stay (in which case it is preferable to have physicians notified before the public), but this "experiment", as DeVita called it, should be discouraged when patient care is at issue.

One ideally should have both a complete data set and a prolonged period of follow-up before making a decision as to whether the results of a clinical trial are relevant to the care of one's own patient. However, that is frequently not possible; we are constantly confronted with making the best decision based on inadequate information. Given that the "longitudinal" dimension is typically incomplete, shouldn't we at least be shown the "breadth" of the study, with the short-term results described in as complete a fashion as possible? Shouldn't we also have the benefit of peer review, so that the new findings are put in perspective?

REFERENCES

1. Fisher B, Redmond C, Dimitrov NV et al (1989) A randomized clinical trial evaluating sequential methotrexate and fluorouracil in the treatment of patients with node-negative breast cancer who have estrogen receptor-negative tumors. N Engl J Med 320: 473–478
2. Fisher B, Costantino J, Redmond C et al (1989) A randomized clinical trial evaluating tamoxifen in the treatment of patients with node-negative breast cancer who have estrogen receptor-positive tumors. N Engl J Med 320: 479–484
3. Mansour EG, Gray R, Shatila AH et al (1989) Efficacy of adjuvant chemotherapy in high risk node-negative breast cancer, an intergroup study. N Engl J Med 320: 485–490
4. DeVita VT Jr (1988) Letter to the editor. N Engl J Med 319: 948–949
5. Balch CM, Singletary SE (1988) Adjuvant therapy for node-negative breast cancer patients: who benefits? Arch Surg 123: 1189–1190
6. Merz B (1988) Clinical alert gives breast cancer data, revises recommendations. JAMA 260: 153–154
7. Spratt JS, Greenberg RA (1990) Validity of the clinical alert on breast cancer. Am J Surg 159: 195–198
8. Prosnitz LR (1988) Medical legal implications of clinical alert. J Nat Cancer Inst 80: 1574
9. Cady B (1989) Clinical alert re-visited. Am J Clin Oncol 12: 541–542
10. Lee KC (1988) The clinical alert from the National Cancer Institute. N Engl J Med 319: 948
11. Ludwig Breast Cancer Study Group (1989) Prolonged disease-free survival after one course of peri-operative chemotherapy for node-negative breast cancer. N Engl J Med 320: 491–496
12. McGuire WL (1989) Adjuvant therapy of node-negative breast cancer. N Engl J Med 320: 525–527
13. DeVita VT Jr (1989) Breast cancer therapy: exercising all our options. N Engl J Med 320: 527–529
14. Buckman RA, Pritchard KI, Sutherland DJ et al (1989) Adjuvant therapy for node-negative breast cancer. N Engl J Med 321: 471

15. Tannock IF (1989) Adjuvant therapy for node-negative breast cancer. N Engl J Med 321: 471
16. Pritchard KI (1989) Systemic adjuvant therapy for node-negative breast cancer: proven or premature? Ann Intern Med 111: 1–4
17. Wittes RE (1988) Of clinical alerts and peer review. J Nat Cancer Inst 80: 984–985
18. Rosner D, Lane WW (1990) Node-negative minimal invasive breast cancer patients are not candidates for routine systemic adjuvant therapy. Cancer 66: 199–205
19. Fisher B, Redmond C, Wickerham DL et al (1989) Systemic therapy in patients with node-negative breast cancer: a commentary based on two national surgical adjuvant breast and bowel project clinical trials. Ann Intern Med 111: 703–712
20. International Ludwig Breast Cancer Study Group (1990) Prognostic importance of occult axillary lymph node micrometastases from breast cancers. Lancet 335: 1565–1568
21. Clark GM, Dressler LG, Owens MA et al (1989) Prediction of relapse or survival in patients with node-negative breast cancer by DNA flow cytometry. N Engl J Med 320: 627–633
22. Sigurdsson H, Baldetorp B, Borg A et al (1990) Indicators of prognosis in node-negative breast cancer. N Engl J Med 322: 1045–1053
23. Joensuu H, Toikkanen S, Klemi PJ (1990) DNA index and S-phase fraction and their combination as prognostic factors in operable ductal breast carcinoma. Cancer 66: 331–340
24. Lewis WE (1990) Prognostic significance of flow cytometric DNA analysis in node-negative breast cancer patients. Cancer 65: 2315–2320
25. Tandon AK, Clark GM, Chamness GC et al (1990) Cathepsin-D and prognosis in breast cancer. N Engl J Med 322: 297–302
26. Spyratos F, Brouillet JP, Defrenne A et al (1989) Cathepsin-D: an independent prognostic factor for metastasis of breast cancer. Lancet ii: 1115–1118
27. Henry JA, McCarthy AL, Angus B et al (1990) Prognostic significance of the estrogen regulated protein, cathepsin-D in breast cancer: an immuno-histochemical study. Cancer 65: 265–271
28. McGuire WL, Tandon AK, Allred DC et al (1990) How to use prognostic factors in axillary node-negative breast cancer patients. J Nat Cancer Inst 82: 1006–1015
29. Laurie JA, Moertel CG, Flemming TR et al (1989) Surgical adjuvant therapy of large bowel carcinoma: an evaluation of levamisole and the combination of levamisole and fluorouracil: the North Central Cancer Treatment Group and the Mayo Clinic. J Clin Oncol 7: 1447–1456
30. Windle R, Bell PRF, Shaw D (1987) Five-year results of a randomized trial of adjuvant 5-fluorouracil and levamisole in colorectal cancer. Br J Surg 74: 569–572
31. Moertel CG, Flemming TR, McDonald JS et al (1990) Levamisole and fluorouracil for adjuvant therapy of resected colon carcinoma. N Engl J Med 322: 352–358
32. NIH Consensus Conference (1990) Adjuvant therapy for patients with colon and rectal cancer. JAMA 264: 1444–1450
33. Higgins GA, Lee LE, Dwight RW et al (1978) The case for adjuvant 5-fluorouracil in colorectal cancer. Cancer Clin Trials 1: 35–41
34. Wollmark N, Fisher B, Rockette H et al (1988) Post-operative adjuvant chemotherapy or BCG for colon cancer: results from NSABP protocol CO1. J Nat Cancer Inst 80: 30–36

35. Gastrointestinal Tumor Study Group (1984) Adjuvant therapy of colon cancer: results of a prospectively randomized trial. N Engl J Med 310: 737–743
36. Panettiere FJ, Goodman PJ, Costanzi JJ et al (1988) Adjuvant therapy in large bowel adenocarcinoma: long term results of the Southwest Oncology Group Study. J Clin Oncol 6: 947–954
37. Higgins GA, Amadeo JH, McElhinney J et al (1984) Efficacy of prolonged intermittent therapy with combined 5-fluorouracil and methyl CCNU following resection for carcinoma of the large bowel: a Veterans Administration Surgical Oncology Group Report. Cancer 53: 1–8
38. Abdi EA, Hanson J, Harbora DE et al (1989) Adjuvant chemo-immunotherapy and immunotherapy in Dukes' stage B2 and C colorectal carcinoma: a seven-year follow-up analysis. J Surg Oncol 40: 205–213
39. Zelen M (1979) A new design for randomized clinical trials. N Engl J Med 300: 1242–1245
40. Mansour E, Ryan L, Lerner H et al (1989) Lack of effectiveness of 5-FU and methyl CCNU as compared to 5-FU for adjuvant therapy in colon cancer: a randomized trial of the Eastern Cooperative Oncology Group. Proc Am Soc Clin Oncol 8: 115 (Abstract 447)
41. Buyse M, Zeleniuch-Jacquotte A, Chalmers TC (1988) Adjuvant therapy of colorectal cancer: why we still don't know. JAMA 259: 3571–3578
42. Hood DL, Petras RE, Edinger M et al (1990) DNA ploidy and cell cycle analysis of colorectal carcinoma by flow cytometry. Am J Clin Pathol 93: 615–620
43. Wiggers T, Arends JW, Schutte B et al (1988) A multivariate analysis of pathologic prognostic indicators in large bowel cancer. Cancer 61: 386–395
44. Kern SE, Fearon ER, Tersmette K et al (1989) Allelic loss in colorectal carcinoma. JAMA 261: 3099–3103
45. Laurie J, Moertel C, Flemming T et al (1986) Surgical adjuvant therapy of poor prognosis colorectal cancer with levamisole alone or combined levamisole and 5-fluorouracil. Proc Am Soc Clin Oncol 5: 81 (Abstract 316)
46. Henderson IC (1990) Shouldn't we see the white flag before we cry victory? J Nat Cancer Inst 82: 103–109

ABOUT THE AUTHOR

Dr George Omura is a native of New York City who graduated from Columbia University magna cum laude; he received his MD degree in 1962 from Cornell University Medical College, where he was elected to Alpha Omega Alpha Honorary Medical Society. After housestaff training at Bellevue Hospital and active duty in the US Navy, he completed fellowships in medical oncology and in hematology at Memorial Sloan-Kettering Cancer Center. Since 1970 he has been on the faculty of the University of Alabama at Birmingham, where he is currently Professor of Medicine and Senior Scientist in the Comprehensive Cancer Centre. His major interest over the past 20 years has been in cancer clinical trials. He has served on various committees of the Southeastern Cancer Study Group, Gynecologic Oncology Group and Cancer and Leukemia Group B. From 1983 to 1987 he served as the Group Chairman of the Southeastern Cancer Study Group.

30 Achieving a Consensus on Cancer Treatment

TONY SMITH

In the USA, Britain and other Western countries treatment given to most cancer patients is a matter of chance determined largely by geography. Take as an example a woman with breast cancer. Where she lives is likely to determine the surgeon to whom she may be referred; and unless she and her general practitioner discuss the matter beforehand (a rare event) she will have no advance idea of the attitudes to treatment held by the surgeon she sees.

And these are very variable. A survey of the treatment of primary breast cancer by British surgeons found substantial differences in the choice of surgical procedure and whether or not treatment was recommended with adjuvant chemotherapy or radiotherapy or both [1]. Only one surgeon in four saw more than 50 patients with breast cancer in a year. Most considered mastectomy the treatment of choice, and many referred these patients for radiotherapy too, but others were willing to treat women by local excision alone. In general the more patients a surgeon saw the less radical the treatment he offered. Around three-quarters of the surgeons sometimes recommended adjuvant chemotherapy, but 32 of 454 said their patients never received it.

The authors concluded that "with the prevalence and diversity of breast cancer and the complexities of the many options for treatment perhaps the time has come to encourage treatment by specialized breast units. This would permit conformity of management of the disease and facilitate research into new modes of treatment."

Well-publicized variations of this kind are disquieting for patients and the public at large, who believe that there must be a clearly defined optimum management for any individual woman. This belief is reinforced by the publicity given to consensus conferences and other apparently authoritative statements setting out treatment guidelines. Is this belief correct? Are there optimum treatments for most cancer patients—in this example all categories of women with breast cancer—and is it true that many women receive treatment that is less than optimum?

To answer these questions we need to examine the origin and purposes of consensus conferences. They were originally introduced at the US National Institutes of Health (NIH) not so much to settle therapeutic

Introducing New Treatments for Cancer: Practical, Ethical and Legal Problems. Edited by C. J. Williams
© 1992 John Wiley & Sons Ltd

controversies as to allay disquiet about the possibly over-enthusiastic adoption of high-technology medical and surgical techniques (the first conference, in 1977, was provoked by fears that the radiation hazards of mammography were being underestimated).

At that time technological and therapeutic innovations in medicine were seen to follow a predictable life cycle, described by several commentators and usefully summarized by Jennet [2]. The first promising reports of small numbers of patients treated successfully are usually uncontrolled and anecdotal—but are often given prominent press publicity. (Research charities should accept much of the blame for these premature ejaculations: all too often the reports are based on press handouts issued by public relations consultants retained by the charities.)

Next, the new treatment/technology is adopted by other groups or institutions either from scientific interest or in the belief that it will improve the care of patients. This is soon followed by public acceptance that the innovation is valuable and should be available to patients. Pressure groups and lobbyists now begin their work (and in the USA the critical decision is whether or not the innovation is accepted for third-party payment). In Britain fund-raising appeals may be launched, often aided by enthusiastic doctors and encouraged by manufacturers or pharmaceutical companies.

Before much longer, if all is going well, the procedure may be promoted by its supporters and enthusiasts as "standard"—which implies that other clinicians may use it without going to the trouble of enrolling their patients into any sort of clinical trial. The amount of evidence available to support such an assessment is highly variable. In the case of mechanical technologies such as scanners, prostheses and so on, the only reports published in peer review journals may be anecdotal and uncontrolled. Published reports of drug trials are of variable quality—but even the most impressive sometimes turn out (years later) to have been defective or even fraudulent. There is, says Jennet, usually little enthusiasm at this stage to mount the large-scale, long-term trials that are really needed. Those who have already invested time, energy and finance in a particular development may, indeed, fear that the results of such well-designed controlled trials may signal the first warning notes that the product is "not the panacea that its promoters hoped (or even claimed)".

Nevertheless, trials are usually mounted and their early results given wide publicity, though depressingly few ever seem to generate the long-term, late results that would provide a convincing verdict. At this stage professional denunciation begins—a confrontation between the champions of the innovation and its opponents, who may be the organizers of the controlled trials or may be commentators on those trials who have drawn attention to their defects and reanalysed their data.

Confusion reigns, and in an attempt to allay it and produce some clear guidance for the great mass of clinicians who are non-participants in the confrontation a consensus conference may be arranged.

CONSENSUS CONFERENCES

When these conferences were first introduced at the NIH the Director, Dr Donald S. Frederickson, saw them as meetings which would bring together medical experts from a wide variety of disciplines who could then assess the whole body of research evidence and distil from it an agreed verdict. From the beginning US consensus conferences recognized the importance of consumer interests, and patients, ethicists, philosophers and economists were added to the panels to widen the range of issues discussed and on which expert opinion would be available.

The first meeting—on the value and risks of methods currently available for screening for breast cancer—took place at the NIH in 1977 and many more followed. By 1984, when the first consensus conference was organized in Britain [4] (on coronary artery bypass grafting) the Americans had organized and reported on nearly 50 topics, and other European countries had already climbed on to the bandwagon.

Unfortunately as the conferences proliferated their initial enthusiastic reception became muted and sceptics began to question their value. The influential editor of the *New England Journal of Medicine*, Dr Arnold Relman, commented cynically that "an assessment of current knowledge, no matter how sophisticated and rigorous, cannot go beyond that knowledge and rarely generates any new information. What was unknown before the review remains unknown afterwards. Major controversies are rarely resolved [5]". Another journalistic assessment, by Dr Drummond Rennie, concluded that most consensus statements were bland generalities that represented the lowest common denominator of a debate—"the only points on which those experts can wholeheartedly agree [6]". These points, said Rennie, were a long way from the cutting edge of progress and might, indeed, be a dead hand discouraging thought.

Another criticism sometimes made is that the medical members of the consensus may be chosen by the organizers to represent one school of thought. The original concept required the panel to be authoritative and to include both supporters and critics of a specific technology, with enough uncommitted members to act as a jury. The majority decisions of the panel were then seen as verdicts by an informed collection of medical and lay jurors. More recently, however, so-called consensus conferences have been set up by pressure groups or simply by well-meaning enthusiasts for a particular policy of treatment or screening. Such self-styled consensus meetings may be expected to carry little weight with clinicians.

SPECIFIC RECOMMENDATIONS

How far, then, do recent consensus conferences help the clinician uncertain about the therapeutic implications of recent research findings? Do they provide him or her with algorithms setting out clear-cut treatment plans for the great majority of patients?

Unfortunately they do not. Consensus conferences have been valuable in achieving their original objective—defining the place of a technological innovation by assessing its efficacy, safety and costs, and comparing these with the results of earlier techniques. They have been less helpful in defining an agreed therapeutic approach to the major cancers.

Let us stay with the example of breast cancer and look at the report of the King's Fund Forum held in London in 1986 [7] (which came only a few months after an NIH conference in the USA [8] and reached broadly similar conclusions). The King's Fund report covered a vast tract of territory in two pages of the *British Medical Journal*. It gave advice on the initial assessment of women with suspicious symptoms and on the initial local treatment. Here it concluded that mastectomy (or more extensive surgery) gave no survival advantage over local excision, but it pointed out that the smaller procedure carried a risk of local recurrence and that this risk could be reduced by radiotherapy. The statement urged doctors to recognize the arguments in favour of women's participation in treatment decisions, and the clear implication was that the decisions on primary treatment should be agreed between the woman and her surgeon after discussion. In practice, however, this verdict must have left each surgeon to make up his own mind when faced with the patient who asks "What would you do, doctor, if it was your wife?"

Probably the most contentious issue in the treatment of breast cancer is the place of adjuvant chemotherapy in women having primary surgical treatment intended to be curative. What was the King's Forum's advice? It made one clear assessment from the research studies: "the use of a combination of agents (cyclophosphamide, methotrexate and 5-fluorouracil—CMF) in women with affected nodes reduces their risk of death over the subsequent five years from 36% to 27% compared with women who had single-agent or no chemotherapy". But the statement then qualified this advice by saying that "any benefits are substantially less in women over 50. Furthermore these drugs may have unpleasant side effects, so their costs and benefits must be carefully assessed". And a final straw was then offered to the therapeutic nihilist—"a study with a 20-year follow up shows a reduced mortality rate after a six day course of cyclophosphamide"—at the end of a paragraph urging the superiority of multiple over single agents.

A surgeon whose prior assessment of the evidence had been that CMF should be given to pre-menopausal women with affected nodes would be reassured by the statement—but surgeons with more conservative views could read into the same statement enough qualifications to continue their therapeutic nihilism. Furthermore the statement gave no advice on the most contentious aspect of adjuvant chemotherapy—the choice of treatment for women with negative nodes [9].

CONSUMER CHOICE AND SCIENTIFIC RIGOUR

One of the reasons for the lack of unequivocal explicit guidelines in the breast cancer consensus was the wish by the panel to emphasize the importance of each woman making a substantial contribution to choices about her treatment. A second reason for vagueness in consensus guidelines was the lack of clear-cut, convincing evidence from clinical trials. As the critics of consensus conferences have said, such meetings cannot generate new findings—indeed what they commonly do is to point up the defects in the body of published evidence the conference experts have examined. Sometimes, indeed, the conclusion reached by a consensus conference is that no consensus is possible on the evidence currently available, a recent example being the conference on in situ breast cancer organized by the European Organization for Research on Treatment of Cancer [10].

MORE TRIALS NEEDED

At the heart of the problem is the shameful fact that only some 1% of adults with cancer are recruited into phase III clinical trials comparing the efficacy of new treatments with "state-of-the-art" therapy [11]. In part this lack of recruitment reflects the anti-intellectual nature of our times, with science having a poor public image and consumer groups campaigning against the enrolment of patients into any form of clinical trial.

A second negative factor is the reluctance of clinicians to embark on trials of treatment for cancer. Many surgeons believe that participation in a trial will be time consuming, will substantially reduce their clinical freedom to tailor the treatment to the individual patient, and will require many years of effort before any results emerge. There is some justification for these fears. A not untypical protocol for patients with advanced breast cancer is set out in Figure 1 [12]. Twenty-seven institutions in the Federal Republic of Germany participated and between them recruited 347 patients over a period of 24 months—an average of slightly less than 13 patients each. Furthermore half the patients did not comply with the protocol, either because they or their doctors "felt the therapy recommended was not appropriate". Instead of the protocol therapy patients were given treatment of either greater or less intensity.

THE WAY FORWARD

If, then, consensus guidelines are too often insufficiently specific and clinicians are reluctant to participate in trials, what is the way forward? Will patients with cancer continue to be treated according to the beliefs, prejudices

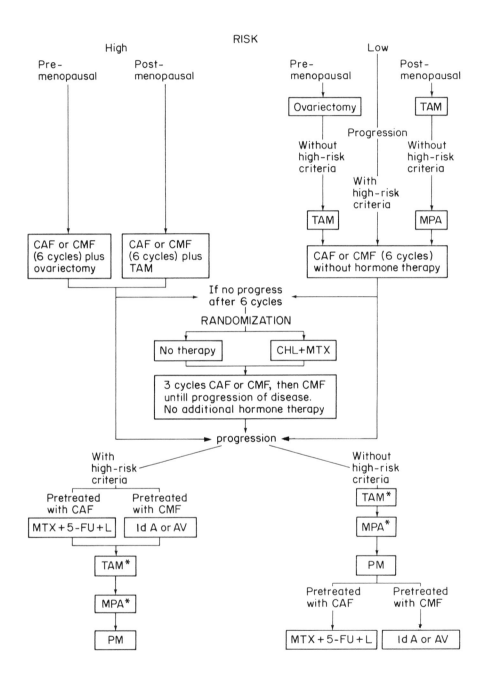

and convictions of individual clinicians? Is there any prospect for patients being given more uniform treatment?

Fortunately the laissez-faire approach that has existed in Britain since the introduction of the National Health Service is about to be changed, by the introduction of medical audit. The central concept of audit is that the outcome of treatment should be systematically assessed and recorded in a cohort of patients, the results analysed, and treatment then modified with the aim of improving outcome in the next cohort. At the very least clinicians engaged in audit will need to decide on basic protocols of treatment for the common conditions they treat and they should be prepared to justify the detailed make-up of those treatments. What are the possible sources for such protocols? In a few cases there may be a consensus statement sufficiently detailed to provide such information, though consensus statements rarely if ever specify details such as doses and duration of drug therapy.

For most conditions, however, clinicians will be left on their own. This presents a real opportunity for oncologists and specialist societies to set up large-scale, broad-spectrum trials of treatment that can be presented to clinicians as packages that will fulfil audit criteria.

Already efforts are being made to find ways of simplifying trials with the intention of making them more acceptable to surgeons and so increasing the numbers of patients recruited. These new-style pragmatic trials are said "to come much closer to daily clinical practice and not to demand more than minimal work from participants". An example is the AXIS trial, designed to settle 30 years' debate about the merits of adjuvant chemotherapy for colorectal cancer [13]. Trial eligibility will be determined by the participants, and while the trial sets out broad guidelines on dose and fractionation clinicians will be given some latitude in adapting the protocol to local practice.

Figure 1. *(opposite)* Protocol for treatment of advanced breast cancer patients. The initial therapies and the consecutive therapies after progression of the disease are shown. The therapies had to be applied for at least two months or two cycles before evaluation of response. If the disease was still progressive the next therapeutic step was applied. If the evaluation confirmed remission or stable disease the therapy was continued until progression. TAM, tamoxifen p.o. 30 mg per day. MPA, medroxy-progesterone acetate p.o. 1000 mg per day. CAF, cyclophosphamide i.v. 500 mg/m^2, day 1 and adriamycin i.v. 50 mg/m^2, day 1 and 5-fluorouracil i.v. 500 mg/m^2, days 1+8. Repeated day 28. CMF, cyclophosphamide p.o. 100 mg/m^2, days 1–14 and methotrexate i.v. 40 mg/m^2, days 1+8 and 5-fluorouracil i.v. 600 mg/m^2, days 1+8. Repeated day 28. CHL+MTX, chlorambucil p.o. 0.1 mg/kg per day and methotrexate p.o. 15 mg weekly. MTX+5 FU+L, methotrexate i.v. 200 mg/m^2, day 1 and 5-fluorouracil i.v. 600 mg/m^2, day 1, 1 h after MTX, and Leucovorin p.o. 10 mg/m^2, six times every 6 h starting 24 h after MTX. Repeated day 21. ldA, low-dose adriamycin i.v. 15 mg/m^2 weekly. AV, adriamycin i.v. 40 mg/m^2 day 1 and vincristine i.v. 1.4 mg/m^2, days 1+8. Repeated day 28. PM, prednimustin p.o. 160 mg/m^2, days 1–5. Repeated day 21.
*Therapy is skipped if patient had not responded to previous application of this drug.

In the new audit era clinicians will, then, need to specify the treatment regimens they intend offering to their patients with cancer. Only in a few cases will there be unequivocal guidance from a consensus statement or some other authoritative source. In other circumstances clinicians should be enrolling as many patients as possible (both above and below 65 years) in well-organized multicentre trials. The challenge for the 1990s is to oncologists, specialist societies and research charities to organize "user-friendly" trials large enough and simple enough to absorb a substantial fraction of all cancer patients. In the future the question for the audit meetings should be "why weren't these patients enrolled in a trial?" Freehand, idiosyncratic treatment (justified by cries of clinical freedom and responsibility to patients) has no place in an era of systematic recording and assessment.

REFERENCES

1. Gazet J-C, Rainsbury RM, Ford HT, Powles TJ, Coombes RC (1985) Survey of treatment of primary breast cancer in Great Britain. Br Med J 290: 1793–1795
2. Jennet B (1983) Managing high technology medicine in the future. In: High technology medicine: benefits and burdens. London: Nuffield Provincial Hospitals Trust, London, pp 187–229
3. Perry S, Kalberer JT (1980) The NIH Consensus-Development Program and the assessment of health-care technologies. N Engl J Med 303: 169–172
4. Anonymous (1984) Consensus development conference: coronary artery bypass grafting. Br Med J 289: 1527–1529
5. Relman AS (1980) Assessment of medical practices: a simple proposal. N Engl J Med 303: 153–154
6. Rennie D (1986) Consensus statements. N Engl J Med 304: 665–666
7. Anonymous (1986) Consensus development conference: treatment of primary breast cancer. Br Med J 293: 946–947
8. Lippman ME (1985) National Institutes of Health consensus development conference on adjuvant chemotherapy and endocrine therapy for breast cancer. In: NCI Monographs. NIH, Bethesda, pp 1–5
9. McGuire W (1989) Adjuvant therapy of node negative breast cancer. N Engl J Med 320: 525–527
10. Dongen JV, Fentiman IS, Harris JR et al (1989) In-situ breast cancer: the EORTC consensus meeting. Lancet ii: 25–27
11. Lawrence W (1990) Introduction to the Workshop on Clinical Trials. Cancer 65: 2369–2370
12. Porzolt F, Meuret G, Kreuzer ED et al (1989) Compliance of physicians and patients with a consensus protocol for treatment of advanced cancer. J Cancer Res Clin Oncol 115: 564–570
13. Taylor I, Northover JMA (1990) Adjuvant therapy in colorectal cancer: the need for a megatrial. Br J Surg 77: 841–842

ABOUT THE AUTHOR

Dr Tony Smith spent six years in clinical medicine before joining the *British Medical Journal* in 1965, and he has worked there ever since, mostly reviewing and referring to outside experts his share of the 5000 papers and articles submitted each year.

As a popular journalist he has written and edited six books on medical topics and has also contributed to *The Times, The Sunday Times, The Observer,* and *The Independent on Sunday*.

The only justification he can advance for having the temerity to contribute to this book is that in recent years he has written quite a lot on the treatment of patients with cancer and on medical audit both in the *British Medical Journal* and elsewhere.

31 Patient Assessment of Adjuvant Treatment in Operable Breast Cancer

ALAN S. COATES and R. JOHN SIMES

Decisions are inseparable from the practice of medicine. They are ultimately taken by the treating doctor, but very often require the consideration of the wishes of the patient. This chapter considers the question of adjuvant cytotoxic therapy for operable breast cancer, in which input from the patient may be crucial to the decision to give or withhold treatment. The views of patients who have experienced such treatment may help to decide whether or not to treat future similar patients.

Some treatments are so clearly beneficial, and have so few side effects, that the decision as to whether they should be used or not is rarely a matter for conscious thought. Pneumococcal pneumonia, a potentially lethal disease with an appalling natural history, responds so well to penicillin that the diagnosis is tantamount to the prescription. It is otherwise with many therapeutic decisions in medical oncology. Even in simple situations, the decision-making process is subliminally present, as would be evident if the patient with pneumonia volunteered a history vaguely suggestive of penicillin allergy, or the bacteriological diagnosis were less than secure. Many factors go into the decision as to whether a particular treatment should be used in a given clinical situation, but they can be boiled down to a balance between the costs and the benefits associated with either the use or the withholding of the treatment. More precisely, the probability and the magnitude of the benefit are weighed against the probability and the severity of the adverse effects, the monetary cost and the social disruption associated with the treatment in question.

Doctors are used to making such decisions, but are less accustomed to quantifying the component factors which go into them. Formal decision theory is lamentably rare in the undergraduate medical curriculum. When alternative therapies involve different practitioners, there is a natural tendency for doctors to exhibit bias in favour of the treatment modality they administer themselves. Arbitrary decisions by doctors bring predictable (and sometimes justified) complaints of paternalism. In an attempt to overcome this charge, some have appealed to the judgment of lay observers. In one important study, Barbara McNeil and colleagues addressed the choice

Introducing New Treatments for Cancer: Practical, Ethical and Legal Problems. Edited by C. J. Williams
© 1992 John Wiley & Sons Ltd

between surgical laryngectomy and radiation therapy for the treatment of carcinoma of the larynx. Healthy volunteers (12 fire-fighters and 25 executives) were informed of the superior survival associated with surgery, and the retention of natural voice with radiation therapy, and asked to choose. About one-fifth of the volunteers indicated a preference for radiation therapy.

The benefits of adjuvant cytotoxic therapy after local treatment for operable breast cancer have been studied in a large number of clinical trials, which were recently the subject of several major overviews conducted by the Early Breast Cancer Trials Group. The results seem quite clear. Beyond reasonable doubt, treatment with several cycles of combination chemotherapy reduces the odds of death by about one-quarter. Benefit is lasting, with further advantage for treated patients becoming evident between five and ten years after treatment. The *proportional* benefit appears largely independent of the risk group. This translates into *absolute* benefits, expressed as differences in percentage alive at a given time after treatment, which are markedly different in groups of varying prognosis. As a rough estimate, the benefit of adjuvant therapy with a combination of cyclophosphamide, methotrexate and 5-fluorouracil (CMF), expressed in difference in five-year survival, is about 10% for patients with stage II disease (metastasis to axillary lymph nodes). The benefit for good-risk stage I patients without nodal involvement is less clear, but may be as little as 1–2%.

The adverse effects of chemotherapy are more difficult to measure. Standard toxicity scales are available for nausea, vomiting, alopecia and other side-effects, but patient self-assessment is more rarely sought. Long-term psychosocial effects of adjuvant chemotherapy were studied by Meyerowitz and colleagues. They interviewed 35 women about two years after treatment, and reported some persisting problems related to chemotherapy in more than half the patients.

The benefits of adjuvant cytotoxic therapy are apparently modest, and the costs real. Who is to decide whether treatment is justifiable?

It is the belief of the present authors that treatment decisions by surrogate decision-makers are fundamentally inappropriate. Healthy volunteers know neither the anxieties of having the disease nor the actual side-effects of treatment. Even when the initial consternation and confusion subside, the values and judgments of a patient with a life-threatening illness are different from those of a healthy person. Furthermore, patients who have not experienced a treatment may tend to make judgments based on the worst possible side-effects, rather than on a reasonable average expectation. The study we conducted was therefore designed to ask the patients themselves.

Between November 1986 and December 1987, women who had received standard cytotoxic chemotherapy comprising at least three 28-day cycles of CMF as adjuvant treatment after local treatment for operable breast cancer were asked to rate the benefit which would make treatment worthwhile.

Patients who, having started such therapy, withdrew from it either by their own choice or by the decision of their doctor were also eligible to participate in the study. Consent was obtained both from the patient and her doctor. Patients with inadequate comprehension of English were ineligible. Of 129 patients considered for participation in the study, 9 were excluded because of insufficient comprehension of English, 5 were considered by their doctors to be too ill to participate, 3 were geographically inaccessible, 2 died before interview and 2 were not asked. Only 4 of those approached failed to participate. Thus 104 patients completed initial interview, and of these 65 completed a retest interview.

All patients underwent a semi-structured interview by one of two observers not connected with their treatment, at least three months after completion of chemotherapy. Baseline data included sociodemographic, disease and treatment variables, listed in Table 1.

TIME TRADE-OFF QUESTIONS

The basic method of the study was to establish the patients' opinion of what additional period of survival with treatment would be worthwhile to justify the adverse experience of the treatment they had received. Patients were presented with hypothetical scenarios, of the general form:

"Suppose that without treatment you would live 5 years. Based on your experience of chemotherapy, what period of survival would make six months of initial treatment worthwhile?"

Two cards were placed on the table, one bearing the five-year period without treatment, and the other card a longer period with initial treatment. The second card was then altered until the patient considered the period to be roughly of equal value to the five years without treatment. To control for framing effects, the sequence in which alternatives were offered was randomly assigned. Patients were initially offered a period of six or 10 years with treatment, versus five years without treatment. In either case, the cards were altered in response to the patient's reply until equivalence was established. This period was referred to as five-year trade-off. A similar sequence was then followed to establish equivalence to an expectation of 15 years survival without treatment, which was referred to as 15-year trade-off.

SURVIVAL RATE QUESTIONS

These were essentially similar to the time trade-off approach, but expressed the outcome of treatment in terms of percentage chance of remaining alive

Table 1. Baseline sociodemographic disease and treatment variables

Patient characteristics

Age at interview	Median 48.5 years, range 25–67
Time between diagnosis and interview	≤1 yr 14%, ≤3.5 yrs 50%, >3.5 yes 50%
Time between last cycle of chemotherapy and interview	≤1 yr 27%, ≤3 yrs 50%, >3 yrs 50%
Educational level	Primary 12%, secondary 63%, tertiary 25%
Employment	Full time 31%, part time 21%, none 48%
Marital status	Married 73%, divorced or separated 16%, widowed 3%, single 9%
Number of cohabitants	None 9%, one 35%, two 22%, three 21%, four or more 13%
Number of children under 15 years of age	None 71%, one 12%, two 11%, three or more 7%
Number of others dependent on patient for support	None 58%, one 26%, two or more 16%
Amount of support required by dependants	Nil 43%, partial 37%, full 20%
Amount of support available to patient	Nil 7%, partial 31%, full 62%

Treatment details

Whether patient completed planned course of chemotherapy	12% did not
Whether patient received radiotherapy as part of initial treatment	18% did
Percentage of full dose received for total planned cycles	≤75%: 41%, >75%: 59%
Percentage of full dose received for cycles actually given	≤75%: 33%, >75%: 67%
Whether concomitant adjuvant endocrine therapy given	18%
Whether disease had relapsed	Local 5%, distant 11%, both 4%
Endocrine therapy for progressive disease	14%
Radiation therapy for progressive disease	11%
Cytotoxic therapy for progressive disease	8%

Treatment toxicities (World Health Organization)

Grade	Nil	Mild	Mod.	Severe
Alopecia	19%	46%	29%	6%
Mucositis	55%	23%	21%	1%
Nausea and vomiting	12%	37%	43%	9%
Haematological toxicity	30%	33%	34%	4%
Other	55%	37%	7%	2%
Maximum non-haematological	3%	20%	62%	15%

at five years. The percentage selected as equivalent to 65% untreated was referred to as SR65, and that equivalent to 85% as SR85. Again, framing effects were assessed by randomly offering initial options at the high or low end of the expected response range.

RISK-POSTURE QUESTIONS

An attempt was made to ascertain whether patients were risk averse, risk seeking or risk neutral. Two hypothetical choices were presented. The first offered a choice between a certain survival of ten years and a 50 : 50 gamble between five and 15 years, while in the second (introduced after the first 12 patients) the certain period was five years and the 50 : 50 gamble between early death (within one month) and a survival of ten years. In each case the period of certain survival was altered until the patient rated it as of equal value to the gamble. Thus risk-neutral patients would accept the mathematically equivalent period first offered, risk-averse patients a shorter and risk-seeking patients a longer period of certain survival as equivalent to the gambles. The results are referred to as 5 : 15 gamble and 1 : 10 gamble respectively.

RETEST INTERVIEWS

Where possible, patients were interviewed three to six months after the initial interview. Twelve patients refused a second interview, 4 had died in the interval and a further 6 were excluded by the interviewer because of poor comprehension or anxiety at the first interview. Seventeen patients initially interviewed by the first observer were not retested by the second. Results of the repeat interviews were used to assess reliability of the measures used, and to determine changes in preference over time.

STATISTICAL METHODS

The results of the time trade-off and survival rate questions were skewed, and no effective normalizing transformation was available. Therefore, the actual scores were replaced by their normal scores whereby the rank of each result was replaced by its expected value in a standard normal distribution. These transformed variables were then used as outcome variables in univariate and multivariate regression analyses. For each patient, the normal scores of the five-year trade-off and 15-year trade-off were added to give a single score (trade-off total), defined a priori as the main outcome for comparing patient groups. Variables from Table 1 for which the frequency of a "yes" category was low were excluded from multivariate analyses.

An individual who is risk averse places more value on early than late survival benefits, while one who is risk neutral would value these equally. Assessment of risk posture was therefore considered relevant to adjuvant chemotherapy, since toxicity occurs early but benefits are delayed.

The risk-posture questions yielded imprecise data in 13 patients, who were unable to define an exact period of equivalence, but merely to decide whether they would accept the initial gamble. For this reason, the outcomes for 1 : 10 gamble and 5 : 15 gamble were recoded to a binary variable: risk averse versus risk neutral or risk seeking. Explanatory variables were then dichotomized, and exact tests performed on the resulting 2×2 tables to investigate associations with risk posture.

RESULTS

RELIABILITY

Test–retest reliability was assessed by Spearman's rank correlation between first and second interview in the 65 patients available. Reasonable correlations (0.63–0.69) were obtained for the main study end-points, the time trade-off and survival rate questions (Table 2), but these figures overestimate reliability, as some patients were excluded from a second interview because they had problems at the first. Reliability of the risk-posture assessment was poor. There was no systematic change in the answers to time trade-off or risk-posture questions, but there was a signficant change to a larger increment in survival rate in second interviews.

FRAMING EFFECTS

No significant difference was observed in any of the end-points selected as a result of the sequence in which alternatives were offered.

Table 2. Test–retest reliability: Spearman's correlation coefficient

	Variable	Size	Coefficient
All test–retests			
	TTO5	65	0.68
	TTO15	63	0.64
	SR65	63	0.63
	SR85	63	0.69
	RA5__15	58	0.25
	RA1__10	48	0.25

Abbreviations: TTO5, TTO15, five and 15-year trade-off; SR65, SR85, survival rate trade-off versus 65% and 85% untreated; RA5__15, 5 versus 15-year gamble; RA1__10, 1-month versus 10-year gamble.

PATIENT PREFERENCES

The major finding of the study was that a large majority of the patients felt that relatively modest improvements in survival duration or in the percentage of five-year survival would justify six months of the treatment they received. This was true both in the relatively optimistic scenarios, with untreated survival of 15 years or five-year survival of 85% and in the less favourable, with untreated expectations of five years and 65%.

Details of the percentage of responding patients accepting that treatment would be worthwhile at various trade-off points are displayed in Table 3 (time trade-off) and Table 4 (survival percentage trade-off). Although chemotherapy lasted about six months in most patients, a substantial minority demanded only this period of extra survival to justify treatment. Thus, 46% of patients considered a survival of five years and six months with treatment equivalent to five years without, and 39% would accept a similar increment even with an expected survival of 15 years (Table 3). Results of the survival percentage trade-off were even more extreme, with almost half the women judging a 1% improvement in five-year survival probability as justifying treatment, whether the expected five-year survival without treatment was 65% or 85%.

The minimum end-points at which a *majority* of patients would accept treatment were five-year trade-off of six years (77% acceptance), 15-year trade-off of 16 years (61% acceptance), SR65 of 67% (53% acceptance) and SR85 of 87% (54% acceptance). Are such increments achievable? A reasonable

Table 3. Time trade-off decision points

Minimum requirement to accept treatment		Number	%	Cumulative %
TTO5 years (1 not obtained)				
	≤ 5.25	28	27	27
	≤ 5.50	19	18	46
	≤ 6.00	32	31	77
	≤ 7.00	13	13	89
	≤ 8.00	3	3	92
	≤10.00	6	6	98
	≤20.00	1	1	99
	>20.00	1	1	–
TTO15 years (2 not obtained)				
	≤15.25	23	23	23
	≤15.50	17	17	39
	≤16.00	22	22	61
	≤17.00	13	13	74
	≤18.00	6	6	79
	≤20.00	12	12	91
	>20.00	9	9	–

Abbreviations: see Table 2.

Table 4. Survival percentage trade-off decision points

Minimum requirement to accept treatment		Number	%	Cumulative %
SR65% chance (5 not obtained)				
	≤ 66	47	47	47
	≤ 67	5	5	53
	≤ 68	5	5	58
	≤ 70	15	15	73
	≤ 75	9	9	82
	≤ 80	9	9	91
	≤ 90	7	7	98
	> 100	2	2	–
SR85% chance (6 not obtained)				
	≤ 86	48	49	49
	≤ 87	5	5	54
	≤ 88	8	8	62
	≤ 90	12	12	74
	≤ 95	8	8	83
	≤ 100	14	14	97
	> 100	3	3	–

Abbreviations: see Table 2.

estimate based on the Early Breast Cancer Trialists Overview of improvement in five-year survival for pre-menopausal node-positive women treated with CMF would be about 10%, which would be acceptable to 82% of the women responding to SR65. If the SR85 scenario is taken to correspond to moderate-risk node-negative disease, a 3% or 5% absolute increase in survival might be predicted, and would be acceptable to 62% and 74% of women respectively, based on responses to SR85. Similarly, in patients aged 50–60 with involved nodes, a 5% improvement in five-year survival for addition of chemotherapy to tamoxifen as estimated from the overview would be acceptable to 73% of women (Table 4), suggesting that additional adjuvant chemotherapy may be worthwhile for some years after the menopause, and therefore raising the possibility that the widespread current practice of offering such women tamoxifen alone may be out of step with patient preferences.

PATIENT FACTORS AFFECTING PREFERENCES

Support required by dependants of the patient

Support required was categorized as none (46 patients), partial (37) and full (20). This was strongly associated with the time trade-off of end-points selected by the women. Patients whose dependants required full or partial support demanded lesser increments in survival to justify treatment

(Kruskall Wallis p-values were 0.002 for five-year trade-off, 0.0004 for 15-year trade-off and 0.0004 for trade-off total). No such effect was seen in the percentage trade-off values, perhaps because most patients selected similar small percentage increments. This factor remained significant in the main multivariate analysis, based on trade-off total ($p=0.0001$).

Support available to the patient

Patients to whom full support was available from others accepted lesser increments in survival as justifying treatment than those with partial or no support. This was significant for the 15-year trade-off (p-value based on Wilcoxon rank sum $=0.01$) and for trade-off total ($p=0.04$). It remained significant in the multivariate analysis based on trade-off total ($p=0.02$). Conversely, this finding could be described by saying that patients without support from others found chemotherapy more unpleasant or life less worthy of prolongation.

Treatment-related toxicity

Various toxicity scores were recorded (Table 1). Univariate analysis showed significant associations between five-year trade-off and mucositis ($p=0.04$), while for 15-year trade-off haematological toxicity and mucositis were significant (both $p=0.04$). In multivariate analysis based on trade-off total, the summary factor describing any toxicity remained independently significant ($p=0.01$). As expected, patients experiencing toxicity demanded higher incremental survival to justify treatment.

Dosage reduction during chemotherapy

Patients whose chemotherapy dosage was reduced to 75% or less of the total planned demanded longer survival increments than those receiving higher dosage ($p=0.05$ for each of five-year trade-off, 15-year trade-off and trade-off total). This was a factor independent of recorded toxicity in a multivariate analysis ($p=0.02$), but may have reflected unrecorded toxicity. Alternatively, physicians may have been more likely to reduce dosage in a group of patients they assessed as less willing to accept treatment toxicity.

Initial radiotherapy

Patients whose initial adjuvant treatment included radiotherapy as well as chemotherapy required longer increments of survival to justify treatment. This was independent of other factors in the multivariate analysis based on trade-off total ($p=0.01$). Whether it reflects patient selection, assimilation of conservative views from radiotherapists or an increase in unrecorded toxicity of the overall treatment remains unknown.

FACTORS *NOT* PREDICTIVE OF PATIENT PREFERENCES

No association was observed between the trade-off total and patient age, educational level, employment status, the time between treatment and interview, the use of concurrent adjuvant endocrine therapy, the occurrence of relapse, or the use of any particular modality (including further chemotherapy) for the treatment of relapse.

DISCUSSION

Adjuvant chemotherapy clearly has a role in the treatment of many patients with operable breast cancer. The essential question is whether the gains achieved are worthwhile, in view of the adverse effects of treatment. The clear result of this study was to show that, for many patients, very modest gains in outcome, such as seem to be readily achievable, would justify the side-effects of standard cytotoxic therapy as adjuvant therapy for operable breast cancer. It is possible that the group surveyed was unduly resilient or fatalistic. Some patients may have been excluded because they were never referred for consideration of chemotherapy, and perhaps they would have answered differently. It is not possible to assess this, since the reasons for non-referral would be likely to include factors related to the doctor of first contact as well as the patient. Indeed, there is no way to predict the severity of side-effects in patients never exposed to treatment. The results obtained in our series may, however, serve as a guide to the assessment of patients who might be considered for treatment. Having regard to the patients' preference, the indication for treatment might be considered relatively stronger in patients with good support from relatives, those with dependants and those in whom adjuvant radiotherapy is not planned.

If the results were distorted to reflect a group converted to the value of chemotherapy, it might be expected that those whose disease had recurred would be disillusioned and prone to demand greater benefits to justify treatment, but no such effect was seen.

Toxicity observed after the commencement of treatment was significantly associated with a requirement for greater benefits. While such a result is plausible and lends credibility to the methodology, it is not of value in deciding whether or not to embark on treatment.

The study we conducted was concerned only with overall survival. It seems probable that adjuvant cytotoxic therapy significantly delays relapse, and therefore improves the time without symptoms of disease or toxicity and the quality-adjusted survival. To the extent that this factor applies, it would add further weight to the argument in favour of such treatment.

We conclude that it is feasible to obtain patient preferences in the assessment of the trade-off inherent in the decision to use a toxic but effective therapy, that the results are reliable and show evidence of validity, and that subgroups can be identified in which more or less is demanded of treatment by the women concerned. This information should be considered in parallel with evidence of the inherent prognosis of each patient and of the efficacy of therapy in reaching clinical decisions on the use of adjuvant chemotherapy in operable breast cancer.

RECOMMENDED READING

Coates AS, Gebski V, Bishop JF et al (Australia–New Zealand Breast Cancer Trials Group) (1987) Improving the quality of life during chemotherapy for advanced breast cancer: a comparison of intermittent and continuous treatment strategies. N Engl J Med 317: 1490–1495

Early Breast Cancer Trialists Collaborative Group (1988) Effects of adjuvant tamoxifen and of cytotoxic chemotherapy on mortality in early breast cancer. N Engl J Med 319: 1681–1692

Goldhirsch A, Gelber RD, Simes RJ, Glasziou P, Coates AS (1989) Costs and benefits of adjuvant therapy in breast cancer: a quality adjusted survival analysis. J Clin Oncol 7: 36–44

McNeil BJ, Pauker SG, Fox HC, Tvesky A (1982) On elicitation of preferences for alternative therapies. N Engl J Med 306: 1259–1262

Meyerowitz BE, Watkins IK, Sparks FC (1983) Psychosocial implications of adjuvant chemotherapy. Cancer 52: 1541–1545

Simes RJ (1985) Treatment selection for cancer patients: application of statistical decision theory to the treatment of advanced ovarian cancer. J Chronic Dis 38: 171–186

Weinstein MC, Fineberg HV, Elstein AS et al (1980) Clinical decision analysis Saunders, Philadelphia

ABOUT THE AUTHORS

Professor Alan Coates was educated at Wesley College, Melbourne, and the University of Melbourne. Apart from medical studies, he qualified as a Methodist Local Preacher. After graduating in 1966, he trained in general medicine at the Royal Melbourne Hospital, leading to membership of the Royal Australasian College of Physicians in 1970. Postgraduate laboratory work in cellular immunology at the Walter and Eliza Hall Institute for Medical Research led to an MD in 1973. During this period his clinical interests moved increasingly to the medical treatment of cancer, and from 1976 to 1978 he trained in medical oncology at the Wisconsin Clinical Cancer Center, simultaneously setting up a laboratory programme in tumour immunology. On returning to Australia he spent two years as a Staff Specialist in Medical

Oncology at the Prince of Wales Hospital, Sydney, before accepting a position with the Sydney Branch of the Ludwig Institute for Cancer Research at Royal Prince Alfred Hospital. His clinical research interests are breast cancer and melanoma, and involve membership of the Australian New Zealand Breast Cancer Trials Group, the International Breast Cancer Study Group and the World Health Organization Melanoma Group. Since 1978 he has been Medical Oncologist to the Sydney Melanoma Unit, and is now its Research Director.

32 The Expert Surrogate System

WILLIAM J. MACKILLOP, MICHAEL J. PALMER,
BRIAN O'SULLIVAN and CAROL F. QUIRT

THE DILEMMA OF THE CLINICIAN–INVESTIGATOR

Progress in medicine requires clinical research and clinical trials have therefore become an accepted part of the practice of oncology. Clinical researchers, however, face ethical problems which have not yet been fully resolved [1]. Doctors who are involved in clinical research retain their traditional role as caregivers in the service of today's patients but they have also become scientists in the service of future generations. This dual role brings with it a potential conflict of interest because, when doctors become scientists, patients become potential research subjects and may be considered as a means to an end, as well as an end in themselves [1–4]. The profession has recognized this problem and has developed guidelines to protect the interests of both the patient and the doctor in this complex new relationship. Codes of practice for clinical researchers comprise two kinds of rules: (a) those which affirm the patient's basic rights in the context of an experiment; and (b) those which define what constitutes an ethical experiment.

THE PATIENT'S RIGHTS

All ethical codes demand that patients must give their informed consent before they are involved in a clinical experiment. This rule is based on the principle of respect for autonomy which has come to occupy a central position in modern medical ethics. However, people who have recently learned that they are seriously ill may not be psychologically capable of considering the implications of participating in a clinical trial [5], and detailed medical information may, in any case, be of little value to those who have not been trained to interpret it [6]. Many empirical studies have shown that patients who have given their informed consent for treatment or investigation may have little understanding of that to which they have consented. In our own clinic we found that, while cancer patients usually know their diagnosis, they frequently misunderstand the purpose of their treatment and overestimate its potential benefits. Thus, it is unreasonable to assume that every patient is able to carry out the kind of cost–benefit analysis required to reach a rational decision about participation in a clinical

Introducing New Treatments for Cancer: Practical, Ethical and Legal Problems. Edited by C. J. Williams
© 1992 John Wiley & Sons Ltd

trial. This makes it all the more important for the profession to ensure that clinical experiments are ethically acceptable before patients are asked to participate in them.

THE DEFINITION OF AN ETHICAL CLINICAL EXPERIMENT

Rules for the conduct of clinical research were first clearly delineated in the Nuremburg Code and subsequently in the Helsinki Declaration of the World Medical Association (Chapters 1 and 2). These rules are designed to maximize the societal gain from the experiment while minimizing the cost and risk to the patients involved, and are based on the related principles of beneficence and non-maleficence. In simplified form, they may be stated as follows:

(a) the experiment should conform to accepted scientific principles;
(b) it should be based on previous laboratory and animal experiments;
(c) it should be carried out only by scientifically qualified persons;
(d) the importance of the objective should be in proportion to the inherent risk to the subject.

While the intent of these rules is clear, we believe that there are problems in the way they are interpreted and applied. Experts in the field need to be involved in the process because neither the quality of the science nor the potential value of the results can be assessed without specialized knowledge and experience. However, it may not be possible for the doctors who instigate and design clinical trials also to evaluate them objectively. Academic careers in medicine today are built on research publications and this creates a powerful motive for experimentation quite separate from the altruistic motives which are usually thought to drive the process. Barber has provided empirical data to support the contention that the "struggle for scientific recognition exerts pressure on ethical considerations". His group conducted a postal survey of nearly 300 biomedical research institutions in the USA and then an intensive interview study of 350 individual investigators at two institutions. Investigators were asked to give their response to six simulated research protocols designed to measure their degree of concern about informed consent and their willingness to approve of studies involving various levels of risk. The respondents were divided into four categories based on the number of papers that they published and the number of times their work had been cited by others. Accepting the frequency of citation as a good measure of scientific excellence, they called the most cited investigators the "high-quality scientists" and those who had published a great deal but were never cited, the "extreme mass producer scientists". They showed that it was the "extreme mass producers" who were most often engaged in investigations with less favourable risk–benefit ratios, who approved protocols with poorer risk–benefit ratios and who least often expressed awareness of the importance of consent. They concluded that "caught up in the socially structured competitive system of science, unsuccessful in it, but still pursuing the prize of peer recognition, they appear to be more likely to overvalue scientific work as against humane therapy".

Currently, the ethical aspects of clinical trials are first considered by the experts who design them, who are not disinterested parties, and subsequently by reviewers on ethics committees who may be impartial but are usually not experts. This system is fundamentally flawed by the dislocation of the two key elements of impartiality and expertise. Even when experts are included on ethics committees, they are often colleagues of the investigators. This may preclude an impartial judgment despite the best intentions of everyone involved. Furthermore, decisions at both levels are often made by a committee and the individuals involved may feel less responsible for the final verdict than they would if each were acting independently. The peer review process provides an additional level of control when external funds are required to carry out clinical trials, but the growing body of clinical research sponsored by drug companies is, unfortunately, exempt from this.

In practice, ethics committees reach decisions which are not reproducible from one institution to the next (Chapter 7). Multicentre clinical research groups often find that a protocol which is approved by an ethics committee in one instititution is rejected by another committee in a second institution. This is absurd. From an ethical standpoint, it is incompatible with the principle of justice. From a medical standpoint, if it is wrong to rely on a diagnostic test which produces widely varying results, then it is equally wrong to use an unreliable process to make ethical decisions. We have therefore explored alternative approaches to the ethical evaluation of clinical trials. We set out to design a system which would meet the following criteria:

(a) it should consider the views of impartial experts;
(b) it should be based on multiple opinions obtained independently;
(c) it should give reproducible results;
(d) it should be comprehensible to lay people and to doctors;
(e) it should be based on widely accepted moral principles.

THE SURROGATE SYSTEM

Fost developed a new approach for the ethical review of clinical trials based on the premise that people who were well would be better able to assess the risks and benefits of participation in a clinical trial than those who were ill. The essence of his system was to ask individuals who were not candidates for a clinical trial to imagine that they were, and to consider whether or not they would consent to participate in it. He reasoned that the surrogate patients had the opportunity to reflect on the question of the experiment with a clearer mind than real patients, and that their decisions would not be influenced by dependence on the doctor.

One large-scale survey in the UK reported by Kemp and colleagues used this method to find out how non-medically trained people felt about participating in several different randomized clinical trials [7]. There was no evidence of any general antipathy to the concept of randomization: on average, 50% of the surrogate patients would consent to each trial, although consent was lower for two studies involving randomization to greater or lesser surgery. The Danish study by Sauerbrey et al. of medical out-patients' attitudes to medical research also showed a generally positive attitude to clinical trials [8]. One important observation from that study was the very high level of trust which lay people put in the medical profession. More than 80% said they would participate in a clinical trial solely on the recommendation of their doctor. A study of attitudes of patients receiving investigational chemotherapy in the USA conducted by Penman et al. also showed that trust in the physician was the primary reason for accepting treatment [9]. A recent Canadian study (Llewellyn-Thomas et al.), which investigated attitudes toward participating in a clinical trial for early breast cancer, showed that surrogate cancer patients were less likely to participate than real patients [10]. This suggests that people who are ill may find it more difficult to refuse to participate in a trial than they would if their autonomy were not compromised by illness and/or by their dependence on their doctor. If this is so, then surrogate patients may indeed provide information which is not available from the patients themselves.

THE EXPERT SURROGATE SYSTEM

The views of non-medically trained people acting as surrogate patients are useful, but the system proposed by Fost still lacked the essential ingredient of expertise. The rules for assessing the ethical acceptability of a clinical trial outlined above need to be applied by individuals who understand scientific method and who have a knowledge of the background to the study. It is beyond question that all clinical experiments which are poorly designed or poorly executed are unethical. Useless work always has a negative, rather than a neutral quality, if only because it diverts resources from potentially more valuable activities. However, the converse does not hold true. Not all well-designed and well-executed studies are necessarily ethical. The question asked in an ethical clinical trial must be a reasonable one and it must be sufficiently important to justify the potential risk to the subjects.

It is in judging this issue, which has a moral component as well as a scientific one, that the views of impartial experts are essential.

Ingelfinger pointed out that the problem with informed consent is that it is not "educated consent" [6] and Jonas argued that, ultimately, the researchers themselves would make the only ideal research subjects, since it is they who best understand the issues at stake and the risks involved [11]. We have therefore adapted Fost's method by using expert doctors as surrogate patients in the evaluation of clinical trials. This strategy exploits the advantages of the surrogate system but also goes some way toward meeting the demand that consent should be *educated*, or comprehending, as well as informed [6].

THE EXPERT SURROGATE SYSTEM IN ACTION

In our first expert surrogate survey, we asked doctors who treat lung cancer in Ontario whether they would be prepared to be treated as patient–subjects on six clinical trials in non-small-cell lung cancer [12]. One hundred and eighteen members of the clinical staff of the eight cancer clinics in Ontario were each sent a questionnaire which asked: (a) how would *they* wish to be managed if *they* had non-small-cell lung cancer; and (b) if *they* would consent to participate as patient–subjects on each of the six trials.

Column 1 of Table 1 shows that the proportion of doctors who would consent ranged from 64% for the most acceptable trial to 11% for the least acceptable trial. Reasons given for refusal varied, but many doctors felt that certain trials offered unacceptable options for treatment. As shown in columns 2 and 3 of Table 1, the medical oncologists were more positive about participation in each trial than were the radiation oncologists, but both disciplines ranked the six studies in exactly the same order of acceptability. Thus, it appeared that doctors were able to discern differences in acceptability among these trials which were not simply based on prejudices engendered by their specialist training [12].

HOW DO YOU INTERPRET THE RESULTS
OF AN EXPERT SURROGATE SURVEY?

We then sent the results shown in column 1 of Table 1 back to the oncologists who had completed the first questionnaire and asked them: "If the information presented to you now had been available *before* these trials were opened to patients, should any of them have been stopped?" Column 4 of Table 1 shows that, when the majority of expert surrogates consented to a given trial, there was almost unanimous agreement that the trial was acceptable for patients. When, on the other hand, the majority of expert

Table 1. Expert surrogates' attitudes to clinical trials in non-small-cell lung cancer

	Would you consent to this clinical trial?			Should this clinical trial have been stopped?[g]
	1	2	3	4
Study code name	All doctors[h] (%)	Radiation oncologists (%)	Medical oncologists (%)	All doctors (%)
LCSG-821[a]	64	49	86	5
EORTC-08824[b]	57	39	71	0
LCSG-791[c]	31	27	32	41
YALE-LUNG-1[d]	27	21	28	53
SWOG-8241[e]	19	9	23	59
NCCTG-812451[f]	11	8	11	55

[a]LCSG-821: a randomized trial of lobectomy versus segmental resection in early operable lung cancer.
[b]EORTC-08824: a randomized trial of immediate radiation treatment versus treatment delayed until symptoms develop.
[c]LCSG-719: a randomized trial of postoperative radiotherapy versus chemotherapy versus radio-chemotherapy in a group of patients with a high risk of recurrence following surgery.
[d]YALE-LUN-1: a randomized trial of surgery alone versus preoperative intralesional BCG immunotherapy followed by surgery in patients with early operable lung cancer.
[e]SWOG-8241: a randomized trial of five different forms of combination chemotherapy in patients with metastatic disease.
[f]NCCTG-812451: a randomized trial of two forms of chemotherapy open to patients with locally advanced or metastatic disease.
[g]Percentage of doctors who answered "yes" to this question.
[h]The sample included a few respirologists and thoracic surgeons as well as the radiation oncologists and medical oncologists.

surrogates would not consent, between 40% and 60% of the doctors surveyed said that they thought the trial should not have gone ahead. In two subsequent surveys doctors and non-medically trained people were explicitly asked what proportion of expert surrogate patients should be prepared to participate in a clinical trial before it was opened to real patients [13, 14]. Figure 1 shows their answers expressed in the form of cumulative frequency distributions. These data show that clinical trials to which more than two-thirds of expert surrogates would consent are perceived as ethically acceptable by most doctors and also by most people who are not medically trained.

As well as looking at the proportion of expert surrogates who consent, the reasons given by those who refuse must be considered in interpreting these data. If some doctors refuse to participate because they regard one arm of a randomized trial as unacceptable, while others refuse to participate because they regard the other arm as unacceptable, then a low overall frequency of consent may simply reflect the *clinical equipoise* which Freedman suggests defines the circumstances in which a randomized trial is most

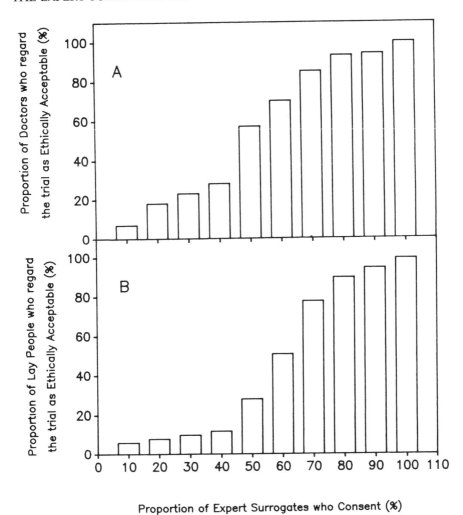

Figure 1. Cumulative frequency distribution showing the proportion of expert doctors (A) and lay people (B) who would consider a clinical trial ethically acceptable as a function of the proportion of expert surrogate patients who would consent to participate in the clinical trial

ethical and most necessary [15]. In the lung cancer expert surrogate study, we found evidence of clinical equipoise only in an EORTC trial, which compared immediate radiotherapy treatment with no treatment until symptoms developed [12]. Some doctors would refuse to participate because of a strong personal preference for immediate radiotherapy, while others would refuse because they wanted no immediate treatment and regarded radiotherapy as futile and/or potentially toxic. Thus, the reasons these two groups gave for refusing to participate in this trial simply reiterate the controversy which it was designed to address.

Reasons for refusing to participate in the other five trials fell into two patterns, neither of which provided any evidence of controversy. Either the doctors rejected the experimental arm alone, as in the randomized trial of preoperative immunotherapy followed by surgery versus surgery alone (YALE-LUN-1), or they rejected all arms of the study, as in the trial of five different kinds of chemotherapy (SWOG-8241). Under these circumstances, a low frequency of consent by expert surrogates can be taken at face value as evidence of unacceptable risk–benefit ratios associated with one or more of the treatment options.

It is our view that a clinical trial in which less than 50% of experts in the field would be willing to participate should be considered unethical except where clinical equipoise is demonstrated.

WHY ASK DOCTORS RATHER THAN PATIENTS?

As a group, doctors who treat lung cancer are evidently able to distinguish trials which are acceptable from those which are not. But couldn't patients make the same distinctions for themselves? Since at least a few doctors would be prepared to consent to any one of these clinical trials, isn't it perfectly reasonable to leave it to the patients to decide if the trial is acceptable or not?

We addressed this question in another survey in which people who were not medically trained were asked about two of the clinical trials included in the expert surrogate survey [14]. The descriptions of the clinical situations and the clinical trials were rewritten to avoid medical terminology and expanded to include an explanation of the nature of the illness, the forms of treatment available, the therapeutic intent, the prognosis, the purpose of the trial and the nature of randomization. The scenarios were reviewed by a panel of oncologists to ensure that the trials had been fairly described, and by a group of non-medically trained people to ensure that they were comprehensible.

Four hundred non-medically trained people were then asked if they would participate in each of these trials if they developed lung cancer. Fifty per cent would consent to the trial of lobectomy versus segmentectomy (LCSG-821), compared to 64% of doctors, while 48% would consent to the trial of five different forms of chemotherapy (SWOG-8241), compared to 19% of doctors [14]. Thus, non-medically trained people appear unable to discern differences in the acceptability of trials which are significantly different in their acceptability to expert doctors. Our respondents' decisions regarding participation were not predetermined by their general attitude to the clinical trials process. There was no association between consent to the surgery trial and consent to the chemotherapy trial. Forty-six per cent of the respondents who consented to the surgical trial also consented to the chemotherapy trial, and 50% of the respondents who did not consent to the surgical trial consented to the chemotherapy trial [14].

Subsequently, the non-medically trained respondents were told the proportion of doctors who would consent to participate in each trial, and asked if this information would modify their previous decisions. There was no change in the proportion that would consent to the surgical trial, but the proportion that would consent to the chemotherapy trial decreased, suggesting that the results of an expert surrogate survey may be considered as material information to which patients should have access in reaching their own decisions. We also explicitly asked these non-medically trained people if they thought that the expert surrogate system was useful. Most of our respondents (74%) believed that cancer specialists should be asked if they would be willing to participate in clinical trials before the trials were opened to patients. Eighty-three per cent stated that they would personally wish to know the views of expert surrogates before deciding whether to consent to participate in a clinical trial if they had cancer and 79% thought that any cancer patient should be given this type of information before being asked to consent to participate in a clinical trial [14].

CONCLUSIONS FROM THE EXPERT SURROGATE STUDIES OF CLINICAL TRIALS IN LUNG CANCER

From the first expert surrogate survey, we concluded that many patients with non-small-cell lung cancer are currently being asked to participate in clinical trials that offer treatment options which the majority of experts in the field would not be prepared to accept for themselves because of their high risk–benefit ratios [12]. Thus, the existing system for protecting the patients' interests in the context of clinical research does not appear to achieve its objectives.

From the subsequent survey of non-medically trained surrogates, we concluded that even highly educated people, who are well, are unable to discern differences in the acceptability of trials which are obvious to experts [14]. Thus, patients cannot always be expected to recognize unacceptable experiments for themselves.

From the combined results of these two surveys, we concluded that a better system for reviewing the ethical acceptability of clinical trials is necessary and that the expert surrogate system meets most of the criteria given above. It is based on the views of impartial experts, it avoids the problem of "groupthink" associated with committee decisions, and it produces results which are interpreted similarly by the majority of physicians and non-medically trained people.

THE USE OF EXPERT SURROGATES TO DEFINE MANAGEMENT CONTROVERSIES

In addition to its role in the ethical evaluation of clinical research, the expert surrogate system may be used to define controversies in patient management and to identify questions which should be addressed in clinical trials. We recently asked doctors in Canada and in the USA: (a) how they would wish to be managed if they had non-small-cell lung cancer; and (b) what treatment they usually recommended for their patients in the same circumstances [13]. Column 1 of Table 2 shows the answers of 222 doctors who were asked how they would want to be treated if they had non-small-cell lung cancer with extensive mediastinal node involvement but no evidence of distant metastases. The variation in these doctors' choices of management is very striking. Some would choose to have an operation followed by radiation therapy and chemotherapy, while others wanted no treatment until

Table 2. Doctors' treatment preferences for non-small-cell lung cancer with extensive mediastinal node involvement

Personal management choice	All doctors $n=222$ Personal choice (%)	All doctors $n=222$ Usual recommendation (%)	Canadian $n=59$ Personal choice (%)	American $n=95$ Personal choice (%)	Authors of articles on lung cancer Personal choice (%)
Radiotherapy alone	38	38	37	41	35
Radiotherapy and chemo-therapy	19	18	14	22	21
No immediate treatment	17	13	37	12	6
Radiotherapy, surgery, and chemotherapy	9	8	2	3	22
Radiotherapy and surgery	8	8	3	12	7
Surgery alone	4	4	0	7	1
Surgery and chemotherapy	0.5	0.5	0	0	1
Chemotherapy alone	0	0.5	0	0	0
Clinical trial	1.5	3	0	1	3
No answer	3	3	7	2	4
Explain options to patients	n/a	4	n/a	n/a	n/a
Total	100	100	100	100	100

Table 3. Doctors' personal choice of management for non-small-cell lung cancer with extensive mediastinal node involvement as a function of specialty

Personal choice of treatment	All doctors[a] (n=222) (%)	Medical oncology (n=55) (%)	Radiation oncology (n=46) (%)	Thoracic surgery (n=48) (%)	Respirology (n=41) (%)	Hematology oncology (n=26) (%)
Radiotherapy ± other treatment	74	71	86	85	56	66
Chemotherapy ± other treatment	28.5	40	19	35	14	27
Surgery ± other treatment	21.5	17	6	48	17	12
No immediate treatment	17	20	11	8	29	15

[a]Six doctors belonged to disciplines not represented in this table.

symptoms developed. Column 2 of Table 3 shows the treatment which these doctors usually recommended for patients in this situation. The vast majority would recommend for their patients the same treatment which they chose for themselves [13].

We also attempted to define the factors which influence these personal preferences. As shown in column 3 of Table 2, the two most frequent choices of Canadian doctors were either radiotherapy alone or no immediate antitumor treatment. However, as shown in column 4 of Table 2, very few American doctors wanted no active treatment and a higher proportion elected to have surgery and/or chemotherapy as part of their management. A group of doctors who had recently published articles on non-small-cell lung cancer made choices closer to those of the Michigan doctors, although a higher proportion opted for aggressive multimodality treatment. Table 3 shows that doctors' personal management preferences were associated with their specialist training. For example, almost half the surgeons would want to have an operation in this situation compared to about one in 20 radio-therapists [13].

Similar variations in practice have since been observed by other investigators using the expert surrogate system. Moore and his colleagues asked urologists, radiotherapists and chemotherapists who practice genito-urinary oncology how they would wish to be treated if they developed genitourinary cancer [16]. In each of the six clinical situations studied, the variation in their treatment preferences was remarkable. For example, 40% of respondents wanted prostatectomy for localized prostate cancer while 39% wanted radiotherapy. Treatment preferences varied geographically. For example, when British urologists were asked how they would want to be treated for a high-grade invasive bladder cancer, they most frequently chose radiotherapy alone whereas not one of the North American urologists made this choice. Preferences were also influenced by doctors' specialty. For example, radiation oncologists more frequently chose radiotherapy alone for invasive bladder cancer than either of the other disciplines.

We have also found wide variations in the management preferences of doctors who treat head and neck cancer and in those of doctors who treat ocular tumors (O'Sullivan et al., Palmer et al.; unpublished data). We are forced to conclude that the way in which patients with cancer actually end up being treated depends to a very large extent on accidents of geography and patterns of referral. It might be argued that different treatments in the hands of different doctors could produce similar results, but this does not explain or justify our observations with lung cancer. The policy of no immediate treatment and that of aggressive multimodality therapy might give similar five-year survival figures, but it does not require a formal cost–benefit analysis to make it clear that there are other ways in which these two approaches really do differ. Either some patients are being grossly over-treated, or others are being grossly under-treated, and this has ethical as well as medical implications.

The related ethical principles of beneficence and non-maleficence demand that we provide our patients with the best available medical care, but the observed variations in practice are so wide that we must collectively acknowledge that this is not the case at present, although we may each be privately satisfied with our own decisions. Furthermore, the principle of justice demands fair distribution of good medical care and the observed unsystematic variations in treatment are inconsistent with this. Variations in practice based on patients' needs are acceptable, but those based only on the bias of individual doctors are not.

VARIATIONS IN PRACTICE: THE PROBLEM AND POTENTIAL SOLUTIONS

The credibility of clinical medicine as a scientific discipline hinges on the claim that knowledge guides practice, but our data suggest that in oncology it is personal beliefs rather than universal knowledge which guide therapeutic decisions. It has been suggested recently that rationality in medical decision making should be added to the list of rules of medical ethics, and that the profession as a whole is under an ethical obligation to define the boundaries of acceptable practice. The first step toward rationalizing decision making is to determine why competent doctors reach different decisions in identical situations. Research will be required to answer the following questions.

(a) Is there simply insufficient information to permit a rational decision?
(b) Do different doctors have different information at their disposal?
(c) Do different doctors maintain different beliefs in the face of identical information?
(d) Do doctors agree about the probability of treatment outcomes but disagree about the value, or utility, of these outcomes?
(e) Do doctors integrate information differently from one another and, therefore, reach different conclusions despite having identical information?
(f) To what extent are doctors' decisions, beliefs, values and thought processes influenced by their education, by what they read, by their colleagues, and by their own personal experience?

The appropriate strategies to improve the quality of medical decisions will depend on the answers to these questions. If it transpires that the observed variations in practice are caused by an absolute lack of information about the outcome of certain treatments, then specific clinical trials may be required to compare alternative therapies. A formal description of a decision problem is useful in defining the missing information and can define the treatment strategies which should be compared and the outcomes which should be measured. If, on the other hand, it turns out that some doctors are simply unaware of important information about the disease, then we should be working on programs of continuing education for medical specialists specifically designed to fill the most important gaps in their knowledge. It is also possible that variation in the perceived value of certain health states is responsible for variation in decisions and, if this is the case, the challenge will be to generate measures of utility which are reliable, stable and valid as well as credible and comprehensible to physicians. One final possibility is that doctors agree about the facts and their relative importance, but integrate the information differently, thus arriving at different conclusions. If this is demonstrated, then a stronger case can be made for the development of expert systems to assist in medical decision making.

Some of the variations in practice we have observed may be due to a simple lack of information. Most of the controversies in the management of non-small-cell lung cancer identified in our surveys have not been, and are not being, addressed in any clinical trials. For example, in Canada the major controversy regarding the management of non-small-cell lung cancer with extensive mediastinal node involvement in the absence of distant metastases is whether any active treatment is indicated at all. The number of Canadian doctors who wanted no immediate treatment equalled the number who wished immediate radiotherapy. This is classical clinical equipoise, but the question of whether any treatment is better than watchful waiting has yet to be adequately addressed in a randomized clinical trial. On the other hand, some current clinical trials focus on areas where we found no evidence of controversy. Many current trials compare the activities of different multidrug regimens without radiotherapy in patients with advance intrathoracic disease, although not one of the 222 doctors that we surveyed would wish to have chemotherapy alone in this situation. We did find evidence of a major controversy in North America surrounding the role of chemotherapy in patients with distant metastases, but the vast majority of North American clinical trials did not ask if chemotherapy is useful but, rather, asked which form of chemotherapy was best.

Variation in the management of patients with lung cancer may also occur, not because doctors disagree about the likely outcome of treatment, but because they disagree about its value. For example, a recent Canadian study demonstrated a modest increase in the life expectancy of patients with metastatic non-small-cell lung cancer treated with chemotherapy, but this has not led to uniform acceptance of chemotherapy as standard treatment in this context. The Ontario Cancer Foundation (OCTRF) Kingston Clinic still does not use chemotherapy in this situation, while at its sister clinic in Ottawa chemotherapy is now considered routine therapy. This disparity in practice is not due to ignorance of the results of the clinical trial, which was in fact co-ordinated in Kingston, but to a difference in the perceived value of the demonstrated increase in life expectancy among Ontario Cancer Foundation's medical oncologists.

THE ROLE OF SELF-REFERENCE IN CLINICAL PRACTICE

A consistent observation made by ourselves, and by others who have used the expert surrogate system, is that doctors recommend for their patients the treatment they would choose for themselves under the same circumstances. In using self-reference to guide our conduct in relation to others we are acting in accordance with a very old moral principle, often called the *golden rule.*

The positive, or prescriptive, form of the golden rule *do to others as you would have them do to you* is usually attributed to Jesus of Nazareth, but the concept is not exclusively Christian. The negative, or proscriptive, form of the rule *never do to others what you would not like them to do to you* is, in fact, much older and has its origins in Eastern philosophy [17]. In either form, the essence of the rule is a demand for moral consistency, and in that sense it has merit regardless of how it is phrased. There are, however, well-known defects in the golden rule as a general guide to human actions [18] and we agree with the prevailing view of medial ethicists that the prescriptive form of the golden rule is a poor guide to individual treatment decisions and that it can be frankly dangerous if taken too literally [18]. Nonetheless, we believe that the prospective form of the rule is entirely valid when it is used at the collective level to define the boundaries of acceptable research. A brief review of the golden rule from the ethical perspective will demonstrate why its use in the expert surrogate system is not vulnerable to the usual criticisms.

Critics of the golden rule argue that it provides no external standard by which to reach moral judgments and that it suggests that "the individual has only to consult his own tastes and needs to discover how he ought to behave to other people". Marcus Singer, however, points out that this criticism only applies to what he calls the *particular* interpretation of the golden rule, that we should do to other people exactly *what* we would want them to do to us, but does not apply to the *general* interpretation of the rule, which demands that we should treat other people *as* we would wish them to treat us [19]. What Singer suggests is that the golden rule is intended to be used as a moral principle rather than as a rule to guide individual actions. Far from demanding that we should inflict our values on other people, his general interpretation merely asks that "if I would have others take account of my interests and wishes in their treatment of me, even though my interests and wishes may differ considerably from their own, then . . . I should take account of the interests and wishes of others in my treatment of them". Blackstone [20] suggested that we should consider the golden rule neither as a moral rule nor as a moral principle but as a way of defining what some philosophers have called *the moral point of view*. It tells us that "any judgement in which the agent denies himself a privileged position, and in which he applies the same standards or rules or principles of evaluation to others as he would have them apply in their treatment of him, is a moral judgement" [20]. Gould, however, has pointed out that the abstract interpretations of the golden rule suggested by Singer and Blackstone are a far cry from the intentions of its original proponents. He says that the rule was meant to be taken literally and that "if one interprets the golden rule as a general rule then one dismisses it as being meaningful to the ordinary person" [21].

Thus, the positive form of the rule can be dangerously misleading if interpreted literally, whereas in its abstract form it is more valid but may be of less practical value. The negative form of the golden rule can, however, be defended without the need for abstraction. The presumption that what is good for you is also good for others, which underlies the particular interpretation of the positive form of the golden rule, does not apply to the negative form of the rule. Allinson suggests that this assumption would be at odds with the basic Confucian attitudes of modesty and humility and that it is no accident that the Eastern form of the rule is stated negatively. All we are asked by the negative formulation is to avoid doing things to others which we would not want them to do to us.

Unfortunately, if we were to use even the negative form of the rule as the basis for making individual treatment decisions in medicine, it would still involve unwarranted assumptions. It is not necessarily true that a doctor should never treat a patient in a way he would not want to be treated himself. For example, individuals differ in their willingness to run risks and it is not necessarily right for a doctor who is highly averse to risk taking to assume that his patient has a similar constitution, and to limit the therapeutic options accordingly. But the assumption which underlies the application of the negative form of the golden rule in the expert surrogate system for evaluating clinical trials is quite different. The rule is being used here to govern the way in which one group of individuals interacts with another group. For the golden rule to be valid in this situation, all that we need to assume is that doctors as a group do not differ fundamentally from the rest of the community.

CONCLUSIONS

We believe that the expert surrogate system is a useful way of exploring management controversies and that it also provides a valid approach to the ethical evaluation of clinical trials. Clinical research is undoubtedly an important part of oncology today. Clinical trials have already resolved many long-standing controversies and now ensure that new forms of therapy are evaluated fairly and cautiously before they become accepted into routine practice. It is vitally important, therefore, that the medical community should set high and consistent standards for the practice of clinical research. In the long term, the number of patients available and willing to participate in clinical experiments will depend on the credibility of the research community. Further attempts to refine the process of reviewing ethical standards in clinical research are not merely important to protect the interests of today's patients but also to protect the integrity of a process which promises great benefits for future generations of patients.

ACKNOWLEDGMENTS

This work was supported by a grant from the National Cancer Institute of Canada. The authors are grateful to Beverley J. Shortt for her assistance in the preparation of this manuscript.

REFERENCES

1. Mackillop WJ, Johnston PA (1986) Ethical problems in clinical research: the need for empirical studies of the clinical trials process. J Chronic Dis 39: 177–188
2. Fried C (1974) Medical experimentation: personal integrity and social policy. North-Holland, Amsterdam
3. Fost N (1979) The ethics of randomized clinical trials: two perspectives. N Engl J Med 300: 1272–1275
4. Barber B (1976) The ethics of experimentation with human subjects. Sci Am 234: 25–31
5. Fost N (1975) A surrogate system for informed consent. JAMA 233: 800–803
6. Ingelfinger FJ (1972) Informed (but uneducated) consent. N Engl J Med 287: 465–466
7. Kemp N, Skinner E, Toms J (1984) Randomized clinical trials of cancer treatment: a public opinion survey. Clin Oncol 10: 849–855
8. Sauerbrey N, Jensen J, Rasmussen PE, Giorup T, Guldager H, Riis P (1984) Danish patients' attitudes to scientific–ethical questions. Acta Med Scand 215: 99–104
9. Penman DT, Holland JC, Bahna GF et al (1984) Informed consent for investigational chemotherapy: patients and physicians' perceptions. J Clin Oncol 2: 849–855
10. Llewellyn-Thomas HA, Thiel EC, Clark RM (1989) Patients versus surrogates: whose opinion counts on ethics review panels? Clin Res 3763: 501–505
11. Jonas H (1969) Philosophical reflections on experimenting with human subjects. Daedalus J Am Acad Arts Sci 98: 219
12. Mackillop WJ, Ward GK, O'Sullivan B (1986) The use of expert surrogates to evaluate clinical trials in non-small cell lung cancer. Br J Cancer 54: 661–667
13. Palmer MJ, O'Sullivan B, Steele R, Mackillop WJ (1990) Controversies in the management of non-small cell lung cancer: the results of an expert surrogate study. Radiat Oncol 19: 17–28

14. Mackillop WJ, Palmer MJ, O'Sullivan B, Ward GK, Steele R, Dotsikas G (1988) Clinical trials in cancer: the role of surrogate patients in defining what constitutes an ethically acceptable clinical experiment. Br J Cancer 59: 388–395
15. Freedman B (1987) Equipoise and the ethics of clinical research. N Engl J Med 317: 141–145
16. Moore MJ, O'Sullivan B, Tannock IF (1988) How expert physicians would wish to be treated if they had genitourinary cancer. J Clin Oncol 6: 1736–1745
17. Allinson RE (1985) The Confucian golden rule: a negative formulation. J Clin Phil 12: 305–315
18. Engelhardt HT (1986) The foundation of bioethics. Oxford University Press, New York
19. Singer M (1963) The golden rule. Philosophy 38: 293–314
20. Blackstone WT (1965) The golden rule: a defence. S J Phil 3: 172–177
21. Gould JA (1983) The golden rule. Am J Theol Phil 4: 73–79

ABOUT THE AUTHORS

Dr Mackillop graduated in medicine from the University of Glasgow in 1975. He trained as a radiation oncologist at the Princess Margaret Hospital in Toronto, and has since worked at McGill University, Montreal, and at the University of Edinburgh, Scotland. He is currently Professor of Oncology at Queen's University, and Head of Radiation Oncology at the Ontario Cancer Research and Treatment Foundation's Kingston Clinic. His research interests include decision-making in oncology and ethical aspects of clinical research.

Michael J. Palmer received his MSc in Community Health and Epidemiology from Queen's University, Kingston, Canada, in 1988. His research interests include the management of non-small-cell lung cancer and clinical trials in oncology. He currently works as a Study Co-ordinator for the National Cancer Institute of Canada Clinical Trials Group in Kingston, Canada.

Dr O'Sullivan received his medical degree from University College, Dublin, Ireland, in June 1976. After initially undergoing training in internal medicine and medical oncology in Dublin and in Toronto, Canada, he subsequently trained in radiation oncology at the Princess Margaret Hospital, Toronto. He joined the radiation oncology staff as a member of faculty at McGill University, Montreal, Canada, in January 1984. In July 1985, he assumed his current position as a Radiation Oncologist at the Princess Margaret Hospital, and holds the rank of Assistant Professor in the Department of Radiation Oncology at the University of Toronto. In addition to teaching commitments at the undergraduate and postgraduate level, he has research interests which include studies of the application of clinical radiotherapy, clinical decision analysis, and the conduct of clinical trials in oncology. Clinical specialty interests in oncology include the management of head and neck cancer, bone and soft tissue sarcomas, and gastrointestinal malignancies.

Carol F. Quirt received her MSc in Biochemistry from Queen's University, Kingston, Canada in 1984. She instructed chemistry at Trent University, then worked as a researcher at the Ontario Cancer Research and Treatment Foundation's Kingston Cancer Clinic. She became a Lecturer in the Department of Oncology at Queen's University in 1990, and is currently in her first year of law school at Queen's University. Her research interests include the process and quality of decision making in oncology and health law.

Index

Index compiled by June Morrison